T0130879

Vascular Access for Hemodialysis—IX

Vascular Access for Hemodialysis—IX

MITCHELL L. HENRY, M.D.

W. L. Gore & Associates, Inc.

Bonus Books

© 2005 by W.L. Gore & Associates, Inc., and Bonus Books
All Rights Reserved

Except for appropriate use in critical reviews or works of scholarship, the reproduction or use of this work in any form or by any electronic, mechanical or other means now known or hereafter invented, including photocopying and recording, and in any information storage and retrieval system is forbidden without the written permission of the publisher.

Library of Congress Cataloging-in-Publication Data
Vascular access for hemodialysis IX / [edited by] Mitchell L. Henry.
    p. ; cm.
Includes bibliographical references.
  ISBN 1-56625-292-X
  1. Hemodialysis. 2. Arterial catheterization. 3. Arteriovenous shunts, Surgical. I. Henry, Mitchell L. II. Title: Vascular access for hemo-dialysis 9. III. Title: Vascular access for hemodialysis nine.
   [DNLM: 1. Renal Dialysis—methods—Congresses. 2. Arteriovenous Shunt, Surgical—Congresses. 3. Catheters, Indwelling—Congresses. 4. Graft Occlusion, Vascular—prevention & control—Congresses. 5. Kidney Failure, Chronic—therapy—Congresses. 6. Vascular Surgical
  Procedures—Congresses.   WJ 378 V33092 2005]
  RC901.7.H45V375 2005
  617.4'61059—dc22

                       2005020785

05 04 03 02 01   5 4 3 2 1

GORE-TEX, GORE-TEX Vascular Graft, and GORE-TEX Suture are registered trademarks of W.L. Gore & Associates, Inc.

Bonus Books, Inc.
9255 Sunset Blvd. Suite 717
Los Angeles, CA 90069
www.bonusbooks.com

Printed in the United States of America

CONTENTS

PREFACE

V ascular Access for Hemodialysis IX proved to be another successful gathering of a broad cross-section of health care providers dedicated to improving the delivery of dialysis, specifically as it pertains to the creation and maintenance of hemodialysis access. The diversity of these individuals continues to give a broad perspective on the problems and solutions of vascular access care. A variety of topics presented at the conference are contained herein, and address how we do it and how we can improve upon it. In addition, there was lively and candid discussion by the audience and presenters that once again proved to be valuable. We remain dedicated to improving the care and outcomes of those suffering from end stage renal disease.

ACKNOWLEDGMENTS

This conference and subsequent book is the result of efforts by a number of people. W.L. Gore, again, provided exceptional support, both from their enthusiasm and resources. Don Lass, Ron Hron, Susan Boothe, and Marty Sylvain from Gore continue to be strong advocates of the principles of access care. Dr. Skip Campbell was invaluable as the co-host of the meeting and helped to facilitate many of the organizational aspects of the meeting. Sheila Zirkle from The Ohio State Medical Center helped sort out many of the details. Terri Rojas and BostonBased did a great job with the meeting arrangements. Our thanks go out to the presenters and participants, and hope that this biennial activity can continue uninterrupted as we strive to be caregivers and innovators to this patient population.

ABOUT THE EDITOR

Mitchell L. Henry, M.D. is the Chief of The Division of Transplantation at The Ohio State University Medical Center, Columbus, and is a Professor in the Department of Surgery and Veterinary Clinical Science. He has been a staff member of the university's Division of Transplantation since 1985. Dr. Henry's other professional appointments include associate attending surgeon at The James Cancer Hospital and Research Institute, Columbus; associate medical director and executive board member of Lifeline of Ohio Organ Procurement; and associate attending surgeon, Children's Hospital, Columbus.

Dr. Henry's undergraduate and medical degrees are from the University of Nebraska where he graduated with high distinction in 1976 and 1979, respectively. His internship and residency in general surgery and fellowship in transplant were at The Ohio State University Hospitals.

As one of the originators of a series of biennial conference on vascular access for hemodialysis begun in 1988, Dr. Henry has served as co-editor of the books based on the meetings and is editor of this ninth of the series. He has published widely in medical specialty journals, authoring or co-authoring more than 170 articles, has contributed chapters to 25 books on vascular access and organ transplantation, and has presented papers at many conferences on these and related fields both nationally and internationally.

CONTRIBUTORS

Casandra A. Anderson, MD
Hennepin County Medical Center
Minneapolis, Minnesota

Selcuk Baktiroglu, MD
General Surgeon, Medical Faculty of Istanbul Istanbul University
Department of General Surgery
Istanbul, Turkey

David Beckett
Departments of Radiology and Vascular Surgery
Birmingham Heartlands Hospital
Birmingham, United Kingdom

Marcello Borzatta, MD, FACS
Vascular Surgeon
Mission Vascular Regional Center
Mission Hospital Medical Center
Mission Viejo, California

Pierre Bourquelot, MD
Clinique Jouvenet
Angioacccess Department
Paris, France

Deborah Brouwer, RN, CNN
Dialysis Nurse
Renal Solutions
Warrendale, Pennsylvania

Ingemar J. Davidson, MD, PhD, FACS
UT Southwestern Medical Center
Dallas, Texas

Charles M. Fisher, FRACS
Royal North Shore Hospital
St. Leonards, Australia

Marc H. Glickman, MD
Vascular and Transplant Specialists
Norfolk, Virginia

Wayne S. Gradman, MD
Cedars-Sinai Medical Center
Beverly Hills, California

Brian W. Haag, MD
Methodist Hospital
Indianapolis, Indiana

Stephen L. Hill, MD, FACS
Roanoke, Virginia

Thomas S. Huber, MD
Division of Vascular and Endovascular Therapy Department of Surgery
University of Florida College of Medicine Gainesville, Florida

Howard E. Katzman, MD
Surgical Group of Miami
Miami, Florida

Andra Konya, MD, PhD
Section of Vascular and Interventional Radiology
Division of Diagnostic Imaging
University of Texas M.D. Anderson Cancer Center
Houston, Texas

Cate Lewis, RN, BSN, CNN
Chair, Patient and Family Council National Kidney Foundation
Moscow, Pennsylvania

Ewan Macaulay
Department of Vascular Surgery
Aberdeen Royal Infirmary
Aberdeen, Scotland

Melody Mulaik, MSHS, CPC, RCC
Coding Strategies, Inc.
Powder Springs, Georgia

David D. Oakes, MD, FACS
Santa Clara Valley Medical Center
San Jose, California

C. Keith Ozaki, MD
University of Florida College of Medicine
Gainesville, Florida

Aslam Pervez, MD
Assistant Professor
Section of Nephrology and Hypertension Louisiana State University Health Sciences Center Shreveport, Louisiana

Rhonda C. Quick, MD
The Southern Arizona Vascular Institute
Tucson, Arizona

P.P.G.M. Rooijens, MD
Medical Center Rijnmond Zuid
Department of Surgery
Rotterdam, The Netherlands

John R. Ross, MD
General Surgery
Bamberg, South Carolina

A. Frederick Schild, MD, FACS
Professor of Surgery
Vascular Access Surgery
University of Miami School of Medicine
Jackson Memorial Hospital
Miami, Florida

Earl Schuman, MD
Portland, Oregon

Daniel A. Siragusa, MD
Chief, Division of Interventional Radiology University of Florida Health Science
Center Jacksonville, Florida

Louis C. Thibodeaux, MD, FACS
General and Vascular Surgical Specialists, Inc.
Cincinnati, Ohio

Candace Walworth, MD
Clinical Assistant Professor, University of Vermont
Lewiston Auburn Kidney Center
Lewiston, Maine

Thomas M. Vesely, MD
Associate Professor of Radiology, Surgery, and Medicine
Washington University School of Medicine St. Louis, Missouri

Fahim Zaman, MD
Assistant Professor of Medicine
Division of Nephrology and Hypertension Department of Medicine
Louisiana State University Health Sciences Center Shreveport, Louisiana

SECTION I
FACULTY PRESENTERS

1

DYNAMIC DUO:
THE CHAIRSIDE PERSPECTIVE OF
THE BUTTONHOLE METHOD
AND SELF-CANNULATION

Cate Lewis RN, BSN, CNN
Chair, Patient and Family Council
National Kidney Foundation
Moscow, Pennsylvania

My 30-year career as a Nephrology nurse was born from a familial diagnosis of Polycystic Kidney Disease (PKD). In 1972, during my senior year of nursing school, my Dad was diagnosed with PKD. I can still remember feeling fear of the unknown when his family physician was not able to offer us information on this disease process and my medical textbook held a one-paragraph description ending with the words "prognosis is poor". In 1974 I was also diagnosed with PKD. As fate would have it, the hospital where I was working, Moses Taylor Hospital in Scranton, Pa had an opening for a RN in the newly opened Renal Unit. It made perfect sense for me to apply for and accept this position, in order to prepare for whatever our family's future should hold. I have never once regretted this decision. I have been asked to share my perspective as both nephrology nurse and Chronic Kidney Disease (CKD) patient regarding vascular access issues.

A Blast from the Past: Home Hemodialysis and Self Care

For those of us who lived through the days of the 70's and 80's we saw the interest in modality options of both in-center self care and home hemodialysis. I had the pleasure of being a Home Training nurse helping several families to complete a 3-month training period including mastering the skill of cannulation. Although the majority of times the training partner would be the cannulator, two of my patients self cannulated. Looking back, these patients had virtually problem-free fistulae with little to no access problems. At least in our experience we saw that no infiltrations and little to no interventions were required. What was the secret to success? I truly believe the key was having the same cannulator, the "expert" performing the venipunctures. To further illustrate this point is the case of one of our patients, "Diane", who began home hemodialysis in 1973, self cannulated her fistula, and continued to self-cannulate upon returning in-center due to changes in stability. Diane's original fistula of 25 years never had a single intervention, not a revision, access study, infection nor aneurysm. Diane was passionate about patients having the choice to take an active role in care, whether home or in-center. As I followed her success throughout the years, I realized the influence that Diane had on me, encouraging my patients to learn as much about his or her care, especially access care in all stages of kidney disease.

When Peritoneal Dialysis became the new home therapy of choice in the mid 80's we saw a major decline in interest for performing home hemodialysis or in-center self care. Unfortunately, we also became complacent about encouraging self-care and self-cannulation to continue within the dialysis unit.

Access Observations

Unfortunately, the decline in native arteriovenous fistula creation and the increase in graft placement became trend. This caused the staff to reach a comfort level with graft cannulation, and as exposure diminished, the art of fistula cannulation suffered. In a 1998 study it was shown that although nephrologists preferred fistulae because of a lower incidence of infection and thrombus, staff preferred forearm grafts because of easier cannulation and better flow.[1] If this poll were repeated in 2004 I would hope that nurses would prefer a fistula as the first permanent access.

In my experience, we have always recognized that the expert cannulators, or as we say, "the sharpshooters", must be called upon to perform venipuncture. We reflect a statement in the medical record such as: *Experienced Staff Only to Cannulate.* Sometimes, however, altered perception interferes with this plan! When a staff member perceives herself or himself as the "experienced person" to cannulate and isn't the best candidate, often an infiltration or unnecessary needle puncture occurs. This is one of my pet peeves, observing this as a nephrology nurse and even more so from the chair side. The other pet peeve was hearing, as a CKD patient, the commonality of these words… "I'll stick you today". Imagine how frightening this initially sounds to a new patient. There becomes an immediate implication and expectation for pain! Simply rephrasing to: "I'll insert your needles today", is a much softer, less traumatizing, sounding statement.

Patient Issues

Fear of painful needle insertions, worry about inability to access sites, disfigurement and the need for additional surgical procedures can all be patient concerns.

When cannulation of a fistula or graft presents as a problem, naturally this can be stressful and anxiety producing for the patient. I have seen a variety of reactions from the patient praying aloud for staff success, becoming extremely angered to the point of threatening to notify the renal administrator, filing a Network grievance or simply refusing to stay for the treatment. A patient may begin to refuse certain staff the opportunity to cannulate and request another staff person. Reasons might include having a previous bad experience with that particular individual or just the fear of seeing a new face approach. Initially, this might be a cause for resentment or hard feelings depending on the staff person's level of maturity. Then, there is the passive unaffected patient, or the person who apologizes to the staff member(s) having difficulty performing the venipuncture, and continues to offer his or her arm to anyone requiring cannulation experience. These patients who willingly volunteer his or her access for "experience" purposes are truly the unsung heroes.

Patients, sadly, have refused to travel when plagued with access problems, especially if needle insertion difficulties are occurring. I've heard worries stated such as, "What if no one can get in and I can't have a treatment on that day?" Concerns that the family's vacation will be strained because of wasted time, or worse yet, the need for a trip to the hospital for intervention can make the difference in travel decisions. Again, the case for buttonhole sites, or even better, self-cannulation of buttonholes, can become advantageous and provide self-confidence.

Personal Early Decisions

Throughout the years I have become aware of the research of Dr. Zyblut Twardowski regarding the "constant site" method of needle insertion. Originally, in 1977 Dr. Twardowski published his first article referring to this technique. In 1993 he returned to his homeland of Poland and observed a patient with continued success of 20 years cannulating constant sites of his original native fistula.[2]

I also became aware of a successful long-term home hemodialysis patient, George Harper of Rome, Georgia, USA, who has self-cannulated buttonhole sites since 1980. His mentor was the late Dr. Peter Lundin, a nephrologist and CKD patient for close to 30 years. Dr. Lundin self cannulated his own established buttonhole sites after his mentor, the late Dr. Belding Scribner, introduced him to this cannulation method.[3]

Despite the skepticism from my nephrologist and staff, buttonhole self-cannulation made perfect sense to me and became part of the plan. Validations from Dr. Twardowski, Dr. Lundin, Dr. Scribner and George Harper were enough for me!

Reality

In May 1999 my kidneys failed and hemodialysis became a reality. Although my plans were well intended, having a fistula created in November 1998 at a serum creatinine level of 4.0 and hoping to dialyze via CAPD, this wasn't meant to be. In mid May, during PD catheter insertion my transverse colon was accidentally nicked thus causing peritonitis, bowel repair and removal of the catheter. Due to sepsis, the creatinine peaked to 9.0 and an urgent HD treatment was necessary. Unfortunately, my fistula had not matured correctly and was developing distally into the hand veins. Another trip to the OR was required for a Tesio catheter insertion. This experience opened up my eyes to several issues that our patients' may face. These include the patient's disappointment when a selected modality is not an option, feeling the concerns of additional access surgery and dealing with catheter issues. My fistula eventually required a branch ligation to correct the flow. The lesson I share with others is that sometimes the best plans backfire. We can encourage our patients' to remain hopeful that other options will be available.

Although eager to use my fistula and have the catheter removed, I could honestly understand the absolute need for catheters to be only a bridge device and not the initial first access. Easy on/off is appealing to a patient and having no delay holding sites post treatment appears to be an advantage. The most obvious reason why catheters are appealing to patients is no needles. If a catheter is the first and only access a security blanket phenomena may occur.

In our experience, we have often had the challenge convincing the patient of the need to begin to access the fistula since the patient has reached such a comfort level with a catheter. Worse yet is the patient refusing fistula or graft creation because the catheter "works fine" in the patient's eyes, yet access infections and adequacy issues were major concerns. All disciplines must collaborate and begin early education, during various stages of CKD, to emphasize that catheters must only be a temporary stepping-stone while the fistula is maturing, or the graft is placed. There are certainly opportunities for the primary care physician, nephrologists, vascular access surgeon, interventionalists and dialysis staff to echo the same messages: save veins, strive for fistula creation with adequate maturation time, and that catheters are not going to be the permanent access. Another strategy to help promote the importance of a fistula versus a catheter is to tap into the expertise and willingness to share success stories from one patient to another. It's a common sense approach to have a good patient advocate, one with a healthy functioning fistula and preferably not a fistula that is frightening in appearance, to meet with the patient fearful of either access surgery or any part of the access concept. One patient becomes the cheerleader and educator, at the same time, and is "listened to" uniquely because each share a common bond through experience. This approach has been very successful in our practice. Patients can be our best resource, and there are so many who would find the opportunity to help another so gratifying, yet this option is often overlooked.

Another eye-opener and complete surprise to me was how protective I became with my fistula. I self cannulated with buttonholes immediately and never once offered my arm to a new staff member to gain cannulation experience. Throughout the years I planned to be supportive by letting new staff cannulate my arm but I never had the courage to do this when the time came. All the same "what if's" became forefront in my thought process. For this reason I traveled with Buttonhole needles for any transient treatments. I was once initially refused the opportunity to self-cannulate because a particular dialysis facility had never heard of this practice. I patiently waited 45 minutes until the medical director could be notified to get his permission to self-cannulate and my dilemma was resolved.

For the first two years of self-cannulation via buttonhole sites sharp needles were the only needles available. Other than putting up with slight bleeding around the needle puncture sites, there were no infiltrations and no problems. In May 2001 I had the good fortune again, as fate would allow, to meet Pat Peterson RN, CNN. Pat at that time was the Manager of Professional Services, Medisystems Corporation, Seattle, WA. Pat introduced me to dull buttonhole needles, about to be FDA approved and as soon as this product was available to me there was an end to bleeding puncture sites. (Buttonhole™ Needle sets, Medisystems Corporation, Seattle, WA).

My nephrologist was soon convinced that this technique worked and began writing orders to initiate buttonhole sites on several of his patients experiencing cannulation concerns due to either limited sites or fragile fistulae.

The challenge faced, especially in our "seasoned staff" with longevity, was to understand the deviation from rotating sites. After all, this had always been drilled into us, and the American Nephrology Nurses Association (ANNA) text did not discuss buttonhole cannulation and continued to stress site rotation. No new articles were being written about this technique so it was even harder to get "buy in" from our staff despite my success and testimonials. In April 2002 Pat Peterson's article called: *Fistula Cannulation: The Buttonhole Technique* was published. Finally, more support for this technique and better yet for nephrology nurses, was published in the ANNA journal for all to read.[4]

Buttonhole Cannulation

In addition to the creation of easily accessible sites, the "constant site" technique provides an essentially pain free venipuncture experience, reduces or may even eliminate infiltrations and helps to promote a long fistula life.

A study performed by G. Kronung demonstrated that needle punctures performed in the same area, also called "one-site-itis", in contrast to the constant site, will cause aneurysmal dilatations and cause stenosis to develop in adjacent areas of the fistula. When the "rope-ladder" puncture technique was used, punctures were equally spaced along the fistulas' entire length. Small dilatations developed over the length of the fistula but not of an aneurysmatic nature. He found that the best technique was the "constant site" method as neither of these problems developed. Kronung renamed the "constant site" method to the "Buttonhole Puncture" technique.[5]

Buttonhole Initiation

Medisystems Corporation has a Buttonhole Starter Kit information pack that includes a complete description of the technique, common questions and answers and a step-by-step guide to the creation and maintenance of the sites. Initial sites selected should be based on the ease of cannulation (especially if the patient is cannulating) where the venous and arterial pressures are within range limits.

Here are some tips:

1. Sites are cannulated by the same person with a sharp needle for six venipunctures (six treatments)
2. If scheduling does not permit the same person to cannulate for these six treatments, another cannulator can initiate an alternative set of sites. This would allow staff person "A" to develop a set of sites and staff person "B" to develop another set. It is important that the same angle and needle depth is used during establishment of the tunnel, thus the reason for the *same* cannulator during the creation phase.[6] To expedite the process the patient might also select the option of daily cannulation for six days. I regret that I only established one set of buttonholes because during the last few months of dialysis, prior to transplant, I occasionally had difficulty accessing the venous site.
3. The scab that forms as each site heals must be lifted prior to venipuncture in order to visualize and access the exact needle puncture. I found that it helped to gently scrub the sites with a soapy washcloth during bathing. Then at the time of cannulation I used an alcohol wipe and 2x2 gauze to further remove the scab. The use of tweezers is also a recommended practice.
4. At the seventh treatment a Medisystems Dull Needle can be used since the tunnel has formed. I can only describe the feeling by referring to inserting an earring into a pierced ear. The post follows the established tract and slides in. If resistance is met gentle rotation of the needle is required to get the needle to slide through the tunnel, exactly as one would wiggle a pierced earring if there was resistance.

The Universal Wish List

Nephrology nurses share common concerns and hopes to continuously improve the quality of life for our patients. Our wish list directly relates to the vascular access and includes the following:

- There would be early referrals to the nephrologist and vascular access surgeon. More fistulae with adequate maturation periods would be created and a major reduction in bridge accesses would result.

- The vascular access cannulates easily, achieves prescribed blood flow rates, and promotes adequacy.

- The vascular access surgeon is committed to all efforts to create a fistula as the first and permanent access. In the ideal world there would be a relationship of collegiality and collaboration between the vascular access surgeon and the renal staff. The surgeon would not question cannulation skills because skills were at expert level. Proactive monitoring of venous and arterial pressures and early recognition of "trouble signs" would decrease access failure.

- Vascular access education of staff and patients would be ongoing and considered the priority component of staff education.

Fortunately we now have improvement projects of both the National Kidney Foundations' (NKF) Disease Outcomes Quality Initiative Guidelines (K/DOQI) and the National Vascular Access Improvement Initiative (NVAII) Fistula First Project sponsored through the Centers for Medicare and Medicaid Services (CMS). This is definitely another Dynamic Duo.

Lesson Learned

We need to encourage our patients to take an active participation in knowledge of his or her access and protecting this lifeline. This could be as simple as prepping sites to the ultimate, self-cannulation. Talking with the patient about specifics of needle depth or angle of insertion helps to get the patient involved. This also encourages self- confidence. A collaborative multi-disciplinary team and/or a vascular access coordinator are quality practice approaches to vascular access management.

The importance of vascular access education for the dialysis team must never be underestimated and must be considered the most important component of staff education. An outstanding teaching tool for all dialysis staff has been developed by Deborah Brouwer RN and is entitled: ***Cannulation Camp.***[7] Ideally, the concepts of this thorough reference would be incorporated in all phases of staff education, not only during orientation but throughout the ongoing competency reinforcement process.

I can't stress enough how important and necessary it is to identify staff members to be the cheerleader advocates for not only buttonhole cannulation but for self-cannulation. It has taken five years but we now have approximately 12 patients with successful buttonhole sites and three self-cannulation patients. Patient testimonials certainly help to spread the word about the ease of needle insertion and this painless technique. Enthusiasm breeds enthusiasm and good news will travel quickly about this DYNAMIC DUO!

References

1. Bay W. H., Van Cleef S., Owens M. The hemodialysis access: preferences and concerns of patients, dialysis nurses and technicians, and physicians. *Am J Nephrol* 1998;18:379–383.
2. Twardowski Z. Constant site (buttonhole) method of needle insertion for hemodialysis. *Dial and Transpl* 1995; Vol. 24, No. 10.
3. Harper G. Buttonhole needle insertion. A patient's experience. 1st International Symposium on Daily Home Hemodialysis. XVth Annual Conference on Peritoneal Dialysis. Baltimore, MD, Feb 13, 1995.
4. Peterson P. Fistula cannulation—the buttonhole technique. *Nephrol Nurs J* 2002; 29. 195.
5. Kronung G. Plastic deformation of cimino fistula by repeated puncture. *Dial Transpl* 1984; 13:635-638.
6. Medisystems Constant-Site Technique Procedure Card, Medisystems Corp., Seattle, WASH.
7. Brouwer D. Cannulation camp: basic needle training for dialysis staff, *Dial and Transpl* 1995; 24 (11): 606-612.

DISCUSSION

Vascular Access for Hemodialysis IX
May 6–7, 2004
Lake Buena Vista, Florida

May 6, 2004
Faculty Presentations
Lewis

Question for Ms Lewis on the buttonhole technique: We have been trying it at our unit. We have been putting all the new fistula patients on it, our results have not been as good as you have described. About half of the patients have requested stopping, primarily for pain. The nurses were in-serviced by the company before starting, we were waiting three to four weeks before changing from the sharp to the dull needles. But the most common complaint we would get was that it was painful, especially in the older patients. The younger patients seem to do well. It was also somewhat difficult to push the needle through the opening even though we did remove the scab. I was curious if you had any comments on that?

Lewis: We had one patient that complained of pain and she was an elderly patient and she asked us if we would switch back to sharp needles in her buttonhole sites. I do not have any other experience with that phenomena. It seems with everyone we have cannulated they have no problem with pain, and think it is an improvement. As far as the pushing, it is the same phenomenon that occurs with a pierced earing. Sometimes the track just might develop a little resistance in there and you have to rotate the needle a little bit, just gentle wiggling of the needle will make it go in. Not forcefully pushing it. But it did happen in my particular situation a lot where I feel a little resistance in there and just gentle pull back on the needle, reposition it a little bit, and wiggle it a little bit and it would slide right in. So that is a common phenomena that you might have to do that. As far as the pain, I do not have any experience with that.

Question: I noticed that you use the sharp needle yourself for a couple of years. Did you have any problems with bleeding around the needle?

Lewis: Yes, and that is the common problem. There was constant oozing around the needle site because typically you will nick the needle track with the sharp needle. That was the only problem. I just had to deal with the constant oozing. I did not have any other problem with that. As soon as I switched over to the dull needle that oozing stopped completely.

Question: What about the buttonhole technique? I have had some experience where we have tried to establish the buttonhole. In those people where we can establish it works great and no doubt about it. But then there is a fair amount of complications including aneurysms and bleeding from us trying to establish this. So I was wondering whether if someone has looked into it?

Lewis: The last studies that I am aware of it were two studies in 2000 and 2001 and Pat Peterson in ANNA. There are not a lot of recent studies about buttonhole cannulation.

2

ENDOVASCULAR PROCEDURES:
NEW TECHNIQUES
AND NEW TECHNOLOGY

Thomas M. Vesely, M.D.
Associate Professor of Radiology, Surgery, and Medicine
Mallinckrodt Institute of Radiology
Washington University School of Medicine
Saint Louis, Missouri

Address correspondence to:
T.M. Vesely, Mallinckrodt Institute of Radiology,
510 South Kingshighway Blvd, Saint Louis, MO 63110

Vascular Access Surveillance

Implementation of a vascular access surveillance program is the single most effective strategy for optimizing the performance and longevity of hemodialysis grafts and fistulae. The fundamental tenet of vascular access surveillance is that routine, periodic monitoring of grafts and fistulae will lead to the early detection of developing venous stenoses. Early detection, combined with expeditious treatment of hemodynamically significant lesions, will decrease the incidence of vascular access thrombosis.

According to the K/DOQI Clinical Practice Guidelines, hemodialysis grafts and fistulae should be monitored by performing a physical exam of the access every week and a quantitative assessment once a month.[1] Routine, periodic assessments of the vascular access, and the subsequent analysis of trends, are more predictive of a developing stenosis than a single, isolated assessment.[2] Unfortunately, due to the

13

cost of surveillance, and the lack of reimbursement for these programs, the majority of hemodialysis units in the United States have not yet implemented vascular access surveillance programs.

Several studies have demonstrated that the prevention of graft thrombosis will increase the overall lifespan of the vascular access.[3–6] Besarab reported an increase in average graft age from 1.97 years to 2.98 years following the implementation of a vascular access surveillance program.[4] Another important benefit of a surveillance program is a reduction in the total cost of maintaining the vascular access. Although frequent angioplasty is often necessary to maintain continued patency, the cost of an angioplasty is less than the cost of a thrombectomy procedure. Preservation of vascular access patency leads to substantial savings by reducing the costs of hospitalization, decreasing the need for temporary hemodialysis catheters, and decreasing the number of missed hemodialysis treatments. A recent study demonstrated a 48% reduction in the annual cost of vascular access services as a result of a surveillance program.[3]

One additional benefit of a surveillance program is improved performance of the vascular access. The early identification and treatment of hemodynamically significant stenoses minimizes intraaccess recirculation and maintains high extracorporeal blood flow, thereby optimizing the efficiency of hemodialysis treatment.

Vascular access surveillance is performed in the hemodialysis unit while the patient is connected to the hemodialysis machine. Since this is a covert activity the majority of radiologists and surgeons remain unaware of this critically important task.

Surveillance Methods.   The development of a venous stenosis will increase intraaccess pressure and decrease blood flow within a hemodialysis graft. Quantitative measurements of these two parameters are the foundation for vascular access surveillance. Clinical studies have demonstrated that the two most sensitive and specific methods for detecting venous stenoses are static venous pressure measurements and intraaccess blood flow monitoring.[7–9]

In a landmark series of clinical investigations and ensuing publications the team of Kevin Sullivan and Anatole Besarab described the hemodynamic relationship between the severity of a stenosis and the increase in pressure within a hemodialysis graft.[4, 10–12] This relationship is the basis for the use of venous pressure measurements for the detection of hemodialysis graft-related stenoses. In their clinical studies, Sullivan and Besarab demonstrated that the increase in intraaccess pressure was dependent on both the severity and the location of the stenosis.

A detailed description of the static venous pressure technique is described in Guideline 10 of K/DOQI.[1] In summary, a static venous pressure is a meticulous measurement of intragraft pressure when the blood pump on the hemodialysis machine is turned off. This measurement (VP0) is divided by the mean arterial pressure to correct for variability in blood pressure. It is important to understand that a static venous pressure measurement reflects the resistance of the vascular circuit that is downstream from the venous needle. Since the majority of stenoses are located near the venous anastomosis or within the native venous outflow tract this method is effective in detecting these lesions. However, access-related problems that are located proximal to the venous needle, such as poor arterial inflow or midgraft stenoses, will often go undetected using this method.[8]

Blood flow within a vascular access is related to the patient's blood pressure and the total resistance of the vascular access circuit.[13] Several clinical studies have demonstrated that the arterial inflow resistance, not the venous outflow resistance, is the most significant component of total graft resistance.[14, 15] Since the arterial inflow component is not assessed using static venous pressure measurements, a more useful surveillance method would be one that reflects the total resistance of the vascular access circuit. Comparative studies of different surveillance methods have shown that routine monitoring of intraaccess blood flow is the most sensitive and specific method for the detection of access-related stenoses.[7, 13]

There are several noninvasive techniques for measuring intraaccess blood flow including Doppler ultrasound, ultrasound dilution, hematocrit dilution, thermal dilution, and differential conductivity. The most widely used technique is the ultrasound dilution method using the Transonics HD01 system. Using this system, the measurement of intraaccess blood flow is performed while the patient is connected to the hemodialysis machine. The measurements should be obtained during the first hour of a hemodialysis treatment so that the results are unaffected by the decrease in cardiac output that often occurs following prolonged ultrafiltration. Hemodialysis treatment is stopped and the arterial and venous blood lines are reversed from their normal position. Flow sensors, which are connected to a laptop computer, are clipped onto the reversed arterial and venous blood lines. The hemodialysis blood pump is restarted at a fixed blood flow, usually 200ml/min, and a saline bolus (5ml) is injected into the venous blood line. The saline mixes with the blood flowing through the access and is detected by the sensor on the arterial line. The data is collected in the laptop computer and blood flow values are automatically calculated and recorded. Two blood flow measurements are typically obtained. If the values differ by more than 10% a third measurement should be performed.

The routine measurement of intragraft blood flow has provided new insights into the hemodynamics of vascular access. Intragraft blood flow is significantly higher than many physicians would have imagined. Prior to the creation of a vascular access in the upper extremity, the blood flow in the brachial artery is approximately 50-150ml/min. This dramatically increases to 800-2000ml/min following placement of a vascular access. Although there is substantial variability from patient to patient, a well-functioning graft typically has a blood flow of 1000-1500ml/min. An unpublished survey of blood flows obtained from 100 hemodialysis patients with PTFE grafts revealed a mean blood flow of 1000ml/min, with a range of 120ml/min to 3300ml/min. The average blood flow in a normal arteriovenous fistulae is slightly lower (700-900ml/min) than in a PTFE graft.

A baseline measurement of blood flow should be obtained and recorded when the access is first used for hemodialysis. As previously mentioned, the analysis of sequential blood flow measurements is important because both the magnitude and the rate of decrease in blood flow are predictive of impending thrombosis. According to the K/DOQI Guidelines, a patient should be referred for a fistulogram if the access flow is less than 600ml/min, or if the access flow is less than 1000ml/min and has decreased by more than 25% over a four-month period. However, it may be prudent to modify this recommendation for certain patients. This would include patients with an initial intraaccess blood flow that is less than normal (i.e. 600-800ml/min) or for patients who have undergone multiple interventions and have persistent, untreatable problems.

Endovascular Treatment of Stenoses

Angioplasty. Angioplasty continues to be the primary endovascular technique for the treatment of vascular access-related stenoses. Several studies have correlated the effectiveness of angioplasty to the patency of a hemodialysis graft. Lilly et al. reported a median graft survival of 6.9 months if there was no residual stenosis following an elective angioplasty procedure.[16] However, if there was a residual stenosis after angioplasty then the median survival was reduced to 4.6 months. These same investigators reported similar findings following combined percutaneous thrombectomy and angioplasty procedures; the median survival was 2.5 months when there was no residual stenosis, 1.6 months if there was a mild residual stenosis, and 0.3 months when there was a moderate or severe residual stenosis. Interestingly, in a retrospective analysis of 65 patients with native fistulae, Clark et al. reported that there was no difference in long-term patency when comparing patients who had a successful angioplasty (<30% residual stenosis) to those who had a residual stenosis of >30%.[17]

Zuckerman et al. measured intragraft blood flow both before and after angioplasty procedures and reported that a more effective dilatation (less residual stenosis) provided superior intragraft blood flow.[18] Furthermore, these investigators also reported that patients who had at least a 50% improvement in blood flow following angioplasty had significantly better long-term graft survival.

The use of high-pressure (>20 atm) and ultra-high pressure (>30 atm) angioplasty balloons has improved our ability to successfully dilate the majority of vascular-access related stenoses. Arnold reported a 96% success rate using an ultra-high pressure angioplasty balloon to treat 25 resistant stenoses that could not be dilated with a standard balloon (22 atm).[19] Similarly, Trerotola reported the successful use of an ultra-high pressure angioplasty balloon to treat seven resistant stenoses that had failed to respond to 27 atmospheres of dilating force using a conventional high-pressure balloon.[20]

The peripheral cutting balloon (Boston Scientific) was designed to provide effective dilatation while simultaneously minimizing the vascular trauma that is associated with conventional angioplasty. A cutting balloon consists of four atherotomes (microsurgical blades) that are mounted longitudinally along the external surface of a non-compliant angioplasty balloon. These cutting blades measure 0.011 – 0.013 inches high and 0.004 – 0.006 inches thick. The balloon material is designed to cover the atherotomes until the balloon is inflated. As the cutting balloon expands the four atherotomes incise the stenotic lesion and facilitate dilatation. Using this technology an effective angioplasty can be performed using low dilating forces (6 atm), thus minimizing trauma to the normal vascular wall adjacent to the stenosis. Several years ago Vorwerk et al. utilized the coronary cutting balloon to treat 14 patients with hemodialysis-related venous stenoses.[21] The reported primary patency rates were 86% at three months and 64% at six months. However, it must be noted that the coronary cutting balloon that was used for these procedures was only 4mm in diameter. Recently, the peripheral cutting balloon has become available for investigative use and is available in diameters ranging from 5mm to 8mm in diameter. Several investigators have reported the successful use of the new peripheral cutting balloon to treat hemodialysis-related stenoses but they did not report the long-term patency rates.[22, 23]

Cryoplasty.   A novel technique, "Cryoplasty", has recently been used to treat atherosclerotic stenoses in the peripheral arteries. The PolarCath angioplasty balloon (CryoVascular) is used to simultaneously freeze (-10C) and dilate the stenosis. Liquid nitrous oxide changes into a gaseous form as it enters the PolarCath balloon. As the liquid changes into a gas it inflates the balloon and freezes the adjacent tissue. Treatment time is about 1 minute. By freezing the vascular tissue, Cryoplasty is thought to work by inciting a more benign healing process instead of a proliferative response. The PolarCath balloon is available in 4mm – 7mm diameters and utilizes a 0.035 inch guidewire. However, to date, this interesting device has not yet been utilized for vascular access-related stenoses.

Brachytherapy.   Ionizing radiation has also been used to prevent the growth of neointimal hyperplastic tissue following angioplasty. Radiation treatment is thought to damage DNA with subsequent inhibition of smooth muscle cell proliferation, a primary component of the restenotic lesion. Radiation therapy can be delivered using external beam techniques or locally delivered (brachytherapy) using either radioactive stents or radioactive liquids within angioplasty balloons. Although both gamma and beta emitters have been used, beta radiation is currently the most common form of radiation for the treatment of endovascular restenosis. The majority of clinical trials have used radiation for the treatment of atherosclerotic stenoses, restenosis of atherosclerotic lesions, or instent restenosis. Several studies have reported the results of using external beam radiation for the treatment of vascular access stenoses but the results have been unremarkable. A more practical and clinically feasible approach would be the use of brachytherapy to treat venous anastomotic stenoses. The Corona brachytherapy system (Novoste) is FDA-approved for treatment of coronary artery stenoses and is currently in clinical trial for the treatment of hemodialysis graft stenoses. The Corona system utilizes a radioactive (Sr/Y-90) wire inserted through a proprietary angioplasty balloon catheter, which is filled with CO_2, to deliver radiation to the venous stenosis. Hopefully, the results of this clinical trial will be more successful than previous studies.

Endovascular Stents.   Endovascular stents would seem to be an ideal method to treat angioplasty failures. Stents can oppose elastic recoil and optimize endoluminal dimensions, thereby improving intragraft blood flow and prolonging graft patency. However, the majority of clinical studies have reported that the routine use of stents does not provide any additional benefit when compared to angioplasty alone.[24, 25] The neointimal hyperplastic tissue continues to grow unabated through the meshwork of the metallic stent. For these reasons the use of endovascular stents to treat hemodialysis-related stenoses continues to be a controversial subject.

Interestingly, a recent report has suggested that S.M.A.R.T. stents (Cordis) are substantially more effective than Wallstents (Boston Scientific) when used to treat hemodialysis-related stenoses. Vogel et al. reported a series of 86 hemodialysis patients; 65 patients received S.M.A.R.T. stents and 21 patients received Wallstents.[26] When used in central veins the median survival time was 16.3 months for S.M.A.R.T stents and 3.9 months for Wallstents. When used in peripheral veins the median survival time was 6.4 months for S.M.A.R.T. stents and 2.0 months for Wallstents. These investigators did not speculate as to the reasons for this dramatic difference in long-term patency. More recently, Vogel compared the results of angioplasty to the use of S.M.A.R.T. stents for the treatment of angioplasty failures.[27] The median primary patency after angioplasty was 130 days and 325 days after stent placement.

Stent Grafts.   As previously mentioned, the primary mode of stent failure is ingrowth of intimal hyperplasic tissue through the mesh of a metallic stent. Therefore, the use of covered stents, or stent-grafts, would seem to be a logical choice to prevent this problem. Early European investigations utilized the Cragg Endopro and Passenger stent-grafts to treat vascular access-related stenoses.[28, 29] Both of these stents-grafts consist of a self-expanding nitinol stent with a woven polyethylene terephthalate (PET) (Dacron) cover. The results of these early investigations were unremarkable, the use of the stent-graft did not provide better results when compared to those obtained using angioplasty alone.

More recently, the preliminary results of two different clinical trials that utilized stent-grafts to treat hemodialysis-related stenoses have been reported. However, the results reported for the aSpire covered stent (Vascular Architects) were worse than those for conventional angioplasty alone.[30] The recent results reported following use of the IMPRA stent graft (Bard) were slightly better than those expected for angioplasty alone.[31] The primary patency at two months was 87% and at six months was 61%. A common mode of failure for both of these devices was the development of new stenoses immediately adjacent to the end of the covered stent. Improvements in stent design, or the use of drug eluting stents, may provide better long-term results. And finally, several clinical reports have described an alternative use for endovascular stent grafts, the treatment of vascular access-related pseudoaneurysms.[32–34]

Of note, there is an important technical factor to consider when using standard metallic stents, or stent-grafts, to treat hemodialysis-related stenoses. Prior to stent deployment the lesion must be successfully pre-dilated using angioplasty. Furthermore, the lesion must be fully dilated, with no residual stenosis, prior to stent insertion. Inability to completely dilate the lesion is a relative contraindication to stent, or stent-graft, placement.

It was hoped that the use of all of these more sophisticated endovascular devices would provide superior long-term results for the treatment vascular access-related stenoses. Unfortunately, the use of these newer technologies has not yet proven to be more effective than conventional angioplasty.

References

1. National Kidney Foundation. K/DOQI Clinical Practice Guidelines for Vascular Access. *Am J Kid Dis* 2001; 37(suppl 1):S137-S181.
2. Neyra NR, Ikizler TA, May RE, Himmelfarb J, Schulman G, Shyr Y, Hakim RM. Change in access blood flow over time predicts vascular access thrombosis. *Kid Int* 1998; 54:1714-1719.

3. McCarley P, Wingard RL, Shyr Y, Pettus W, Hakim RM, Ikizler TA. Vascular access blood flow monitoring reduces access morbidity and costs. *Kid Int* 2001; 60:1164-1172.

4. Besarab A, Sullivan KL, Ross RP, Moritz MJ. Utility of intra-access pressure monitoring in detecting and correcting venous outlet stenoses prior to thrombosis. *Kid Int* 1995; 47:1364-1373.

5. Sands JJ, Miranda CL. Prolongation of hemodialysis access survival with elective revision. *Clin Nephrol* 1995; 44:329-333.

6. Roberts AB, Kahn MB, Bradford S, Lee J, Ahmed Z, Fitzsimmons J, Ball D. Graft surveillance and angioplasty prolongs dialysis graft patency. *J Am Coll Surg* 1996; 183:486-492.

7. May RE, Himmelfarb J, Yenicesu M, Knights S, Ikizler TA, Schulman G, Hernanz-Schuman M, Shyr Y, Hakim R. Predictive measures of vascular access thrombosis. A prospective study. *Kid Int* 1997; 52:1656-1662.

8. Bosman PJ, Boereboom FT, Eikelboom BC, Koomans HA, Blankestijn PJ. Graft flow as a predictor of thrombosis in hemodialysis grafts. *Kid Int* 1998; 54:1726-1730.

9. Smits JHM, van der Linden J, Hagen EC, Modderkolk-Cammeraat EC, Feith GW, Koomans HA, van den Dorpel MA, Blankestijn PJ. Grafts surveillance: venous pressure, access flow, or the combination? *Kid Int* 2001; 59:1551-1558.

10. Sullivan KL, Besarab A, Bonn J, Shapiro MJ, Gardiner GA, Moritz MJ. Hemodynamics of failing dialysis grafts. *Radiology* 1993; 186:867-872.

11. Sullivan KL, Besarab A, Dorrell S, Moritz MJ. The relationship between dialysis graft pressure and stenosis. *Invest Radiol* 1992; 27:352-355.

12. Sullivan KL, Besarab A. Hemodynamic screening and early percutaneous intervention reduce hemodialysis access thrombosis and increase graft longevity. *J Vasc Interv Radiol* 1997; 8:163-170.
    Gray RJ. Percutaneous intervention for permanent hemodialysis access: a review. *J Vasc Interv Radiol* 1997; 8:313-327.

13. Blankestijn PJ, Smits JHM. How to identify the hemodialysis access at risk of thrombosis? Are flow measurements the answer? *Nephrol Dial Transplant* 1999; 14:1068-1071.

14. Bosman PJ, Boereboom FT, Smits HF, Eikelboom BC, Koomans HA, Blankestijn PJ. Pressure or flow recordings for the surveillance of hemodialysis grafts. *Kid Int* 1997; 52:1084-1088.

15. Van Stone JC, Jones M, Van Stone J. Detection of hemodialysis access outlet stenosis by measuring outlet resistance. *Am J Kid Dis* 1994; 23:562-568.

16. Lilly RZ, Carlton D, Barker J, Saddekni S, Hamrick K, Oser R, Westfall AO, Allon M. Predictors of arteriovenous graft patency after radiologic intervention in hemodialysis patients. *Am J Kid Dis* 2001; 37:945-953.

17. Clark TW, Hirsch DA, Jindal KJ, Veugelers PJ, LeBlanc J. Outcome and prognostic factors of restenosis after percutaneous treatment of native hemodialysis fistulas. *J Vasc Interv Radiol* 2002; 13:51-59.

18. Zuckerman DA, Alspaugh JP, Faiyaz R, Duncan HJ, Munda R, Roy-Chaudhury P, et al. Increase in vascular access blood flow following venous angioplasty: a determinant of graft survival. *J Vasc Interv Radiol* 2002; 13(suppl): S37.

19. Arnold WP. A current approach to the endovascular treatment of resistant venous stenosis in hemodialysis vascular access. *J Vasc Interv Radiol* 2003; 14:S120 (abstr).

20. Trerotola SO, Stavropoulos SW, Shlansky-Goldberg R, Tuite CM, Kobrin S, Rudnick MR. Hemodialysis-related venous stenosis: treatment with ultrahigh-pressure angioplasty balloons. *Radiology* 2004; 231(1): 259–62.

21. Vorwerk D, Adam G, Muller-Leisse C, Guenther RW. Hemodialysis fistulas and grafts: use of cutting balloons to dilate venous stenoses. *Radiology* 1996; 864-867.

22. Aarts JC, Meier M, Vermeij C, Elsman B. Peripheral cutting balloon: initial experience in hemodialysis fistulas. *J Vasc Interv Radiol* 2003; 14:S119 (abstr).

23. McBride K, Cookson D, Warren M, Goddard J. Use of a cutting balloon to treat recurrent and resistant stenoses of native hemodialysis arteriovenous fistulas. *J Vasc Interv Radiol* 2003; 14:S28 (abstr).

24. Patel RI, Peck SH, Cooper SG, Epstein DM, Sofocleous CT, Schur I, Falk A. Patency of Wallstents placed across the venous anastomosis of hemodialysis grafts after percutaneous recanalization. *Radiology* 1998; 209:365-370.

25. Hoffer EK, Borsa J, Santulli P, Bloch R, Fontaine AB. Prospective randomized trial of a metallic intravascular stent in hemodialysis graft maintenance. *J Vasc Interv Radiol* 1997; 8:965-973.

26. Vogel PM. Hemodialysis access venous stenosis: Wallstent vs. SMART stent. *J Vasc Interv Radiol* 2002; 13:S38 (abstr).

27. Vogel PM. SMART stent use following angioplasty failure in dialysis access venous stenoses. *J Vasc Interv Radiol* 2003; 14:S28 (abstr).

28. Sapoval MR, Turmel-Rodriques LA, Raynaud AC, Bourquelot P, Rodrigue H, Gaux JC. Cragg covered stents in hemodialysis access: initial and midterm results. *J Vasc Interv Radiol* 1996; 7:335-342.

29. Farber A, Barbey MM, Grunert JH, Gmelin E. Access related venous stenoses and occlusions: treatment with percutaneous transluminal angioplasty and dacron covered stents. *Cardiovasc Intervent Radiol* 1999; 22:214-218.

30. Vesely TM. Use of the aSpire covered stent for treatment of hemodialysis graft related stenoses. *J Vasc Interv Radiol* 2002; 13:S38.

31. Haskal ZJ, Vesley T, Schuman E, McLennan G, Rivera F, Berman S, et al. Multicenter phase I results of the Bard PTFE stent graft trial for hemodialysis venous anastomotic graft stenoses. *J Vasc Interv Radiol* 2003; 14:S25 (abstr).

32. Rabindranauth P, Shindelman L. Transluminal stent-graft repair for pseudoaneurysm of PTFE hemodialysis grafts. *J Endovasc Surg* 1998; 5:138-141.

33. Hausegger KA, Tiessenhausen K, Klimpfinger M, Raith J, Hauser H, Tauss J. Aneurysms of hemodialysis access grafts: treatment with covered stents. A report of three cases. *Cardiovasc Intervent Radiol* 1998; 21:334-337.

34. Ryan JM, Smith TP. Use of a covered stent (Wallgraft) for treatment of pseudoaneurysms of dialysis grafts and fistulae. *J Vasc Interv Radiol* 2003; 14:S119 (abstr).

DISCUSSION

Vascular Access for Hemodialysis IX
May 6-7, 2004
Lake Buena Vista, Florida

May 6, 2004
Faculty Presentations
Vesely

Question to Dr. Vesely: In doing the full measurements, are you able to get any information relative to the location of lesions?

Vesely: There is no location involved. That is the good part and bad part about it. You can measure the flow anywhere in the circuit and it will tell you that there is something wrong with the circuit and then you have to go find it. That is where I have really had to change my practice in looking at subtle lesions. Subtle lesions can be a lot more significant than I ever thought before. Things that I knew years ago, I was blowing off. Now I don't blow them off. I can measure them and I can get everything else fixed and the blood flow is still only 500. Then I start looking more carefully. I really look critically at little subtle things. Let me take a balloon and just touch that area up and then re-measure the pressure and, boom, a flow of one thousand. I didn't know that was it. So I'm learning a lot. If nothing else measuring blood flow is good for that purpose. Use it for a couple of months and you realize what kinds of things you are missing. Arterial anastomotic stenoses are the single most important flow determinant of the entire vascular access. But the arterial anastomosis, just because it is not a 50% stenosis, does not mean it is not affecting blood flow. A subtle stenosis at 20-30% stenosis at the arterial anastomosis can be pretty significant.

Question: Every vascular access goes from aortic arterial pressure to central venous pressure that is from 140 over 190 down to about 4 over zero. The way they should run is it should smoothly decline in pressure throughout the whole length. I thank you for emphasizing the circuit. Do you think we are going to come to the time when clinicians will take over this pull-back pressure and look at it? Is there a lesion at one point? It does strike me that the intravascular ultrasound folks are finding lesions that look very serious that are very hard to see on the angiogram and vice versa. It depends on how you look at a lesion.

Vesely: Yes, you have touched on a lot of points there and I think I agree with all of them. Measurement of a pull-back gradient across the stenosis is a very good thing to do. I would not ever discourage anyone from doing that. Among interventional radiologists I did a very informal pole and I would say about 25% of them do it routinely. I actually do not. Although if I had a question of a lesion I would do that. I would measure that. It only tells you information about that one thing. If you had an arterial anastomotic stenosis that was substantially decreasing the pressure head into your graft and then you would measure pressure gradients across a venous anastomotic stenosis, it could be falsely negative because of your arterial anasto-motic stenosis which has decreased the over all pressure head. Intravascular ultra-sound, as far as I am concerned, is the gold standard. My point of a lot of my talk is that angiography does not work. Angiography gives you pictures but they are very coarse pictures of really what is going on. It is not that good. Intravascular ultra-sound is super sensitive. It gives you an incredible look at these lesions and actual-ly allows you to characterize them into three dimensions by doing pull-back ultra-sound. It is incredible. The trouble is it is very operator dependant, very expensive to do, and you have to do it at multiple locations around the graft so it becomes time extensive as well. If that is what you are into that is great. But it would probably take me two hours to do. It clearly is the gold standard.

Question: As dialysis patients get older and they are placed in the nursing homes, I see that they are coming out and no one has looked at their blood pressure med-ications. They come to you with a thrombosed graft and their blood pressure is 60 to 80. You know that their secondary patency rates are going to be limited by that. I would like to know how you are handling that?

Vesely: I agree with you. I am just learning about the fact that the pump is so important. It is only now over the last year that I have discovered that a lot of the chronic problems, the frequent flyers, who are having continuous graft thrombosis everything is fine and it is really their heart problem. I am not really sure what to do, basically I just call up the nephrologist and tell them to take care of that heart please. There is nothing I can do about that. I think they are starting to develop man-agement plans and things like that. We have not had a lot of patients like that and we are also working under the presumption that that is the problem. The subtle stuff becomes important and it is only by a process of exclusion that we then blame the pump and that is not that many patients.

Comment: I would like to introduce a note of caution about the holy grail of rou-tine transonic monitoring of graft flow triggering interventions. Perhaps because of the probability of damage to the vessel as a result of angiography that Dr. Chaudhury raised. A recent double blind study in the Journal of American Society of Nephrology by Moist demonstrated no benefit of the intervention triggered by routine transonic. The graft flows were followed and then interventions were triggered by the routine ones in the treatment group and the control group got them triggered only by the rou-tine clinical indications as before, independent of the graft flow data.

Veseley: Awesome paper. But the things to take away from the Moist paper are that, if you read the discussion carefully, their take home message is that they use their cannula and they use the value of 650 blood flow. Their conclusions were that the use of a 650 mls per minute blood flow is an excellent predictor of the presence of a stenosis. It is sensitive and it is specific. They said just because you can identi-fy a stenosis, that does not translate into better long term patency or durability of the graft. So they said, the use of transonics did not increase the patency of the graft. That is your point and that is very well taken. But lets take that a little bit further. Their conclusion was, that interventional radiology is failing because they do not have the technology to treat the stenoses, which the blood flow measurement techniques identify and that is true. I will not disagree with that. We know that from my talk. I have no tools to make this really better. One of the things I can do is try to optimize the blood flow and make it as best as I can when I am done with the tools I have and that is the result of the Moist paper.

Question: That is an excellent concept of looking at the circuit. I think it makes sense because when we talk about 30% stenosis we are just looking at it relative to the existing vessel. So once you treat one stenosis, the second stenosis down stream might become more significant. I think it is a great concept and I think the pull-back pressures are something to be looked into. Things that look insignificant in the beginning might get significant half way through the procedure. With the changing flows I think what we are achieving is that we are just trying to compress this tissue, which has grown there to the wall. Is this tissue recoiling or is it something like deposition of platelets, which appears as a recoil? Have you gone back and tried to open this up when you see this recoil after ten minutes?

Veseley: The way I think of it is the classic elastic recoil. These are muscular arteries. I do not think it is any new acute platelet deposition. I think it is simply the vessel wall expanding. Like you said all we do with angioplasty is controlled injury. All we do is squish the stuff away and hope it does not come back. Like Prabir showed, there is good remodeling and bad remodeling, and elastic recoil is acute bad remodeling. I think it is the muscular contractions that have reacted against it.

Question: One of the things that we have been doing is measuring flow in the access in the angio suite. We have also been using pressure measurements. This has led us to what we call our "Milwaukee special". We have a combination inflow/outflow stenosis. Your pressure measurements might be normal but as soon as you angioplasty the inflow, your pressure measurement goes sky high indicating there is an outflow stenosis. You angioplasty the outflow stenosis and now you are back at where you started with a normal pressure measurement. We use that in combination with the transonic flow catheter. If we don't get a result that we are expecting, then we just keep going back and looking to see what is going on.

Veseley: That is great. You are measuring pressures and blood flow. There is certainly a direct relationship between those two but I think if you are using both in combination clearly you have a pretty good idea to figure out what is wrong with that vascular access.

Question: So you would not necessarily recommend the cutting balloon?

Veseley: I think that the cutting balloon will be helpful to prevent elastic recoil. I was keeping track of elastic recoil. I would do my angioplasty and I would wait 15 minutes. Then I would repeat an angiogram. My guess had been that it was going to be about 15% of lesions would actually elastic recoil. It was not that high. It was only about eight or nine percent. So ten or 12 percent would benefit from a cutting balloon. I think a cutting balloon would help prevent elastic recoil.

3

ARTERIOVENOUS BRIDGE FISTULA PLACEMENT AND ITS EARLY USE

Dr. Selcuk Baktiroglu
Istanbul University, Istanbul Medical Faculty,
Department of General Surgery

Introduction

In our practice, we rarely use (9% of the time) prosthetic grafts for arteriovenous fistula (avf) construction.[1] The main indications for their use are:

1. Exhaustion of all native usable veins
2. Fat, diabetic, old patients
3. Bridging the two ends of a problematic segment (aneurysm, stenosis, obstruction, etc)
4. Prompt need for dialysis

In all of these indications (with perhaps the exception of number 2) these accesses are being used as soon as possible. In this paper, our experience with a-v bridge fistulas with prosthetic grafts in a specific location, namely in the distal forearm, and their early use is going to be presented.

Patients requiring dialysis access may be stratified into three groups according to the urgency of the situation:[2]

1. Those in need of emergency dialysis (within hours)
2. Those in need of prompt dialysis (within 48 hours)
3. Those whose dialysis need is anticipated within several months

The first group of patients in need of immediate dialysis should have percutaneous dialysis catheter placed. Patients in the third group are prepared for future dialysis by placement of an a-v fistula. In today's practice, catheters are also placed in the patients in the second group. We are all aware of the possible complications of percutaneous catheters.[3]

Because of the fear of possible complications of percutaneous catheters and in the light of previous reports[4, 5] and our limited experience with our own cases regarding the safety of early cannulation of PTFE grafts, we decided to perform a-v bridge graft fistula at the wrist between the radial artery and cephalic vein.

By doing this, our expectations are threefold:

1. Patients can be dialyzed as soon as possible (within 48 hours).
2. Complications that may occur can easily be managed because the bridge fistula is superficial and short and easily be accessed.
3. If we cannot save the bridge fistula because of a complication, we can still make a Cimino avf right above the venous anastomosis, because the vein is already matured after a couple of weeks. The patient can be dialyzed from this autogenous fistula without missing a dialysis session.

Technique

We perform a bridge fistula between the distal radial artery and cephalic vein by using a 10 – 12 cm x 6 mm Polytetrafluoroethylene stretch dialysis graft (Goretex, WL Gore and Associates, Flagstaff, Arizona). All operations were done under local anesthesia (1% lidocaine). One gram Cefazolin was given one half hour before the operation for perioperative prophylaxis. Heparin-saline solution (1%) was used liberally for flushing the vein and the graft during the operation.

In five patients, we used the distal radial artery as the inflow vessel and made the arterial anastomosis first, and then turned the graft back in a subcutaneuos tunnel with a wide U shape to about 6-7 cm proximally. We then made the venous anastomosis to the cephalic vein (Figure 1).

In three patients (5th, 6th, 7th) we did the arterial anastomosis proximally and venous anastomosis distally because:

1. Better flow characteristics with antegrade flow
2. We observed we have had almost all the problems in or around venous anastomosis, so if we have a problem in this anastomosis (thrombosis due to intimal hyperplasia) we can make a new one 1-2 cm proximally and spare much of patient's outflow vein (Figure 2).

Not all of the patients are good candidates for this operation. Because of anatomical variations, previous vein cannulations and unsuccessful or occluded previous av fistulas, performing the operation may not be possible.

First, a very careful physical examination should be done. In some cases a doppler ultrasound examination may be needed.

After the operation the patients are advised to keep their arms elevated because of the fear of hematoma formation.

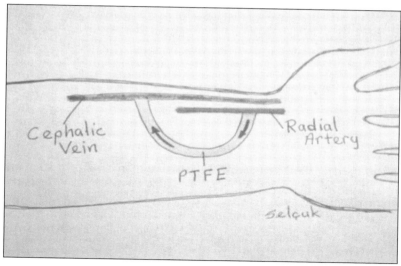

Figure 1

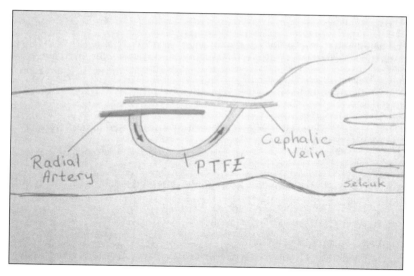

Figure 2

Material

From December 2001 to April 2004 we have applied this technique to 8 patients who were in need of prompt dialysis. Six patients were male and two were female . The mean age was 53 (29-75) years. Effective hemodialysis was achieved in all of the patients within a mean of 43.2 hours (16-91 hours) of access creation.

Our previous reports described time to use was 34.4 hours.[6] Our sixth patient could not reach the dialysis unit because of very bad weather conditions although he was scheduled to be dialyzed in about 36 hours instead of 91 hours. The seventh patient was scheduled for dialysis in 24 hours, but waited one more day on his own,

Results

Patient-1: 45, F, diabetic

The patient was operated on December 2001. Her graft thrombosed 3 times at the 6th, 10th and 12th month, and was salvaged. The last one was because of a tear during accessing the graft. The torn segment in the graft was excised and the graft thrombectomized. At the 14th month the graft thrombosed again and could not be salvaged. A new radial–cephalic fistula was done 2 cm proximal to the arterial anastomosis. She is being dialyzed via this fistula since that time.

Patient-2: 46, M

The operation was done in February 2002. He has had 3 dialysis in our institution and turned back to the city where he came from without a problem. He is lost to follow up.

Patient-3: 67, M, diabetic

The patient was operated in February 2002. At the 7th month the graft thrombosed, but thrombectomy was not successful. A 4-5 cm jump graft was interposed between the graft and the proximal cephalic vein. He died of sepsis following his second above the knee amputation on April 2003 with functioning fistula.

Patient-4: 49, M

Fourth operation was done in August 2002. The graft thrombosed at the 7th month. He refused further intervention and was lost to follow up.

Patient-5: 53, F, diabetic

The operation was done in November 2002 with the antegrade technique. She is still being dialyzed via this bridge fistula.

Patient-6: 29, M

This operation was accomplishd with the antegrade technique on January 2004. He could not be dialyzed until 91 hours post access creation because of very bad weather conditions. He is being dialyzed via this access.

Patient-7: 75, M

The operation was done on January 2004 by the antegrade technique. His graft thrombosed on the 98th day in another city. The problem was in the proximal needling area, and there was no intimal hyperplasia in or around the venous anastomosis. After thrombectomy he had dialysis via this access in less than 24 hours postop.

Patient-8: 61, M

The operation was done on March 2004 by the retrograde technique because his cephalic vein distal to the dorsal branch was rudimentary. The venous anastomosis was done to a dorsal branch. He was first dialyzed 43 hours after the operation and still being dialyzed via this graft.

Discussion

In common practice a-v grafts are being used at least 2-3 weeks after the operation. In 1985 Taucher reported safe, early use of the a-v grafts created by a new tunneler within 2-4 days. He stated "it seems apparent that application of the tunneler has greately facilitated the immediate use of the graft a-v fistulas".[4]

In his prospective, nonrandomised trial, Hakaim concluded that "early cannulation of prosthetic dialysis grafts does not increase perioperative morbidity rate or decrease 12 month cumulative primary patency rates".[5] He also used a tunneling device.

In recent years we have had a limited experience with early use of a-v grafts in different locations. Our experience encouraged us about the safety of early cannulation. Besides we could still make an autogenous fistula right above the venous anastomosis if we cannot salvage the a-v graft in this specific location. We now prefer the antegrade technique whenever possible. We do not use tunneling devices.

The earliest complication (thrombosis) occurred at 98th day in our seventh patient. The critical period is 3-6 weeks. During this time, the outflow vein matures and a new autogenous fistula (Cimino) can be created without missing a dialysis session. Our patients always prefer their grafts to be salvaged because they are taught they have limited access sites and the operation (thrombectomy) is easy and simple. Hence, we create a Cimino avf only when we cannot salvage the graft as in our first case. In our third patient we used the jump graft because the intimal hyperplasia at the venous anastomosis was very dense and this operation was easier than performing an a-v fistula.

We did not encounter any infectious or other extremity or life threatening complications.

Conclusions

With this technique, effective hemodialysis was achieved in all of our patients in a mean duration of 43.2 (16-91) hours.

We saved our patients from possible complications of percutaneous catheters.

We did not encounter any life or extremity threatening complications. The complications that occurred (thrombosis) could easily be managed and the patients did not miss any single dialysis session.

In patients with grafts that could not be salvaged, we were able to create a Cimino fistula right above the venous anastomosis without missing dialysis.

References

1. Dilege S, Genc FA, Baktiroglu S, Kalayci G: Hemodiyaliz amaçli sentetik greft interpozisyonlari. VI. Ulusal Gögüs Kalp Damar Cerrahisi Kongresi, Ekim 2000, Antalya.
2. Gelabert HA, Freischlag JA: Hemodialysis access. In Vascular Surgery, Rutherford Vth edition Saunders vol: 2, p: 1466-77, 2000.

3. Starting Management of Vascular Access. In Management of The Renal Patient: Clinical Algorithms on Vascular Access For Haemodialysis. Bakran A, Mickley V, Passlick-Deetjen J eds, Pabst Science Publishers, p: 16.

4. Taucher LA: Immediate, safe hemodialysis into arteriovenous fistulas created with a new tunneler. An 11 year experience. Am J Surg 1985; 150 (2): 212-215.

5. Hakaim AG, Scott TE: Durability of early prosthetic dialysis graft cannulation: Results of a prospective, nonrandomized clinical trial. J Vasc Surg 1997; 25 (6): 1002-1005.

6. Baktiroglu S, Aksoy M: Wrist arteriovenous graft fistulas for early hemodialysis cannulation. Oral presentation; 3rd International Congress of Vascular Access Society, 21-23 May 2003, Lisbon-Portugal.

DISCUSSION

Vascular Access for Hemodialysis IX
May 6-7, 2004
Lake Buena Vista, Florida

May 6, 2004
Faculty Presentations
Baktiroglu

Question to Dr. Baktiroglu: Do you do any study of the radial artery or the cephalic vein prior to putting in the bridge fistula?

Baktiroglu: Yes, sometimes we do only Doppler examination. We did not do any angiography before putting these special placements.

SECTION II
ABSTRACT PRESENTERS

4

CHANGES IN HEMODIALYSIS ACCESS OVER THE PAST TWENTY YEARS

Stephen L. Hill, M.D., F.A.C.S.
Antonio T. Donato, M.D., F.A.C.S.

Corresponding author:
Stephen L. Hill, M.D., F.A.C.S.
1125 South Jefferson Street
Roanoke, Virginia 24016
Phone-540-982-1141
Fax-540-982-5802
e-mail: stoverhill@aol.com

Introduction

Procedures and trends in hemodialysis access, as in many aspects of medicine, will change from year to year with new techniques, innovations, and products. It is only with retrospective evaluations over a long period of time that it becomes apparent which of the changes are significant and long lasting. We have chosen to review our results over the past twenty years in order to evaluate these changes. During this twenty-year period there have been changes in catheters, graft materials, and techniques for declotting grafts. There was also a change in emphasis back to autogenous fistulae as the ideal type of access as advocated by the National Kidney Foundation Dialysis Outcomes Quality Initiative in 1997. In addition, the development of the vascular laboratory and its impact on the field of hemodialysis in identifying veins for possible fistula construction, detecting significant stenoses, and its use in surveillance of hemodialysis access grafts has changed the manner in which we approach the patient with renal failure. All of these changes will be reviewed and evaluated to see which, if any, may be of significance over the next twenty years.

Methods

All patients referred for hemodialysis access to a two man surgical practice over the past twenty years were evaluated. The fact that only two surgeons were involved provided consistency in evaluation, work-up, surgical technique, and treatment of complications. Patients were followed for any complications, occlusions, or infections of their access. Their age, etiology of renal failure, and type of graft were documented. Their length of survival were followed as best could be for this type of population. The primary patency and cumulative patency were calculated as well as the number of different locations and grafts used in each patient. Changes that occurred through the years, including the use of the vascular laboratory, interventional radiology, the introduction of tunneled dialysis catheters and surgical technique were documented and followed.

Results

There were a total of 1,120 procedures performed on 366 patients in this study which ran from July, 1983 until March 2004. All patients were referred for hemodialysis, and access was obtained by a variety of means depending on the acuity, anatomy, and need for long term or acute dialysis. The types of access varied through this long time period with alterations between autogenous fistulae vs. prosthetic grafts, catheters vs. cuffed catheters and location varying between the jugular, subclavian, and femoral vein. The average age of the patient was 60.3 years with 177 males and 189 females. There were a total of 49 patients (13%) who were lost to follow-up. The etiology of the renal failure varied, as to be expected, with 51% due to hypertension, 29% due to diabetes mellitus, 12% due to acute tubular necrosis, 4% due to glomerulonephritis, 2% due to polycystic kidney disease and 1% due to drug overdose. Multiple other diseases such as phenylketonuria, toxemia of pregnancy, ITP, oxalate nephropathy, Good-pasture's Syndrome, and leukemia were some of the remaining causes of the renal failure.

There were a total of 213 patients who received 314 expanded polytetrafluoroethylene (ePFTE) grafts for hemodialysis during this study. There were 129 of these patients who received only one prosthetic graft, however the vast majority of these patients either died during the study or were lost to follow-up. Most patients with prosthetic grafts had multiple grafts and multiple procedures in order to continue with dialysis. There were only ten patients (4.5%) who had long term patency with a prosthetic graft without revisions or replacements. The remaining patients required an additional 202 operative procedures (excluding temporary dialysis catheters used to continue dialysis while the graft was being repaired, or replaced) to maintain patency, giving rise to a total of 516 operative procedures in this prosthetic group. In the later years of the study (approximately the last ten years), interventional radiology played a larger role in declotting grafts as opposed to an operative approach. In the 202 procedures required to maintain patency, interventional radiology performed the procedure 49 times, while an operative approach was used the remaining times (153).

The prosthetic grafts had an average primary patency of 14.6 months with an average cumulative patency of 19.8 months. Operative procedures to open a graft after its first occlusion increased patency an average of 8.1 months; after its second occlusion an average of 4.4 months was gained. Primary patency ranged from hours to 208 months while cumulative patency ranged from one month to 208 months. There were 97 patients who died during the study with a functioning PFTE graft and the average patency at the time of their death was 18.9 months. There were 13 patients who at the end of the study had a functioning PFTE graft and the average patency of this group of patients was 26 months. The vast majority (93.4%) were upper arm grafts, with a small number of forearm grafts (4.7%). In only six patients (1.9 %) did we have to resort to the femoral approach for hemodialysis access with a prosthetic graft. No patient died from lack of access in this study over the twenty-year period and only one patient died during the performance of an access procedure due to cardiac causes.

Temporary and tunneled catheters were used extensively throughout this study. In the earlier years of the study, before the hazards of subclavian vein stenoses were recognized, the subclavian vein was used extensively for temporary dialysis access; likewise the internal jugular route was used for temporary catheters before the tunneled catheters were available. There were a total of 119 femoral lines placed, 190 jugular lines and 188 subclavian lines for acute and subacute access. In the later years of the study the use of the subclavian vein for dialysis essentially stopped. The use of the femoral vein increased mainly for its use in emergent access and the use of the internal jugular veins increased due to its use for the tunneled dialysis catheters for temporary and chronic use. (FIGURE 1)

There were 43 patients who received only temporary catheters, with no placement of a graft or fistula. The femoral route was used 19 times, while the subclavian or jugular route was used (in the earlier part of the study) 24 times. There were 20 patients who received just a tunneled catheter for long term dialysis. Over this twenty-year period and 366 patients there were 13 patients (3.6%) who had exhausted all possible areas for hemodialysis access and could only receive dialysis permanently through a tunneled dialysis catheter.

There were 123 patients who had placement of an autogenous fistula. Fifty patients had 52 attempts of a Cimino fistula with 28 being successfully used for dialysis (58%). They had an average primary patency of 60.7 months and an average cumulative patency of 70.4 months

There were 73 patients who had 76 attempts at a brachial-cephalic fistula. A total of fifty-eight fistulae (78%) were successful and used for dialysis. The brachial – cephalic fistulae were constructed late in the study and therefore their long-term statistics were far shorter than for Cimino fistulae. The average primary patency was 17.3 months, with a cumulative patency of 21 months.

In looking at the numbers of fistulae constructed through the years compared to the use of prosthetic grafts (FIGURE 2) there is a significant increase beginning about 1996. It occurred when the vascular laboratory began to be used extensively

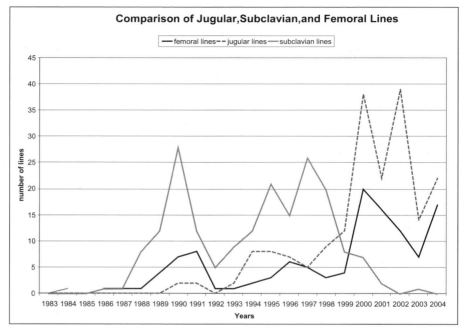

Figure 1

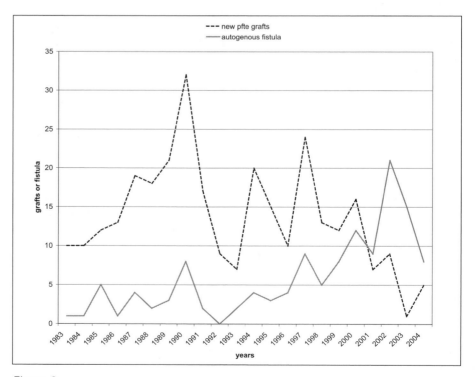

Figure 2

in dialysis access work and the recommendations of the National Kidney Foundation for dialysis access became prominent.

As expected, thrombosis was the main complication in this study, and thus gave rise to the limited patency in the prosthetic grafts and required multiple procedures to maintain patency. In this group of 213 patients who received a prosthetic graft, there was a subgroup (18 patients) that was particularly susceptible to thrombosis and infection, requiring an excessive number of procedures to continue dialysis. These eighteen patients required a total of 255 procedures including multiple temporary catheters to continue to receive dialysis. The autogenous fistulae, as has been shown in the past, had better and longer patency periods. There were only a total of 21 additional procedures performed in the autogenous fistula group to maintain patency. The cumulative patency for the Cimino fistula was 70.4 months compared to the prosthetic grafts 19.8 months; the brachiocephalic (21 months) group show a trend toward much better patency rates but they are too recent in this study to prove to be significantly better than the prosthetic graft. Another follow up study will have to be done in the future to determine the true primary and cumulative patency of the brachiocephalic fistula in this group of patients.

There were 43 patients who had both an autogenous fistula and a prosthetic graft. Twenty-nine failed an attempt at an autogenous fistula and then had a prosthetic graft placed. Five patients had a prolonged period of a functioning fistula (9-102 months) prior to occlusion and then placement of a prosthetic graft. There were nine patients who first had a prosthetic graft and when it occluded had a successful autogenous fistula placed.

Infections were the next most common complication. It occurred in 23 patients out of the total group of patients 213 patients (10.8%) who received a prosthetic graft. There were 30 infections in these patients who had had a total of 516 operative procedures giving rise to an incidence of infection of 5.8% in the prosthetic group. In the autogenous group there were no infections in the Cimino group of fistulae and only occurred in 5 in the brachiocephalic group. There were 128 procedures performed in 123 patients. Infection occurred in 4.1% of patients and 3.9% of procedures. It is of note that in two of the five autogenous fistulae infections the infection was controlled and the access salvaged. This never occurred in the prosthetic group.

The steal syndrome occurred in both groups. In the prosthetic group, it occurred 10 times in 9 patients for an incidence of 4.2% and could be repaired in three patients by making the arterial anastomosis smaller. In the autogenous fistulae group the steal syndrome occurred three times in three different patients for an incidence of 2.5%. In this group the steal syndrome was eradicated in one patient, again by making the arterial anastomosis smaller. It is of note that in all thirteen cases of the steal syndrome the patients were insulin dependent diabetics and 75%[10] were female.

Aneurysm formation was a problem in both groups due to repetitive cannulations in the same location, however in the prosthetic group it led to infection and replacement. In the prosthetic group there were 15 patients (7%) who developed pseudoaneuysms of the graft which necessitated removal. In the autogenous fistula group there were only two patients (2.3%) who developed significant pseudoaneuysms (both in the brachiocephalic group) which precluded dialysis and required surgical attention; one could be repaired and the other was infected requiring ligation.

Discussion

Hemodialysis access continues to be a recurring problem in the chronic renal failure population. Complications of dialysis access alone account for twenty per cent of the hospitalizations for patients with renal failure.[1, 2] There has never been a perfect, long lasting access that works for all patients. The closest we have come to the best hemodialysis access for the most patients has been the Cimino radiocephalic fistula. Unfortunately, many patients do not have an adequate cephalic vein for a Cimino fistula either due to anatomy, thrombosis, or sclerosis after many intravenous lines during previous hospitalizations. The perfect prosthetic graft has been sought but never found. Reports have stated that long term patency of synthetic grafts rarely exceed 50% due to thrombosis.[3, 4] The problems with prosthetics are all too well known, including infections, pseudointimal hyperplasia causing occlusion, aneurysmal dilatation and occlusions due to low flow. Dialysis catheters have intermittently been used for both emergent temporary use as well as long-term use in selected individuals who cannot have hemodialysis access by a graft or fistula; unfortunately these, too, have numerous complications including infection, malfunction, and stenosis with obstruction of surrounding veins. Consequently, through the years, there have been innovations, new catheters, graft materials and suggestions to deal with these vexing, recurring problems. It was the purpose of this paper to look at the changes and innovations that have occurred and determine their lasting or fleeting effect.

Expanded polytetrafluoroethylene (ePFTE) grafts have been used over the past twenty years and appeared to have withstood the test of time. They are durable, reliable, and an adequate conduit for hemodialysis access in those individuals who have no native vein that can be used for an autogenous access. The results in this paper would indicate that their results are variable – excellent in some segments of the population and miserable in other segments with persistent and frequent clotting. Numerous studies in the literature have published similar results describing only fifty per cent patency rate with prosthetic grafts and certain groups of patients having recurrent infections and clotting with prosthetic grafts.[3–6] Infections, aneurysm formation, and steal are more common than in an autogenous fistula (TABLE 1). One of their strong points is their ability to be opened after thrombosis, first intraoperatively by embolectomy in the early phases of this study, and in the past several years by interventional radiology. In most cases it is often necessary to treat the outflow tract, revisions including patch angioplasty or a jump graft in the operative phase, or a dilatation by interventional radiology. In our hands, ePFTE is the graft of choice after an exhaustive search for an adequate cephalic vein. A good cephalic vein is always chosen over a prosthetic, but a poor vein (less than 2 millimeters or sclerotic) is not better than a prosthetic. Our current treatment regimen when a prosthetic graft comes in occluded includes interventional radiology attempts to declot the graft and dilate the outflow vein, if necessary. If there is not an obvious reason for the occlusion such as a stenosis, the patient will occasionally be placed on coumadin with the assumption that his blood pressure gets too low on dialysis or immediately after a treatment. If the patient has an occlusion more than three times in a six month period, operative intervention is then perfomed to revise the venous anastomosis or perform a jump graft over the venous stenosis.

Table 1.

Type of Graft	Number of Patients	Primary Patency (Months)	Cumulative Patency (Months)	% Patent 12 Months	% Patent 24 Months	Infections %	Steal %
ePFTE	213	14.6	19.8	37%	21%	10.8%	4.2%
Autogenous	128					3.9%	2.5%
Cimino	52	60.7	70.4	82%	61%	0.0%	1.9%
Brachiocephalic	76	17.2	21	47%	32%	6.6%	2.6%

All patients who require emergent dialysis undergo femoral catherization with a percutaneous dialysis catheter. This does not require an operative procedure and does not limit or affect future options. Placing a percutaneous dialysis catheter in the subclavian veins risks causing a significant stenosis of the subclavian vein that essentially prevents ever using that extremity for dialysis access. This has been reported several times in the literature.[6, 7] Use of the jugular vein for a temporary percutaneous dialysis catheter jeopardizes a stenosis and limits choices for a longer term tunneled dialysis catheter. The advantage of the percutaneous femoral dialysis catheter is that it allows immediate access and then affords the ability to place a tunneled catheter in either jugular vein if time is needed for maturation of an autogenous fistula or a prosthetic graft. After presentation of a patient with need for hemodialysis access, whether they be a new patient or an old patient with a failing graft, an extensive search is done by the vascular lab evaluating the upper and lower arm cephalic veins, as well as the patency and condition of the subclavian and internal jugular veins. Decisions are then made concerning the feasibility of an autogenous fistula. A tunneled dialysis catheter is placed to allow the six to ten week period needed for maturation of an autogenous fistula. If an autogenous fistula is not possible, then a prosthetic graft is placed in the arm that provides the best artery and a deep vein. There is a portion of the renal failure population who have no areas for possible hemodialysis access due to previous surgeries, jugular and subclavian vein occlusion and are forced to use a tunneled dialysis catheter for the rest of their life or until they can receive a transplant. In this retrospective study, this group comprised 3.6% of the total and compares favorably to the Clinical Practice Guidelines advocated by the National Kidney Foundation Dialysis Outcomes Quality Initiative.[8] We have found that there is a segment of the renal failure population who do not tolerate the tunneled dialysis catheters very well. We have seen several severe complications of these tunneled catheters such as innominate and subclavian vein occlusion both with and without an infection. This then gives rise to significant edema of the upper extremities and/ or neck areas which may take months to resolve; if the patient has a dialysis graft or fistula in the affected extremity it will either thrombose or exacerbate the situation due to the increased venous pressure.

One of the other changes, as stated above, is the use of the vascular lab to search for veins for possible autogenous fistula. The upper arm cephalic vein has been shown to be a good source for an autogenous fistula but is rarely used because it is not as obvious as the cephalic vein at the wrist.[9–11] Unlike the cephalic vein at the wrist, is often spared intravenous lines and therefore not sclerotic. If the vein is equal or greater than two millimeters, it can serve as an excellent autogenous fistula. The operative procedure only requires one anastomosis and the cephalic vein remains relatively superficial throughout its course in the upper arm. Occasionally in obese patients, a transposition of the vein to a more superficial location is necessary initially or in a follow-up operation.[6, 12, 13]

The search for an autogenous fistula does not only occur when the patient first presents for dialysis, but instead every time there is a problem with hemodialysis access. There were many times during this study that an autogenous fistula was constructed after the patients prosthetic graft had occluded. Similarly, when an autogenous access occludes it may be necessary to move on to a prosthetic graft for access, if there are no more autogenous sites available. In fact, sometimes a forearm graft or a Cimino fistula will over time dilate a cephalic vein in the upper arm which initially had appeared too small to mature into an adequate size vein amenable to dialysis.

The vascular laboratory can also be used prior to the placement of tunneled dialysis catheters. It is used to assess the patency of the internal jugular and subclavian veins to avoid attempts at trying to identify and cannulate occluded or stenotic central veins. Many of the patients with renal failure have had multiple previous hospitalizations with central lines and could have an occluded or stenotic subclavian or jugular vein.[7]

The steal syndrome, though relatively uncommon, can cause significant morbidity with pain, necrosis, and loss of a functioning access graft. It is more common in patients with prosthetic hemodialysis access grafts (4.2%) than in patients with autogenous fistula (2.4%). Similar numbers have been previously reported in the literature.[13] We have also found it to occur most commonly in female diabetics, and this is corroborated by other studies in the literature.[14] The theory behind it is that the significant peripheral vascular disease and the calcifications in the brachial and/or radial artery do not allow the vessel to dilate and supply the extremity with more blood for the fistula and the extremity. The presence of the distal disease with multiple stenoses and obstructions cause the blood to go the path of least resistance through the fistula - thus causing a painful ischemic extremity.[15] We have found the only way to correct this and salvage the fistula or graft was to make the arterial anastomosis smaller, encouraging the flow to continue down the arterial vasculature rather than the fistula. This approach was successful in approximately 30% in both the prosthetic group and the autogenous group in salvaging the fistula/graft and relieving the symptoms.

It is through extensive reviews and evaluation of new techniques that the many and varied problems encountered in the chronic dialysis population can be painstakingly studied and solved. We have made many changes through the years that have increased our success rate and lessened the complication rate. We have once again, reaffirmed the superiority of the autogenous dialysis access graft with its higher long-term patency rate and decreased complication rate of thrombosis and infection. The non-invasive vascular laboratory has allowed us to find cephalic veins in the upper arm for autogenous fistulae. The introduction of superior tunneled dialysis catheters have allowed us the opportunity to seek out autogenous fistulae and provided time for adequate maturation. The lessons learned about subclavian stenosis have made us avoid the subclavian vein and instead use the internal jugular vein.

It is with retrospective studies such as these which can direct us in the future, with the full understanding that there will be numerous changes which may show us that these innovations were only fleeting and not durable. Technology and medicine have been successful in prolonging the life of the renal failure patient we must respond by prolonging their dialysis access.

Bibliography

1. Feldman HI, Held PJ, Hutchinson J T, et al. Hemodialysis vascular access morbidity in the United States. *Kidney Int* 1993; 43:1091-6.
2. Feldman HI, Kobrin S, Wasserstein A. Hemodialysis vascular access morbidity *J Am Soc Nephrol* 1996; 7: 523-35.
3. Palder SB, Kirkman RL, Whittemore AD, et al. Vascular access for hemodialysis: patency rates and results of revision. *Ann Surg* 1985; 202:235-9.
4. Sullivan KL, Besarb A, Bonn J. et al. Hemodynamics of failing grafts. *Radiology* 1993; 186:867-72.
5. Arnold WP. Frequent failure patients in hemodialysis access thrombosis – an ongoing problem. *Abstract presentation SCVIR 2000,* SS%, March 26, 2000.
6. Huber TS, Seeger J. Approach to patients with "Complex" hemodialysis access problems. *Semin Dial* 2003;16: 22-29.
7. Surratt RS, Picus D, Hicks ME. The importance of preoperative evaluation of the subclavian vein in dialysis access planning. *Am J Roentgenol* 1991 ; 156: 623-625.
8. The Vascular Access Work Group NKF-DOQI Clinical Practice Guidelines for Vascular Access. *Am J Kidney Dis* 1997; 30: (Suppl 3) 5: 150-91.
9. Rubens F, Wellington JL. Brachiocephalic Fistula: a useful alternative for vascular access in chronic hemodialysis. *Cardiovasc Surg* 1993; 1: 128-130.
10. Nazzal MMS, Neglen P, Naseem J, et al. The brachiocephalic fistula : a successful secondary vascular access procedure. *VASA* 1990; 19:326-329.
11. Bender MH, Bruyninckx CMA, Gerlag PGG. The brachiocephalic elbow fistula: a useful alternative angioaccess for permanent hemodialysis. *J Vasc Surg* 1994; 20:808-813.
12. Cull DL, Taylor SM, Carsten CG, et al. The fistula elevation procedure: A valuable technique for maximizing arteriovenous fistula utilization. *Ann Vasc Surg 2002;* 16: 84-88.
13. Ascher E, Gade P, Hingorani A, et al. Changes in the practice of angioaccess surgery: Impact of dialysis outcome and quality initiative recommendations. *J Vasc Surg 2000;* 31:84-92.
14. Redfern AB, Zimmerman NB. Neurologic and ischemic complications of upper extremity vascular access for dialysis. *J Hand Surg (AM)* 1995; 20 : 199-204
15. Konner K. Vascular Access in the 21st Century. *J Nephrol* 2002; 15 (suppl 5): S28-S32.

5

AUTOGENOUS RADIAL-CEPHALIC OR PROSTHETIC BRACHIAL-ANTECUBITAL FOREARM LOOP AVF? A RANDOMIZED PROSPECTIVE MULTICENTER STUDY OF THE PATENCY OF PRIMARY HEMODIALYSIS VASCULAR ACCESS

Rooijens P.P.G.M., M.D.[1]*, Burgmans J.P.J., M.D.*[1]*,*
Tordoir J.H.M., M.D., Ph.D.[2]*, Smet de A.A.E.A., M.D., Ph.D.*[1]*,*
Fritchy W.M., M.D., Ph.D.[3]*, Groot de H.G.W., M.D.*[4]*,*
Burger H., M.D., Ph.D.[5]*, Yo T.I., M.D., Ph.D.*[1]

Address of correspondence:
Patrick P.G.M. Rooijens, Department of Surgery,
Medical Center Rijnmond Zuid,
location Clara, Olympiaweg 350, 3078 HT
Rotterdam, The Netherlands, E-mail: prooijens@hotmail.com,
phone: 00 31 102911283, fax: 00 31 104323481

1. Medical Center Rijnmond Zuid, Location Clara, Department of Surgery, Rotterdam, The Netherlands
2. University Hospital Maastricht, Department of Surgery, Maastricht, The Netherlands
3. Isala Clinics, Location Weezenlanden, Department of Surgery, Zwolle, The Netherlands
4. Amphia Hospital, Location Molengracht, Department of Surgery, Breda, The Netherlands
5. Albert Schweitzer Hospital, Location Dordwijk, Department of Surgery, Dordrecht, The Netherlands.

Introduction

A well-functioning vascular access remains the lifeline of end stage renal disease patients needing chronic intermittent hemodialysis. DOQI and European guidelines propose the construction of an autogenous radial-cephalic wrist arteriovenous fistula (RCAVF) as the primary and best option. However, 10-24% of RCAVF's thrombose postoperatively or do not function adequately due to failure of maturation[1-5]. Usually, arteriovenous fistulae (AVF) thrombosis and non-maturation depend on the quality and size of the vessels used for the arteriovenous anastomosis and the ability of vessel adaptation induced by the augmented blood flow volumes. However, a high percentage of RCAVF failure may be anticipated in patients with small or diseased vessels. These patients probably benefit from the creation of a prosthetic brachial-antecubital forearm loop access. Therefore a randomised prospective study comparing primary RCAVF versus prosthetic (polytetrafluoroethylene - PTFE) implantation in patients with poor vessels was performed.

Methods

Preoperative duplex-derived parameters and physical examination were used for patient selection. When the total score for the cephalic vein was 1 or 2 (Table 1) and/or the diameter of the radial artery was ≥ 1 mm and < 2 mm (measured by duplex), patients were randomised either for a RCAVF at the wrist or a forearm loop PTFE- AVF. The number of complications and interventions were registered and primary and secondary patencies were calculated by the life-table method.

Statistical analysis. Patient characteristics of RCAVFs and loop PTFE AVFs were compared with the Student's t-test. Functional patencies were determined by the Kaplan-Meier survival analysis and compared with the Log-rank method. A p-value <0.05 was considered statistically significant.

Results

During a 3½ yrs period, a total of 182 patients (97 men / 85 females; mean age 59 yrs) were randomised for a RCAVF (n=93) or prosthetic graft implant (n=89).

Table 1.   Preoperative duplex score table for patient selection.

Cephalic vein	Diameter	≤ 1.6 mm	0
		> 1.6 mm	1
	Continuity	poor: = 10 cm, many collaterals	0
		average: > 10 cm, not to the elbow, collaterals	1
		good: to the deep system, few collaterals, no stenosis	2

Patient characteristics of both groups are shown in Table 2. Sixty-nine percent of the RCAVFs (i.e. 31% primary failures) and 99% of prosthetic graft AVFs were functional for dialysis treatment.

Patients with RCAVFs developed a total of 109 versus 118 (p=0.242) complications in the prosthetic AVFs. Thrombosis and infections were significantly higher in the prosthetic graft group (Table 3).

A total of 52 interventions in the RCAVF group and 77 in the prosthetic graft group were needed for access salvage (p=0.046). Significantly more surgical thrombectomies were done in the prosthetic graft group (Table 4).

Primary and secondary one year patency was 30% *vs* 42% (p=0.101) and 54% *vs* 78% (p=0.002) for RCAVF and prosthetic AVF, respectively.

Table 2.   Patient characteristics.

	RCAVF	Loop PTFE AVF	*p*-value
N	93 (%)	89 (%)	
Male	50 (54)	47 (53)	0.449
Age (years)	58.4	61.9	0.059
Diabetes	28 (30)	27 (30)	0.489
Hypertension	74 (80)	61 (69)	0.045
Ischaemic cardiac disease	12 (13)	17 (19)	0.129
Peripheral vascular disease	15 (16)	20 (22)	0.141
Cerebrovascular disease	9 (10)	12 (13)	0.213

Table 3.   Complications.

	RCAVF	Loop PTFE AVF	*p*-value
N	93	89	
Hematoma	19	12	0.120
Seroma	1	1	0.486
Infection	4	11	0.034
Thrombosis	20	44	0.020
Pseudoaneurysm	2	6	0.091
Steal syndrome	2	4	0.191
Stenosis	29	22	0.262
Non-maturation	16	1	0.0002
Inability to puncture	12	4	0.095
Bleeding	2	3	0.309
Others	2	10	
Total of complications	109	118	0.242

Table 4.   Interventions.

	RCAVF	Loop PTFE AVF	p-value
N	93	89	
PTA	24	24	0.160
Surgical thrombectomy	12	38	0.007
Thrombolysis	1	0	0.160
Stent	0	1	0.160
Surgical revision	9	5	0.152
Other interventions	6	9	
Total of interventions	52	77	0.046

Conclusion

From these results we conclude that patients with poor forearm vessels benefit from implantation of a prosthetic graft and this may a better option than a primary autogenous radial-cephalic direct wrist access.

References

1. Reilly DT, Wood RF, Bell PR. Arteriovenous fistulas for dialysis: blood flow, viscosity, and long-term patency. *World J Surg* 1982; 6:628-633.
2. Tordoir JH, Kwan TS, Herman JM, Carol EJ, Jakimowicz JJ. Primary and secondary access surgery for haemodialysis with the Brescia-Cimino fistula and the polytetrafluoroethylene (PTFE) graft. *Neth J Surg* 1983; 35:8-12
3. Wedgwood KR, Wiggins PA, Guillou PJ. A prospective study of end-to-end vs. end-to-side arteriovenous fistulas for haemodialysis. *Br J Surg* 1984; 71:640-642.
4. Kherlakian GM, Roedersheimer LR, Arbaugh JJ, Newark KJ, King LR. Comparison of autogenous fistula versus expanded polytetrafluoroethylene graft fistula for angioaccess in hemodialysis. *Am J Surg* 1986; 152:238-243
5. Palder SB, Kirkman RL, Whittemore AD, Hakim RM, Lazarus JM, Tilney NL. Vascular access for hemodialysis. Patency rates and results of revision. *Ann Surg* 1985; 202:235-239.

DISCUSSION

Vascular Access for Hemodialysis IX
May 6-7, 2004
Lake Buena Vista, Florida

May 6, 2004
Abstract Session 1

Dr. Rooijens
"Autogenous Radial-Cephalic or Prosthetic Brachial Antecubital Forearm Loop Graft?—A Randomized Prospective Multicenter Study of the Patency of Primary Hemodialysis Vascular Access"

Question: I have some problems with the study. One is that you have selected out patients who are extremely poor candidates from whatever standards we use. You have said your artery diameter of one millimeter and two millimeter in these patients and vein diameter was less than 1.6 for the radial cephalic fistula. I do not think it is fair to say fistulas do poorly and grafts stay open very well. Can you really conclude saying that grafts do better in these people compared to small AV fistulas?

Rooijens: We chose these measurements and 1.6 millimeter as formal investigations and you have to do something else with the people. We have bad vessels at the wrist so we chose for the elbow fistula. So we didn't make any investigations for the diameter in the elbow vessels. We cannot say anything about that.

Question: At looking at your data, I agree with what the previous speaker said. It appears that you compared apples with oranges. If you take out the 30% primary failure rate, your unassisted patency rate in those forearm fistulas was about 60% and it is better than the grafts. The question I would ask is do you think it is better to put in a forearm loop graft after a failed fistula or should the comparison be a forearm loop graft versus either a transposed forearm fistula or a brachial cephalic fistula in the other arm?

Rooijens: When we looked at the patient group there are a lot of old people with multiple diseases with a short life expectancy with hemodialysis. I think it is better to get a functioning graft than wait for the 30% failure rate, requiring another operation.

Question: The only issue with that was when we all did that in the early 90's we created a procedure epidemic that we are still trying to recover.

Question: Just a quick question about the technique you have chosen for the native fistula. Have you used a certain type of magnification, I am talking about the scope or the magnification glasses?

Rooijens: The surgeons who did the operations used the glasses about three times magnification.

6

A SYSTEMATIC REVIEW: EXAMINING THE PATENCY OF UPPER EXTREMITY AUTOGENOUS AND PTFE HEMODIALYSIS ACCESSES

Thomas S. Huber, MD, PhD[1]
Jeffrey W. Carter, BS[2]
Randy L. Carter, PhD[2]
James M. Seeger, MD[1]

Correspondence:
Thomas S. Huber MD, PhD
Division of Vascular Surgery and Endovascular Therapy
Department of Surgery
P.O. Box 100286
University of Florida College of Medicine
Gainesville, Florida 32610-0286
PH: 352-265-0605, FAX: 352-338-9818
E-mail: Huber@surgery.ufl.edu

Departments of Surgery[1] and Statistics,[2] University of Florida College of Medicine, Gainesville, Florida

Introduction

The general consensus among health care providers is that the patency rates for autogenous hemodialysis accesses are superior to their prosthetic counterparts. Indeed, the National Kidney Foundation Clinical Guidelines for Vascular Access (NKF/DOQI) recommend the autogenous radiocephalic and brachiocephalic accesses as the first and second permanent access choices based partly upon their presumed superior patency rates.[1] However, the quality of the evidence supporting the superior patency of autogenous accesses referenced by the NKF/DOQI is limited and includes retrospective case series[2,3] and expert opinions.[4,5] Furthermore, the opinion that the patency rates for autogenous arteriovenous accesses are superior to their prosthetic counterparts is not universal. Notably, Hodges et al.[6] reviewed the outcome of all dialysis access procedures performed over a several year period and reported that the patency rates for autogenous and prosthetic accesses were similar although significantly less that those for peritoneal catheters. It is likely that this uncertainty about patency contributed to the fact that only 17% of new hemodialysis access procedures performed in the United States among Medicare patients during 1996-1997 were autogenous.[7]

This report will review our published systematic review testing the hypothesis that the patency rates for upper extremity autogenous hemodialysis accesses in adults are superior to their polytetrafluoroethylene (PTFE) counterparts.[8]

Methods

The MEDLINE electronic database was searched from 1966 – July 2001 using PubMed (U.S. National Library of Medicine, Bethesda, MD) and the terms *hemodialysis access, arteriovenous fistula, arteriovenous graft, arteriovenous shunt* or *access surgery* in conjunction with the terms *life table* or *Kaplan-Meier.* The titles and available abstracts identified by the MEDLINE search were then reviewed and the relevant articles identified for further in-depth review. The bibliographies of these articles identified by MEDLINE for the further in-depth review, the bibliographies from the clinical practice guidelines from the National Kidney Foundation (NKF/DOQI) and the Canadian Society for Nephrology, and the bibliographies from several hemodialysis accesses, vascular surgical and general surgical textbooks were searched by hand to identify additional relevant articles. These relevant articles identified by the hand search were subsequently found on MEDLINE and similar criteria were used to determine whether they merited further in-depth review. The searches were limited to full-text articles published in English and all searches were performed by a single author (TSH) with the assistance of the health science librarians.

The analysis was restricted to studies that documented the patency of upper extremity autogenous or PTFE arteriovenous accesses using either the life table or Kaplan-Meier method and included the number of patients at risk. Patency was defined as the ability to successfully dialyze through the access. Data reported in both tabular and graphic format were considered acceptable if all the initial patients were accounted for and the data could be converted into the standard life table format.[9] The analysis was limited to studies encompassing predominantly adults (age > 17 years) although no other demographics, comorbidities, or past medical events were factored into the inclusion criteria. All possible upper extremity autogenous and PTFE access configurations were included. Furthermore, all types of PTFE grafts were included regardless of the manufacturer or fabric characteristics although composite vein/prosthetic configurations such as those incorporating a venous anastomotic cuff were excluded. Accesses constructed with biologic grafts, alternative prosthetic grafts, and translocated, autogenous saphenous vein grafts were specifically excluded. Studies confounded by comparisons with these alternative graft types were included although the data extracted was limited to the autogenous and PTFE accesses. Only the most recent publication was included from an institution when serial publications encompassing some of the same patients were identified.

Two reviewers (TSH, JMS) independently evaluated the 211 full-text articles identified by the search for in-depth review to further determine whether they satisfied the inclusion criteria. Data were extracted from the acceptable articles and the differences of opinion between the reviewers were resolved by consensus. Data extracted included details about the study design, access configurations, patient demographics, perioperative outcome, and patency. The perioperative complications were defined using the conventions in the individual articles since no standard reporting system was available at the time of their publication. The patency data extracted comprised the relevant components of the life table and Kaplan-Meier method. Patency data were extracted for all patency assessments (primary, secondary) and anatomic locations (upper arm, forearm) when reported. Primary patency was defined as the functional access patency until any type of intervention while secondary patency was defined as the functional access patency until either final failure or the access was abandoned.

Separate life tables were constructed for every access type (PTFE, autogenous), patency assessment (primary, secondary) and anatomic location (forearm, upper arm) reported in the individual studies (e.g. forearm/PTFE/secondary patency). This required converting the data from Kaplan-Meier to the life table format in a subset of the individual studies. Unfortunately, simple compilation of these separate life tables into larger, aggregate life tables for the various access types/patency assessments/anatomic locations by adding the number of patients at risk, failures and interval withdrawals was not possible because the time intervals used in the individual studies varied with the most common intervals being 3 mos, 6 mos, or 12 mos. To overcome this limitation, the individual studies for the various access/patency assessments/anatomic locations in which the life tables were reported in 3 mos intervals were aggregated into a single 3 mos interval table by adding the number of patients at risk, the interval failures, and the interval withdrawals. The studies for the various access/patency assessments/anatomic locations reporting patency at 6 mos intervals were similarly combined to from a single 6 mos interval life table. Lastly, all the studies for the various access/patency assessments/anatomic locations were similarly used to create a 12 mos interval life table. Failure rates were then calculated over each of the respective time intervals for these aggregate 3 mos, 6 mos, and 12 mos life tables with the failure point between the respective consecutive time intervals assumed to be the midpoint. Based upon these failure rates, the cumulative patencies and standard error were calculated. Comparisons of the cumulative patency curves were made at the various time points by assuming a standard normal distribution and calculating z-statistics. Corrections were made for multiple comparisons using the Bonferroni technique and a p value < .05 was accepted as significant.

Results

The systematic review identified 34 studies that satisfied the inclusion criteria (Table 1). The publication dates ranged from 1972 – 2001 with 76% of the total published after 1990. The experimental design was either a case series or a non-randomized, controlled study in the majority of the reports and the data were collected predominantly in a retrospective fashion. There were five randomized, controlled trials, however, none compared autogenous and PTFE accesses. Rather, they compared different types of grafts (e.g. standard PTFE vs. stretch PTFE), different brands of PTFE grafts or a modification of the PTFE grafts (venous cuff vs. no venous cuff). Indeed, only three of the studies included acceptable patency data for both autogenous and PTFE accesses. The study sample sizes ranged from 15 – 388 patients with a median of 80. The patency rates were reported predominantly using the life table method (vs. Kaplan-Meier), and they were reported in a graphic format in slightly more than half of the reports.

The patient demographics, comorbidities and perioperative outcomes were not always provided in the studies that comprised the review (Table 2). However, the patients in the individual studies tended to be somewhat older (median – 57 years, range 45 - > 70 years), equally distributed by gender (male: median – 50%, range 45 – 64%), and comprised of a relative high percentage of diabetics (median - 47%, range 32 – 68%). The lack of a standard reporting system limited the ability to combine the complications. However, the results from the individual studies suggest that the perioperative mortality rate was essentially 0 (median – 0, range 0 – 1%) while the incidence of hand ischemia (median – 2%, range 0 – 14%) access infection (median – 7%, range 0 – 30%), and aneurysm/pseudoaneurysm formation (median – 4%, range 0 – 6%) were low for both autogenous and PTFE accesses. Notably, the overwhelming majority of the access infections were seen in the PTFE accesses.

The primary and secondary patency rates for the autogenous accesses were significantly greater than those for the PTFE accesses at all time points analyzed with the exception of the initial time point (1.5 mos) for the primary patency comparison (Figure 1 and Table 3). Notably, the primary patency rate for the autogenous accesses was 72% (95% CI: 70 – 74%) at 6 mos and 51% (95% CI: 48 – 53%) at 18 mos while the corresponding primary patencies for the PTFE accesses were 58% (95% CI: 56 - 61%) and 33% (95% CI: 31 – 36%) respectively. Comparable differences were also seen for the secondary patency rates at both 6 mos (autogenous – 86% (95% CI: 84 – 88%) vs. PTFE – 76% (95% CI: 73 – 79%)) and 18 mos (autogenous 77% (95% CI: 74 – 79%) vs. PTFE – 55% (95% CI: 51 – 59%)). Predictably, the secondary patency rates for both the autogenous and PTFE accesses types were significantly greater than their corresponding primary patency rates. Interestingly, the primary patency rates for the autogenous accesses were comparable to the secondary patencies for the PTFE accesses.

Subset analysis of the patients undergoing forearm and upper arm accesses revealed many of the same trends (Table 3). The primary and secondary patency rates for the forearm autogenous accesses were significantly greater than those for the corresponding PTFE accesses at both 6 and 18 mos. The primary patency rates for the autogenous upper arm accesses were also significantly greater than those for PTFE at 6 mos and the difference approached significance at 18 mos (p = .06). Comparison of the secondary patency rates for the upper arm accesses at both 6 and 18 mos was not possible due to insufficient data. Interestingly, the primary patency rates for both the autogenous and PTFE upper arm accesses were significantly greater than the corresponding forearm accesses at both 6 and 18 mos.

Discussion

Our results confirm the prevailing opinion that the patency rates for autogenous upper extremity hemodialysis accesses are significantly better than their PTFE counterparts. The supporting data represent the "best possible evidence" from the literature and are comprised of a meta-analysis of 34 studies in which accesses patency was reported using the life table or Kaplan-Meier method. The strength of these observations and data are reinforced by the large sample size and the fact that they represent an aggregate of access configurations and patient comorbidities without significant selection bias since no *a priori* criteria were incorporated in the study to exclude either configurations or patients potentially at higher risk for access failure.

The superior patency rates suggest that autogenous accesses should be the initial choice for permanent hemodialysis access. However, patency is only one of several determinants that factors into this clinical decision. These additional factors are multiple and include life expectancy, patient preference, cost, the number of revisions to maintain access patency, the duration of time that temporary access catheters are required the duration of time from the operative procedure until the access is sufficient for cannulation, and the postoperative complications. We did attempt to define the complication rates, but were unable to extract data for several of these clinically relevant factors because they were rarely reported. Furthermore, the complication rates reported in the majority of studies were somewhat suspect and not amenable to meta-analysis. Additionally, most of the studies reported the complications rates in terms of their incidence (patients experiencing event/ total number of patients) although this is potentially misleading since it fails to account for the duration that the access was functional. Ideally, the complications should be defined in terms of the number of events per patient year at risk.

The overall quality of the individual studies that comprised the meta-analysis was not very good by Evidence Based Medicine standards with the overwhelming majority representing the lowest level of evidence (case series). Indeed, it is ironic that a large percentage of the included studies were retrospective case reports since the inclusion of similar "marginal" studies as documentation for the superior patency rates of autogenous accesses by the NKF/DOQI Guidelines was one impetus for the review. In our original study design, the search strategy involved a tiered approach that linked the search terms to study qualifiers (e.g. meta-analysis, randomized, controlled trial), and we had hoped to perform a sensitivity analyses based upon the hierarchy of study design or the study characteristics (e.g. publication date). However, this was not feasible due to the limitations of the studies identified.

Table 1.   Study description.

Author	Reference	Study Question	Study Design	Data Collection	Fistula Type Included	Sample Size	Patency Assessment	Source of Patency Data
Ascher	Ann Vasc Surg 2001;15:89	native brachiobasilic vs. brachiocephalic fistula	controlled	retrospective	native	172	Kaplan-Meier	table
Lemson	J Vasc Surg 2000;32:1155	impact of venous anastomotic cuff on PTFE fistulae	randomized, controlled	prospective	PTFE	61	life table	graph
Staramos	Eur J Surg 2000;166:777	native vs. PTFE fistulae in patients >69 yrs	controlled	retrospective	native	68	Kaplan-Meier	table
Matsuura	Ann Vasc Surg 2000;14:50	cadaveric superficial femoral vein vs. PTFE fistula	controlled	retrospective	PTFE	68	life table	table
Kalman	J Vasc Surg 1999;30:727	impact of access program and coordinator	controlled	prospective	native, PTFE	native - 239, PTFE - 215	Kaplan-Meier	graph
Curi	J Vasc Surg 1999;29:608	native vs. PTFE fistulae in patients HIV+/HIV-	controlled	retrospective	native, PTFE	native - 55, PTFE - 57	life table	table
Hurlbert	Cardiovasc Surg 1998;6:652	Gore PTFE vs Impra PTFE fistulae	controlled	prospective	PTFE	190	life table	table
Matsuura	Am J Surg 1998;176:219	native brachiobasilic vs. PTFE brachioaxillary fistulae	controlled	retrospective	native	30	Kaplan-Meier	graph
Lenz	J Vasc Surg 1998;28:464	standard vs. thin wall PTFE fistulae	randomized, controlled	prospective	PTFE	108	life table	table
Silva	J Vasc Surg 1998;27:304	impact of algorithm to increase native fistulae	controlled	prospective	native, PTFE	native - 108, PTFE - 52	life table	table
Silva	J Vasc Surg 1997;26:981	native forearm fistulae	case series	retrospective	native	89	life table	table
Kaufman	J Am Coll Surg 1997;185:74	Gore PTFE vs Impra PTFE fistulae	randomized, controlled	prospective	PTFE	129	life table	table
Hakaim	J Vasc Surg 1997;25:1002	early vs. late cannulation of PTFE fistulae	controlled	prospective	PTFE	79	Kaplan-Meier	table
Miller	Ann Vasc Surg 1997;11:397	impact of algorithm to increase native fistulae	controlled	retrospective	native	75	Kaplan-Meier	table
Yasuhara	Am J Surg 1997;174:83	impact of revision on native radiocephalic fistulae	case series	Retrospective	native	283	life table	graph
Wang	Artif Organs 1996;20:1278	biological vs. PTFE fistulae	controlled	retrospective	PTFE	34	Kaplan-Meier	graph
Leapman	Am Surg 1996;62:652	native radiocephalic fistulae	case series	retrospective	native	150	Kaplan-Meier	graph

Table 1.   Study description. *(Continued)*

Author	Reference	Study Question	Study Design	Data Collection	Fistula Type Included	Sample Size	Patency Assessment	Source of Patency Data
Bender	*Eur J Vasc Endovasc Surg* 1995;10:294	median antecubital vs brachiocephalic native fistulae	controlled	retrospective	native	73	life table	graph
Tordoir	*Eur J Vasc Endovasc Surg* 1995;305	standard vs. stretch PTFE fistulae	randomized, controlled	prospective	PTFE	37	life table	graph
Burger	*Eur J Surg* 1995;161:327	comparison of different hemodialysis accesses	controlled	retrospective	native	208	Kaplan-Meier	graph
Polo	*Artif Organs* 1995;19:1181	brachioaxillary PTFE fistulae	case series	prospective	PTFE	157	life table	graph
Elcheroth	*Br J Surg* 1994;81:982	native arm fistulae	case series	retrospective	native	272	life table	graph
Simoni	*Cardiovasc Surg* 1994;2:63	snuff box vs wrist native radiocephalic fistulae	controlled	retrospective	native	388	Kaplan-Meier	graph
Rivers	*J Vasc Surg* 1993;18:391	native brachiobasilic fistulae	case series	retrospective	native	65	life table	table
Rubens	*Cardiovasc Surg* 1993;1:128	native brachiocephalic fistulae	case series	retrospective	native	16	life table	graph
Hibberd	*Aust N Z J Surg* 1991;61:631	native brachiobasilic fistulae	case series	prospective	native	15	life table	table
Schanzer	*Am J Surg* 1989;158:117	PTFE vs. PTFE-silicone fistulae	controlled	retrospective	PTFE	35	life table	graph
Dunlop	*Ann R Coll Surg Engl* 1986;68:203	native brachiocephalic fistulae	case series	retrospective	native	81	life table	graph
Munda	*JAMA* 1983;249:219	PTFE fistulae	case series	retrospective	PTFE	67	life table	graph
Salmon	*Can J Surg* 1981;24:59	biological vs. Gore PTFE vs. Impra PTFE fistulae	controlled	retrospective	PTFE	42	life table	graph
Rapaport	*Aust N Z J Surg* 1981;51:562	PTFE fistulae	case series	retrospective	PTFE	103	life table	table
Bone	*J Surg Res* 1980;29:223	biological vs. PTFE fistulae	randomized, controlled	prospective	PTFE	20	life table	graph
Haimov	*J Cardiovasc Surg* 1980;21:149	biologic vs. saphenous vs. PTFE fistulae	controlled	retrospective	PTFE	22	life table	table
Haimov	*Proc Eur Dial Transplant Assoc* 1972;9:173	native radiocephalic fistulae	case series	retrospective	native	203	life table	table

(From Huber TS, et al. Patency of autogenous and PTFE upper extremity arteriovenous hemodialysis accesses: a systematic review. J Vasc Surg 2003;38:1005-1011)

Table 2.   Study outcome.

Author	Reference	Fistula Type	Group Size	Age - mean (SD)	Male	Diabetes	Prior Permanent Access	Postop Death	Hand Ischemia	Graft Infection	Aneurysm/pseudoaneurysm
Ascher	Ann Vasc Surg 2001;15:89	arm native - brachiocephalic	109	67 (1.4)	37%	56%			0%	0%	1%
		arm native - brachiobasilic	63	69 (2.0)	40%	65%			5%	5%	0%
Lemson	J Vasc Surg 2000;32:1155	forearm PTFE	61	63 (2)	48%	35%	46%		0%	0.01 pt/yr	0.02 pt/yr
Staramos	Eur J Surg 2000;166:777	forearm/arm native	68	> 70	78%	32%		0%			
Matsuura	Ann Vasc Surg 2000;14:50	arm PTFE	68	62	53%	47%		0%	3%	12%	3%
Kalman	J Vasc Surg 1999;30:727	forearm/arm fistula	239								
		forearm/arm PTFE	215								
Curi	J Vasc Surg 1999;29:608	forearm/arm PTFE - HIV+	27							30%	
		forearm/arm PTFE - HIV-	30							7%	
		forearm/arm native - HIV+	23							9%	
		forearm/arm native - HIV-	32							0%	
Hurlbert	Cardiovasc Surg 1998;6:652	forearm/arm PTFE - Impra	90	63	48%	33%			2%	3%	3%
		forearm/arm PTFE - Gore	100	64	40%	43%			3%	9%	
Matsuura	Am J Surg 1998;176:219	arm native	30	59	47%	64%		0%		0%	
Lenz	J Vasc Surg 1998;28:464	foream PTFE - standard wall	56	54		48%				2%	6%
		forearm PTFE - thin wall	52	55		50%				3%	5%
Silva	J Vasc Surg 1998;27:304	forearm/arm native	108						0%	0%	1%
		forearm/arm PTFE	52						2%	12%	4%
Silva	J Vasc Surg 1997;26:981	forearm native	89	62	60%				0%	0%	0%
Kaufman	J Am Coll Surg 1997;185:74	forearm PTFE - Gore	64						6%	11%	
		forearm PTFE - Impra	65						6%	14%	
Hakaim	J Vasc Surg 1997;25:1002	arm PTFE - early cannulate	48	61(3)	48%	61%	83%	0%			
		arm PTFE - late cannulate	31	62 (4)	100%	55%	81%	0%			
Miller	Ann Vasc Surg 1997;11:397	forearm/arm native	75						1%	1%	
Yasuhara	Am J Surg 1997;174:83	forearm native	283	56	64%						
Wang	Artif Organs 1996;20:1278	forearm PTFE	34								
Leapman	Am Surg 1996;62:652	forearm native	150	50 (16)	73%	34%				0%	5%

Table 2. Study outcome. *(Continued)*

Author	Reference	Fistula Type	Group Size	Age - mean (SD)	Male	Diabetes	Prior Permanent Access	Postop Death	Hand Ischemia	Graft Infection	Aneurysm/pseudoaneurysm
Bender	*Eur J Vasc Endovasc Surg 1995;10:294*	arm native	73	61 (median)	47		53		0%	1%	1%
Tordoir	*Eur J Vasc Endovasc Surg 1995;305*	forearm PTFE - standard wall	20	58	60%	36%		0%	5%	10%	5%
		forearm PTFE - stretch	17	59	29%	43%		0%	6%	6%	0%
Burger	*Eur J Surg 1995;161:327*	forearm native	208								
Polo	*Artif Organs 1995;19:181*	arm PTFE	157	50			83%		1% early 0.01 pt/yr late	1% early, 0.06 pt/yr late	0.02 pt/yr
Elcheroth	*Br J Surg 1994;81:982*	arm native	272		42%		52%		14%	5%	4%
Simoni	*Cardiovasc Surg 1994;2:63*	wrist native	248	53	54%			0%	0%		
		snuffbox native	140	51	65%			0%	0%		
Rivers	*J Vasc Surg 1993;18:391*	arm native	65	47	43%		75%	0%	2%		4%
Rubens	*Cardiovasc Surg 1993;1:128*	arm native	16						6%	6%	
Hibberd	*Aust N Z J Surg 1991;61:631*	arm native	15	54	7%		66%		7%	7%	7%
Schanzer	*Am J Surg 1989;158:117*	arm PTFE	35	57		68%	40%		0%	11%	17%
Dunlop	*Ann R Coll Surg Engl 1986;68:203*	arm native	81	45	48%				4%	2%	4%
Munda	*JAMA 1983;249:219*	forearm/arm PTFE	67	58	31%		85%		3%	25%	8%
Salmon	*Can J Surg 1981;24:59*	forearm shunt - Gore	14	45				0%	0%	7%	7%
		forearm shunt - Impra	28	46				0%	0%	4%	4%
Rapaport	*Aust N Z J Surg 1981;51:562*	forearm/arm PTFE	103	48	61%						
Bone	*J Surg Res 1980;29:223*	forearm PTFE	20	53 (10)	100%	45%				10%	0%
Haimov	*J Cardiovasc Surg 1980;21:149*	forearm PTFE	22								
Haimov	*Proc Eur Dial Transplant Assoc 1972;9:173*	radiocephalic native	203								

(From Huber TS, et al. Patency of autogenous and PTFE upper extremity arteriovenous hemodialysis accesses: a systematic review. *J Vasc Surg* 2003;38:1005-1011)

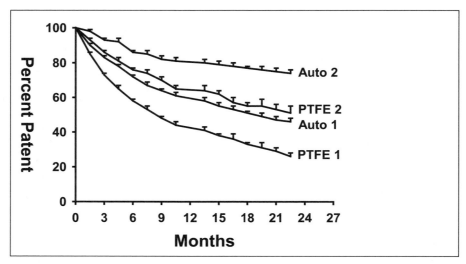

Figure 1:   The patency rates (percent patent) for the autogenous (Auto) and
PTFE (PTFE) upper extremity hemodialysis accesses are plotted
against time (months) with the positive standard error bars. Both
the primary (Auto 1, PTFE 1) and secondary (Auto 2, PTFE 2) patency rates for the two access types are shown. The patency rates for
the autogenous accesses were better than their corresponding
PTFE counterparts with the one exception of the initial (1.5 mos)
time point for the primary patency comparison.

Source: (From Huber TS, et al. Patency of autogenous and PTFE upper extremity arteriovenous hemodialysis accesses: a systematic review. *J Vasc Surg* 2003;38:1005-1011)

Importantly, the requirement that the access patency had to be reported using either
the life table or Kaplan-Meier method with the number of patients at risk partly
overcame the limitations of the overall study quality and lent itself to the meta-
analysis. The life table method is the "gold standard" for reporting patency after
revascularization procedures and allows presentation of data for patients undergoing procedures at different times with different followup durations. Admittedly, the
life table method may overestimate the "true" patency rates since it has been reported that the patients lost to followup do not have as favorable an outcome as those
whose followup is known.[10]

Our search strategy was potentially subject to several criticisms. First, we used
only the Medline electronic database although there are other ones such Embase that
could have been searched. Second, it is possible that the search terms were too strict
and that appropriate articles were not identified because the life table or Kaplan-
Meier terms were not included in the abstract of the article or among the key words.
Lastly, our search was restricted to full-text articles written in English. We would
justify the choice of the electronic database by its overall extent and quality in addition to the more practical points that our library services did not have access to
Embase and the single-user subscription rates were prohibitive. The requirement for
full-text articles was justified by the need to critically appraise the methodology and

Table 3.   Breakdown of autogenous and PTFE hemodialysis accesses by location.

Fistula/Patency Endpoint	Initial Number at Risk	6 Mos Patency (95% CI)	18 Mos Patency (95% CI)
All Autogenous—Primary	1849	72% (70 – 74)*#	51% (48 – 53)*#
All Autogenous—Secondary	1336	86% (84 – 88)#	77% (74 – 79)#
All PTFE—Primary	1245	58% (56 – 61)*	33% (31 – 36)*
All PTFE—Secondary	703	76% (73 – 79)	55% (51 – 59)
Forearm Autogenous—Primary	1325	71% (69 – 73)*#	49% (47 – 52)*#
Forearm Autogenous—Secondary	641	91% (89 – 93)#	86% (83 – 89)#
Forearm PTFE—Primary	537	51% (48 – 54)*	28% (25 – 32)*
Forearm PTFE—Secondary	330	69% (65 – 73)	47% (42 – 52)
Upper arm Autogenous—Primary	286	81% (77 – 85)#&	60% (53 – 67)&
Upper arm Autogenous—Secondary	280	NA@	NA
Upper arm PTFE—Primary	431	69% (66 – 73)&	49% (45 – 54)&
Upper arm PTFE—Secondary	270	NA	NA

* Significant difference between primary/secondary patency for the specific access type.
# Significant difference between autogenous/PTFE for the specific patency assessment.
& Significant difference between upper arm/forearm for the specific access type and patency assessment.
@ NA – not applicable, insufficient data at the specific time point.
(From Huber TS, et al. Patency of autogenous and PTFE upper extremity arteriovenous hemodialysis accesses: a systematic review. *J Vasc Surg* 2003;38:1005-1011)

results of the individual studies in an attempt to determine the suitability of the life table or Kaplan-Meier data. Similarly, the practicality of finding appropriate translators and the associated costs limited our search to articles published in English. Despite these limitations, it is unlikely that our search missed many relevant articles and it is even less likely that including these potentially "missed" articles in our meta-analysis would have impacted our results. It is difficult to imagine that a "definitive" article about hemodialysis access patency was not included in the DOQI Guidelines or one of the hemodialysis texts regardless of the language of origin. Furthermore, the sample sizes in the meta-analysis were so large and the respective standard errors (confidence intervals) so small that even several additional studies would not likely have altered the patency curves.

In conclusion, the patency rates for autogenous, upper extremity hemodialysis accesses appear to be superior to their PTFE counterparts given the "best available evidence" in the literature. However, the overall quality of the studies that comprised the meta-analysis was less than ideal as defined by the standards of Evidence Based Medicine. Randomized, controlled trials comparing autogenous and PTFE hemodialysis accesses are necessary to examine differences in patency and the other relevant outcome measures, and this need is underscored by the magnitude of the clinical problem both in the United States and abroad.

References

1. III. NKF-K/DOQI Clinical Practice Guidelines for Vascular Access: update 2000. *Am J Kidney Dis* 2001; 37:S137-S181.
2. Munda R, First MR, Alexander JW, et al. Polytetrafluoroethylene graft survival in hemodialysis. *JAMA* 1983; 249:219-222.
3. Palder SB, Kirkman RL, Whittemore AD, et al. Vascular access for hemodialysis. Patency rates and results of revision. *Ann Surg* 1985; 202:235-239.
4. Ryan JJ, Dennis MJ. Radiocephalic fistula in vascular access. *Br J Surg* 1990; 77:1321-1322.
5. Windus DW. Permanent vascular access: a nephrologist's view. *Am J Kidney Dis* 1993; 21:457-471.
6. Hodges TC, Fillinger MF, Zwolak RM, Cronenwett JL, et al. Longitudinal comparison of dialysis access methods: risk factors for failure. *J Vasc Surg* 1997; 26:1009-1019.
7. Use of Hemodialysis Access Procedures. In Cronenwett JL, Birkmeyer JD (eds). *The Dartmouth Atlas of Vascular Health Care.* Chicago: Health Forum; 2000:126.
8. Huber TS, Carter JW, Carter RL, et al. Patency of autogenous and PTFE upper extremity arteriovenous hemodialysis accesses: a systematic review. *J Vasc Surg* 2003;38:1005-1011.
9. Rutherford RB, Baker JD, Ernst C, et al. Recommended standards for reports dealing with lower extremity ischemia: revised version. *J Vasc Surg* 1997; 26:517-538.
10. Jensen LP, Nielsen OM, Schroeder TV. The importance of complete follow-up for results after femoro-infrapopliteal vascular surgery. *Eur J Vasc Endovasc Surg* 1996; 12:282-286.

DISCUSSION

Vascular Access for Hemodialysis IX
May 6-7, 2004
Lake Buena Vista, Florida

May 6, 2004
Abstract Session 1

Dr. Thomas Huber
"A Systematic Review: Examining the Patency of Upper Extremity Autogenous and PTFE Hemodialysis Accesses"

Question: After you have reviewed all this material, what is your choice for the next prospective randomized trial in this area?

Huber: I pitched this to the NIH, a randomized controlled study of an autogenous versus prosthetic access and they sent it back to me saying that that is a done deal and there is no interest in that concept. So I am going to go back to them with that same plan. The design I would be PTFE in the upper extremity versus any type of autogenous access.

Comment/Question: The comment goes back to the Dutch study that was just presented as well as Jeff Sands' comments. If we look at this over the last four or five years in the United States, there has been an effort made to create an autogenous fistulas. We are clearly using less adequate veins size and perhaps less adequate arterial inflow, to be creating an increase number of fistulas. I suspect that the patency rates that have been reported in the time frame that you are looking at for autogenous fistulas are based on identifying more optimal veins, and then opting out if the optimal vein is not present to a PTFE graft. If you would re-look at this now and take a cross sectional view of creation of fistulas with our increased efforts, would the outcomes be near the outcomes you report now?

Huber: This data is not very old. I would say this is a year old, there has not been just a randomized controlled studies or quality access studies that have been published within the last year. Since looking at this on a monthly basis, I would say that the data is no different now than it was when we concluded the trial. I think there is a bit of a push back as we felt some pressures as surgeons to do more autogenous accesses and we are trying to push that envelope a little bit. This is in many ways a justification for a trial. I think some of the success rates in these marginal situations are poor. Maybe PTFE is the better accesses in some of those people, if you use a bad artery or bad vein; I think your fistula maturation rate is lower, quite poor. There have been a couple of trials that have come out and have had similar conclusions.

Question: What is the time distribution of the studies in the literature? For example, in 1970 I would suggest to you that we were using three and a half to five millimeter veins at the wrist rather than the 1.5 to 3 millimeter veins that we are using now to push increasing autogenous fistulas. That was my point.

Huber: The majority of the studies, 70 or 75% of the studies, were from 1990 and on.

Question from Indiana: I was curious about the incidence of complications particularly forearm steal syndrome between fistulas and grafts? In your study did you see a difference, and secondly, what is the best way to predict that if you are making an upperarm fistula?

Huber: I can tell you it is difficult to pull that data out of the literature and part of it is because of the way we have traditionally reported. Everyone reports incidence of hand ischemia at varying rates. I guess ideally it should be reported as the incidence per patient per year. Since we started this systematic review, the National Vascular Societies have defined a reporting standard for hand ischemia. It is still not perfect but it is pretty good and at least able us to quantify and qualify what hand ischemia really is. To answer your second question, which is not really part of my talk, I would say the incidence of hand ischemia of a brachial artery based access is probably about ten percent. It is higher at least anecdotally in patients who have an autogenous access rather than a piece of plastic in our own experience. It is difficult to predict and higher in older patients, women, diabetics, people with peripheral vascular occlusive disease, and people with a prior incidence of hand eschemia.

Comment/Question: I am still waiting for someone to do a randomized prospective forearm loop versus basilic vein transposition. Is anyone doing that?

Huber: Not that I am aware of.

7

IMPACT OF A DIALYSIS ACCESS COORDINATOR ON A VASCULAR SURGERY PRACTICE

Rhonda C. Quick, M.D., Alfredo Altamirano, PA,
Andrew T. Gentile, M.D., and Scott S. Berman, M.D.
The Southern Arizona Vascular Institute, Tucson, AZ

Address correspondence to:
Rhonda C. Quick, MD
Southern Arizona Vascular Institute
6080 La Cholla Blvd
Tucson, AZ 85745
(520) 628-1400-phone
(520) 628-4863-fax
rquick@azvasc.com

Introduction

The end stage renal disease population continues to grow yearly by approximately 10%. The Kidney Disease Outcomes Initiative (K-DOQI) has developed guidelines to improve dialysis patients' quality of life. With these guidelines and the expanding patient population, vascular access has become an even larger portion of a vascular surgery practice. This study was undertaken to determine the effect of a dialysis coordinator in the vascular practice on the type and quantity of access procedures performed and whether such an individual is budget neutral for the surgical practice.

Methods

The number of new hemodialysis access procedures performed over a 48-month period were reviewed and divided into two groups based upon the presence (PA group) or absence (NPA group) of the dialysis access coordinator. In the 2nd half of the review period, a physician's assistant functioned as a full-time dialysis access coordinator. The coordinator was responsible for evaluating new dialysis patients for access options, including the use of 1) venous mapping, 2) coordinating an access surveillance program with the nephrologists and the dialysis centers, 3) maintaining an access history database on all new and existing dialysis patients, and 4) placing acute dialysis catheters for patients needing emergent access. The reviewed procedures were also separated into new access procedures and revisions of existing access. Comparisons between the groups were made using Chi square analysis. The reimbursement for the coordinator's services was recorded along with the expenses associated with the coordinator's employment. Expenses included actual values for salary, malpractice and benefits. To protect proprietary information, the economic impact of the coordinator is reported as a ratio of reimbursement to expenses.

Results

Over the 48-month period of review, 1214 access procedures were performed. In the NPA group (no coordinator), 369 new access procedures were performed of which 195 were autogenous and 174 were prosthetic grafts. In the PA group (with coordinator), 454 new access procedures were performed with 261 autogenous and 193 prosthetic grafts. The incidence of autogenous access procedures increased from 52.8% in the NPA groups to 57.5% in the PA group (p-=0.18). In the NPA group, 132 revisions were performed of which only 11 (8%) were percutaneous interventions for failing but patent accesses. This contrasts to the PA group in which 97 (37%) of 259 revisions were percutaneous interventions for failing accesses. Not only did the number of access revisions increase, the incidence of elective and largely percutaneous revision of failing accesses increased significantly with the availability of an access coordinator (p<0.001). (Table 1) Reimbursement to the practice for the coordinator's services exceeded the expense of the position by a factor of 1.2.

Table 1.   Effect of coordinator on access experience.

	Autogenous	Prosthetic	Percutaneous Intervention
PA Group	57.5%	42.5%	37%
NPA Group	52.8%	47.2%	8%
P Value	NS	NS	<0.001

Conclusions

The number of people in the United States with end stage renal disease requiring hemodialysis continues to grow each year with the US Renal Data System reporting an incidence in 2001 of 334 cases per million population.[1] This impact is further compounded by the increasing age of the dialysis patient. As the numbers of end stage renal disease patients continue to grow and the health care expenditures for dialysis related health care escalate, there will be more emphasis on quality outcomes regarding dialysis access.

Improving the quality of life of dialysis patients has become the focus of the National Kidney Foundation Dialysis Outcome and Quality Initiative (DOQI) which first published guidelines in 1997 which were updated in 2000.[2,3] Vascular access is one specific area of interest of DOQI. These guidelines have emphasized the superiority of autogenous accesses recommending that 50% of access procedures be autogenous. They have also recognized the superior results of intervention on failing access prior to thrombosis that can avoid temporary catheter placement. These guidelines and others have brought new emphasis on dialysis access in the vascular surgery practice.

Some have attempted to improve DOQI compliance by establishing dedicated vascular access centers[4] while others have opted for access coordinators. Individuals who function as dialysis coordinators include nurses, nurse practitioners and physician assistants.

Our design uses a physician's assistant as a dialysis coordinator. This individual has been specifically trained by vascular surgeons regarding patient evaluation pre and post access placement as well as trained in placement of temporary non-cuffed catheters.

In our experience, our physician's assistant functioning as dialysis coordinator has improved our ability to meet the DOQI guidelines facilitating earlier consultation between nephrologists and vascular surgeons as well as ensuring that the appropriate measures are taken to protect an extremity for access creation. Although the number did not reach statistical significance, the percentage of autogenous access procedures increased. The increase in intervention on failing accesses was significant and allowed our practice to increase endovascular volume and experience. The coordinator functions as initial contact for nephrologists, dialysis nurses and patients facilitating the timely evaluation and management of the patient.

The costs of a full-time dialysis coordinator can be tangibly recovered through reimbursable services provided to the patients by the coordinator (non-cuffed catheters, consultations, etc). The maintenance of the database affords an easy and quick assessment of the access history of the patient that can streamline decision making and avoid duplication of efforts with diagnostic imaging and attempted intervention. The intangible contribution of the dialysis coordinator involves the efficiency of managing difficult access problems diffusing emergency intervention for the surgeon and delay in appropriate and timely dialysis treatments. By utilizing the dialysis coordinator as a provider in the above functions, there have been no negative financial effects. In the future, we plan to further involve the coordinator in a more aggressive screening program in addition to providing the above described service and maintenance of the database.

References

1. US Renal Data System: USRDS 2003 Annual Data Report. The National Institute of Health, National Institute of Diabetic, Digestive and Kidney Disease, Bethesda, MD 2003.
2. The Vascular Access Work Group. NKF-DOQI clinical practice guidelines for vascular access. *Am J Kidney Dis* 1997; 30. 5150-5191.
3. National Kidney Foundation: K/DOQI clinical practice guidelines for vascular access. *Am J Kidney Dis* 2000; 37. S137-S181,2001 (suppl1)
4. Arnold, WP. Improvement in hemodialysis vascular access outcomes: a dedicated access center. *Sem Dial* 2000 Nov-Dec; 13(6). 359-363.

DISCUSSION

Vascular Access for Hemodialysis IX
May 6-7, 2004
Lake Buena Vista, Florida

May 6, 2004
Abstract Session 1

Dr. Rhonda Quick
"Impact of a Dialysis Access Coordinator on a Vascular Surgery Practice"

Comment/Question: If I proposed to our hospital administrators that we were going to establish a budget neutral position, they would not have a lot of enthusiasm for that. What else can you use for an encouragement to establish this kind of position? Do you think we should do it, is it worthwhile?

Quick: I think it is worthwhile. I think there are a lot of intangible positives that this individual brings. He/she provides streamline care to somewhat complex patients. Maintaining an ongoing database centrally as far as what access procedures they have had before as well as most recent radiographic evaluations of the access, provides improved care. It may increase your patient's satisfaction and decrease your length of stay and your cost of care. I think for this individual the time that we looked at in that 48 month period was the first two years he was in the practice. He also had other duties not just specific to dialysis that was not included in this. Given that he may be dedicating more and more time of his time to just dialysis access may also increase the amount of billing that he generates.

Comment/Question: We have a coordinator in our hospital and it certainly makes life easier for the patients and the doctors and nurses. The establishment of a database could provide regular updates of how we are doing in terms of patency. To me that is really an attractive feature of this. Someone who has the time to do that is focusing on the quality of the effort we are making. I think it would really be an important part of it and it would justify the cost.

Question: You showed increase in interventions, did you show any impact on longevity of the accesses?

Quick: Actually we did not look at this specifically. We looked primarily at the number of procedures generated, not the long term outcomes of the patency of those grafts.

How many of you in the audience have a dialysis access coordinator in your institution?

So the majority have that and would support what you are saying. It is helpful even though you can't necessarily justify it financially.

Question: I would like to ask you a question about that coordinator. Earlier this morning a lady was saying that some of the patients were quite hooked on their catheter because they were quite afraid of having a fistula performed by the surgeons. Do you think that some sort of coordinator may help to convince such reluctant people to have their access performed?

Quick: Yes, I think it will because again it is another individual that establishes a relationship with these patients because of the chronicity of their illness. A lot of people in our practice identify with our dialysis coordinator. They are very familiar with him and they know that he has their best interest in heart as well. I think having an additional person that has a lot of continuity of care with that individual may also convince them that a fistula or prosthetic graft is more in their best interest than a tunneled catheter.

Question: Do you think that when you will improve all of the methods for all the monitoring, you may do some savings in terms of costing type of inpatient admission and complication?

Quick: Yes, I think so and although it would be difficult to pull that data out of the database I think we already have. It helps patients with a thrombosed access, so they are not all necessarily seen in the emergency room or brought emergently to the operative room that day or put in the hospital for temporary access. It may avoid admission or an ER visit. One phone call from the dialysis unit to the dialysis coordinator can engineer whatever intervention they need in a timely fashion.

Comment: I am actually a vascular access coordinator and we have 13 different dialysis units that our patients are at. I cover about 500 dialysis patients who have specifically grafts and fistulas. The point I wanted to make is that it has been said over and over again that the reimbursement for this type of service is not out there yet. They are not reimbursing as much for doing the transonic readings. But I think the amount of time that is spent in the dialysis units versus in the hospital for revisions, we save money in other ways. The bottom line here is looking at the things we are doing for the patients.

Comment: I think by the show of hands that we just saw, that point has been accepted. We believe that it is helpful but it is just hard to measure it.

Question: You kind of glossed over the fact that the people who have the coordinators had a lot more percutaneous interventions than the people who didn't. My understanding is that the coordinators were actually the ones doing these interventions, is that correct?

Quick: No, the coordinator will take the phone call from the dialysis unit that says this patient's flows are X and then he will organize the intervention or diagnostic maneuver on that patient, which is either performed by interventional radiology or by the vascular surgeons in the practice. So in a way, by having the coordinator as part of the vascular surgery practice, may be a financially positive thing for the vascular surgical practice for the number of intervascular interventions as well. But that person was not performing the interventions, no.

Question: And a percutaneous intervention does not mean like an insertion of a temporarily dialysis catheter?

Quick: No, it was all fistulograms with angioplasty or interventional procedures.

8

SAFETY OF CONSCIOUS SEDATION WITH MIDAZOLAM AND FENTANYL IN INTERVENTIONAL NEPHROLOGY: A SINGLE CENTER EXPERIENCE

Fahim Zaman MD, Aslam Pervez MD,
Sara Murphy RN, Kenneth Abreo MD
Departments of Medicine; Division of Nephrology
Louisiana State University Health Sciences Center;
Shreveport LA

Address correspondence to:
Fahim Zaman MD
Department of Medicine
Division of Nephrology
Louisiana State University Health Sciences Center
1501 Kings Highway
Shreveport, LA 71130
Phone: (318) 675 7402
Fax: (318) 675 5913
E mail: fzaman@lsuhsc.edu

Introduction:

Technological advances and economical restraints have given rise to procedures for-merly done as an inpatient to be performed in the outpatient setting. Since invasive procedures cause anxiety and apprehension, the majority of patients require seda-tion. The therapeutic goals of conscious sedation in the interventional nephrology vascular suite at our institution include: (1) reduction or elimination of the pain associated with the invasive procedure, (2) reduction of physiologic stress and anx-iety related to the procedure, (3) amnesia or inability to recall the procedure. Conscious sedation is defined as the use of a combination of pharmacological agents, administered by one or more routes, to produce a minimally depressed level of consciousness and analgesia, without respiratory depression, and with the ability to respond to physical stimulation and verbal commands. Herein, we report our experience with conscious sedation at our institution.

Methods:

The computer database and medical records of all patients who received conscious sedation in the interventional nephrology vascular suite at the Louisiana State University Health Sciences Center, Shreveport, LA between April 2001 and December 2003 were reviewed. Indications and types of procedures requiring conscious sedation are outlined in Table 1.

All the procedures were performed by one of three interventional nephrologists, or by the nephrology fellow under direct supervision of the faculty. Informed consent was obtained prior to administering conscious sedation. The responsible physician

Table 1.   Type of procedure and dose of conscious sedation.

Type of Procedure (n)	Mean Fentanyl Dose (mcg)	Mean Midazolam Dose (mg)
Percutaneous Thrombolysis and Angioplasty of Synthetic Hemodialysis Grafts (203)	100	2.0
Cuffed Tunneled Catheter Placement (551)	100	2.0
Port-a-cath Placement (322)	150	2.0
Lifesite® Hemodialysis Access System Placement (4)	250	4.5
Peritoneal Dialysis Catheter Placement (40)	250	4.0
Port–a -cath Removal (14)	100	1.0
Lifesite® Hemodialysis Access System Removal (4)	250	3.0
Fistulogram with Coil Occlusion of Accessory Veins (17)	100	1.0
Central Vein Angioplasty (6)	150	2.0
Percutaneous Transluminal Angioplasty of Synthetic Hemodialysis Graft or Autogenous Fistula (72)	100	2.0
Central Line Placement (127)	100	1.0

provided the patient with information considered necessary for obtaining an informed consent. The registered nurse (RN) reinforced the physician's explanation prior to and during the procedure. All patients receiving conscious sedation had an intravenous access. A physical examination and review of all medications including allergies was done in every case. Emergency equipment, including a crash cart, and medications were available where the sedation was given. Only RN's or physicians who are trained in Advanced Cardiac Life Support (ACLS) administered sedation. A one-to-one RN to patient ratio was maintained during the entire procedure, with the responsible physician being present throughout its administration. The patient's vital signs, including blood pressure, oxygen saturation, and electrocardiography were monitored continuously and recorded. Data analysis was performed using Stat View software (SAS institute Inc. Cary, North Carolina). Patients were kept in the recovery room post-procedure and monitored.

Results:

Intravenous conscious sedation was administered in 1360 patients from April 2001 to December 2003. The different types of procedures are outlined in Table 1. Mild hypoxemia ($SaO_2 > 80\%$ but $<90\%$) occurred in 27 patients (2%) and was easily reversed with verbal stimulation and increase in O_2 flow. Intravenous flumazenil (Romazicon 0.2 mg) was required in 4 cases (0.3%) for hypoxemia. No patient required naloxone hydrochloride (Narcan) for reversal of sedation. Reversible hypotension (systolic blood pressure <100 mmHg but >80 mmHg) occurred in 20 patients (1.47%) and was easily corrected with intravenous normal saline alone. There were no deaths or adverse outcomes requiring admission to the hospital due to the effects of conscious sedation.

Discussion:

The intravenous (IV) route is preferred for conscious sedation because it has a fast onset of action and the absorption is more predictable than other routes. Response to pharmacological agents is highly individual and therefore all agents and doses are titrated to patient response.

Fentanyl hydrochloride is a potent synthetic opioid. It has short duration of action (as long as 1-2 h) and minimal cardiovascular effects, such as hypotension. Respiratory depression is uncommon, but this effect lasts longer than its analgesic effect. The IV dose is 1-3 mcg/kg (50-200 mcg in adults), titrated in 50-100 mcg increments. It is the preferred drug for analgesia in short procedures because it provides the most reliable pain control. Midazolam (Versed) is a water-soluble short-acting benzodiazepine that is suitable for short-term sedation and anxiolysis, ideally suited for short procedures. The dose in adults is 2-5 mg intravenously, but doses of 0.5-3.0 mg usually are adequate in elderly patients. The onset of action is rapid, with a peak effect in 5 minutes. The duration of action is 60-90 minutes. Midazolam is metabolized by the hepatic microsomal system and is not affected by renal failure making it a good choice in our patient population.

The reversal agents used are naloxone hydrochloride and flumazenil. Flumazenil is a competitive antagonist of the benzodiazepine class of drugs. The onset of action is within 2 minutes after IV administration, with peak effects within 10 minutes. Repeat dosing may be required. The recommended and titration rates for conscious sedation are 0.2-1.0 mg in adults. Caution should be exercised in patients receiving long-term benzodiazepine therapy, because seizures can occur. Naloxone is a competitive antagonist of the opioid class of drugs. The onset of action following IV administration is rapid, with effects appearing within 2-3 minutes. The duration of action is dose related. This antagonist may have shorter duration of action compared with that of the longer-acting opioids, and observation may be required with repeated dosing. The initial dose in adults is 0.4 mg IV, which may be repeated, if necessary, to a total of 2 mg.

Practitioners cannot underestimate the potential for serious trouble during conscious sedation. When given together, sedative, hypnotic, and opioid medications can exert potent synergistic effects that can lead to (1) hypoventilation (2) peripheral vasodilation (3) hypotension. Other potential complications include (1) respiratory obstruction associated with decreased oropharyngeal muscle tone (2) hypoxia (3) hypercapnia (3) cardiopulmonary depression. However, for carefully selected patients, intravenous sedation provides a good alternative to general anesthesia. Its safe track record in various specialties such as oral surgery, cosmetic surgery, cardiology, gastroenterology and radiology has allowed us to safely implement it in our vascular suite. We feel that in experienced hands, with adequate monitoring, it is a very safe and effective form of sedation in our patient population. As can be seen in our large population, conscious sedation can be used safely as an adjunct to interventional procedures on vascular access in an outpatient setting.

References:

1. Hasen KV, Samartzis D, Casas LA, Mustoe TA. An outcome study comparing intravenous sedation with Midazolam /Fentanyl(conscious sedation) versus propofol infusion (deep sedation) for aesthetic surgery. Plast Reconstr Surg 2003; 12(6):1683- 1690
2. Pachulski RT, Adkins DC, Mirza H. Conscious sedation with intermittent Midazolam and Fentanyl in electrophysiology procedures. J Inter Cardiol 2001; 14(2): 143-146
3. Arepally A, Oechsle D, Kirkwood S, Savader SJ. Safety of conscious sedation in interventional radiology. Cardiovasc Intervent Radiol 2001; 24(3): 185-190
4. Trotteur G, Stockx L, Dondelinger RF. Sedation, analgesia and anesthesia for interventional radiological procedures in adults. Part I. Survey of interventional radiological practice in Belgium. JBR-BTR 2000; 83(3): 111-115
5. Venneman I, Lamy M. Sedation, analgesia and anesthesia for interventional radiological procedures in adults. Part II. Recommendations for interventional radiologists. JBR-BTR 2000; 83(3): 116-120
6. McDermott VG, Chapman ME, Gillespie I. Sedation and patient monitoring in vascular and interventional radiology. Br J Radiol 1993; 66(788): 667-671

DISCUSSION

Vascular Access for Hemodialysis IX
May 6-7, 2004
Lake Buena Vista, Florida

May 6, 2004
Abstract Session 1

Dr. Fahim Zaman
"Safety of Conscious Sedation with Midazolam and Fentanyl in Interventional Nephrology: A Single Center Experience"

Question: Let me make sure I understand. When you are doing this in the interventional suite, who is there besides the interventional radiologist?

Zaman: Interventional radiologist, sometimes one fellow who is on the rotation, sometimes two fellows, and we have two RNs.

Question: They have a pulse ox on them and they are taking blood pressures readings?

Zaman: Blood pressure, EKG, pulse ox. One nurse basically monitors the patient, and the other nurse is next to the patient with the fluoro machine. So there are two RNs.

Comment: It is very safe. One of the things we have had a problem with in our hospital and occasionally not necessarily in this context, but Fentanyl because it is in a microgram dose and not a milligram dose. You actually said milligram in your presentation. That is one of the problems we have had with drug overdoses, that is that someone may not be as familiar with the drug makes that mistake.

Question: You did a nice job of showing the safety of your conscious sedation but I wonder if you have monitored the effectiveness. Have you interviewed these patients afterwards about their perceived experience during the intervention?

Zaman: I have talked to them because a lot of those patients will come back to you especially if it is related to access or for dialysis or poor placements in chemo patients because we do their dressing changes. Once those patients have been admitted our nurses will do their dressing changes not the hemo nurses. We have been pleasantly surprised that a lot of those patients have not complained of extensive pain. A lot of patients do get anxious and a lot of times versed is very helpful. But pain control has been adequate. But we have not filled out a questionnaire, if that is what you're asking.

Comment: I think its very important. Our population is so elderly it has been my observation that Fentanyl often is not necessary and it has some serious side effects.

Zaman: Right, we have been lucky because we use smaller doses. Some patients are obviously very big, some of those patients are obese weigh over 100 kgs. They tolerate without major problems. I have put in a foley cath for chemo therapy just with local. It was a 80 year older and she said she didn't want anything.

Question: We use a similar type of sedation although we rely primarily on Versed and use very little Fentanyl and use considerably higher doses of Versed. We do 100% patient survey and we get about a 40% response. This is mailed to the patient rather than given to them at the center. They indicate an excellent or very good response to amnesia at a rate of about 85%.

Comment: In our state we can not do this without a nurse available, a CRNA, and that adds to the expense of the procedure tremendously. This does not allow you to do any of these procedures at a free standing unit because so many nurses and anesthesiologists do not want to do this for the lower reimbursement. I think it is an impediment. I think your studies show that it can be done very safely and very nicely and this is a legislative problem.

9

FIRST VASCULAR ACCESS: THE SURGEON'S VIEWPOINT

Amy L. Friedman, M.D.
Yale University School of Medicine, Department of Surgery
333 Cedar Street, Room FMB 112, New Haven, CT 06520
PH: 203-785-2565, FAX: 203-785-7162
Email: amy.friedman@yale.edu

Douglas Mesler, M.D., M.P.H.
Clinical Director, Renal Section Boston University Medical Center
Evan Biomedical Research Center
650 Albany Street, 5th Floor, Boston, MA 02118
PH: 617-638-7337, FAX: 617-859-7356
Email: dmesler@bu.edu

Cynthia Lambert, R.N., B.S.
Medical Quality Manager, Network of New England
30 Hazel Terrace, Woodbridge, CT 06525
PH: 203-387-9332, FAX: 203-389-9902
Email: clambert@nw1.esrd.net

Connie Hill, R.N., M.S.
Medical Quality Manager, Network of New England
30 Hazel Terrace, Woodbridge, CT 06525
PH: 203-387-9332, FAX: 203-389-9902
Email: chill@nw1.esrd.net

Jenny Kitsen, B.A.
Executive Director, Network of New England
30 Hazel Terrace, Woodbridge, CT 06525
PH: 203-387-9332, FAX: 203-389-9902
Email: jkitsen@nw1.esrd.net

Helen Wander, R.N., C.N.N.
Director of Nursing, Damariscotta Dialysis
4 Edwards Avenue, Damariscotta, ME 04543
PH: 207-563-2601, FAX: 207-563-2605
Email: helen.wander@fmc-na.com

William DeSoi, Ph.D.
Data Consultant
710 Main Street, Lewiston, ME 04240
PH: 207-783-1449, FAX: 207-777-3865
Email: wedesoi@exploremaine.com

Cecilia Meehan, R.N., M.S.N.
Regional Administrator, Gambro Healthcare
29 Elm Ridge Drive, Rocky Hill, CT 06112
PH: 860-916-7105, FAX: 860-242-2239
Email: cecilia.meehan@us.gambro.com

Candace Walworth M.D.
Clinical Assistant Professor, University of Vermont
710 Main Street, Lewiston, ME 04240
PH: 207-783-1449, FAX: 207-777-3865
Email: cwalworth@aol.com

Introduction

Long-term survival of the ESRD patient depends on the availability of durable dialysis options. For hemodialysis, conservative utilization of potential vascular access sites is a fundamental principal of care. The radiocephalic fistula remains the gold standard primary access, although there is considerable controversy regarding the most appropriate algorithm of sequential access selection. The National Kidney Foundation's landmark dialysis outcomes quality initiative guidelines (DOQI) for vascular access state that a primary arterial venous fistula (AVF) should be constructed in at least 50% of all patients electing hemodialysis as their initial treatment.[1] In addition, the wrist fistula is specifically identified as the preferred first choice of access type.

Despite these recommendations, construction of an arteriovenous fistula as the primary vascular access occurs in less than 30% of U.S. hemodialysis patients, (CPM 2001 Report),[2] a rate specifically decried as being "unjustifiably low" in the DOQI guidelines.[1] Within the 18 Networks, the incident AVF experience in 2000 ranged between 17% and 39%, with the Network of New England reporting 29%.[3] This wide variation in experience led Network 1 to investigate those factors controlled by the surgeon (as opposed to clinical medical factors) that might influence ultimate access selection. The Medical Review Board of the Network undertook a prospective analysis of the reasons specific access types and sites were chosen by the vascular access surgeons, who created them in a representative population of ESRD patients undergoing surgical access construction.

Methods

Surgeons at six locations in the New England area agreed to participate in prospective data collection. These centers were selected because each has a small number of surgeons routinely performing a substantial number of vascular access operations and each has a predictable pattern of referring ESRD patients to a small number of outpatient hemodialysis facilities, thereby enhancing collection of outcome data.

All patients brought to the operating room for the purpose of construction of a primary vascular access from 6/15/99 through 12/15/99 were included. Prior catheter placement in any location was not considered an exclusion if the operative procedure reported was the first upper extremity access for that patient. Similarly, a patient undergoing insertion of a catheter, in addition to an arm access, was classified by the type of upper extremity procedure performed. Ten patients of the total 108 in this study had a surgical catheter placement with the intent of it serving as a permanent form of access.

The access surgeon completed a two-page data collection sheet immediately following surgery (Figure 1a & 1b). Demographic data collected included patient age, height, weight and gender. Anatomic data included description of all potential venous sites (cephalic vein in the wrist and forearm, antecubital veins, basilic vein, axillary vein, proximal cephalic vein) as (1) present or absent on physical examination, (2) patent or thrombosed and (3) acceptable caliber or too small to use. The specific site and type of access constructed were collected.

NETWORK OF NEW ENGLAND VASCULAR ACCESS QUALITY IMPROVEMENT PROJECT

Surgeon's Questionnaire

Choice of Vascular Access (To be completed day of vascular access placement)

Medical Center: _____

Surgeon's Name: _____

Referring Nephrologist: _____

Date of Access Placement: _____

Patient Name: _____

Social Security #: _____

Gender: _____ Age: _____

Weight: _____ Height: _____ *cm or inches*

Check all that apply for each of the following categories.

	Exam		Patency		Caliber	
	Present	Absent	Patent	Thrombosed	Acceptable	Too Small to Use
RIGHT SIDE						
Cephalic Vein at Wrist & Forearm						
Antecubital Veins						
Basilic Vein						
Axillary Vein						
Proximal Cephalic Vein						
LEFT SIDE						
Cephalic Vein at Wrist & Forearm						
Antecubital Veins						
Basilic Vein						
Axillary Vein						
Proximal Cephalic Vein						

Comments: _____

Figure 1a

PLEASE CHECK ALL THAT APPLY TO EACH APPLICABLE PROCEDURE:

FISTULA

TYPE:
Wrist Radial-Cephalic _____
Brachio-Cephalic _____
Brachio-Basilic _____
Other _____

LOCATION:
Left-Side _____
Right-Side _____
Dominant _____
Non-Dominant _____

Was a Doppler done prior to
placement? Yes _____ No _____
Was a Venogram done prior to
placement? Yes _____ No _____

Why did you choose this access?
Nephrologist's request _____
Needed immediately _____
Needs time to mature _____
Anatomical limitations _____
Patient's choice _____
Diabetic patient _____
Other (specify) _____

Completed by: _____

Figure 1b

PROSTHETIC GRAFT

TYPE:
Forearm Straight _____
Forearm Loop _____
Upper Arm Brachio-Axillary _____
Thigh Graft _____
Other _____

LOCATION:
Left-Side _____
Right-Side _____
Dominant _____
Non-Dominant _____

Was a Doppler done prior to
placement? Yes _____ No _____
Was a Venogram done prior to
placement? Yes _____ No _____

Why did you choose this access?
Nephrologist's request _____
Needed immediately _____
Needs time to mature _____
Anatomical limitations _____
Patient's choice _____
Diabetic patient _____
Other (specify) _____

CATHETER

TYPE:
Tunneled _____
Tunneled Dual Lumen _____
Non-Tunneled Lumen _____
Tunneled Dual Catheter _____
Other _____

LOCATION:
Left-Side _____
Right-Side _____
Dominant _____
Non-Dominant _____

Was a Doppler done prior to
placement? Yes _____ No _____
Was a Venogram done prior to
placement? Yes _____ No _____

Why did you choose this access?
Nephrologist's request _____
Needed immediately _____
Anatomical limitations _____
Patient's choice _____
Diabetic patient _____
Other (specify) _____

Phone #: _____

Of the 98 patients with accesses placed, 80 were available for follow-up at 6 months (11 lost to follow-up, 7 deaths). Outcome data were collected from the dialysis center actively caring for the patient six months following primary access construction. The need for maintenance dialysis, access patency and the need for any interventions to restore or maintain patency in the primary access were recorded. A total of 12 patients were not yet on dialysis at the time this follow-up data was abstracted.

This study was a baseline survey and was not conceived to have statistical power. Comparisons between groups were performed using Chi Square and Fishers Exact Test. A p-value of less than 0.05 was considered as statistically significant. Analyses were performed using SAS 6.12.

Results

During the six-month enrollment period, 108 patients underwent primary operative access placement for hemodialysis. The mean age of this group was 69.6 +/- 13.8 years and included 55 females (50.9%) and 53 males (49.1%). The mean body mass index (BMI) [weight in kilograms/(height in meters)^2] was 25.9. Diabetes was present in 40.7% (44/108) of patients. The 10 patients undergoing surgical catheter placement did not differ in age or body mass index (BMI) from the other patients in this study. These catheter patients have been removed from the remaining analysis.

The 98 patients with an arm access fall into two groups: 65 received an AVF and 33 received a prosthetic graft. Fistulae were placed primarily in 66% (65/98) of patients, and of these 29.6% (29/98) were radial-cephalic procedures. PTFE grafts were constructed in 33.7% (33/98) of the group. The vast majority of these (29/33, 88%) were placed in the forearm. Figure 2 shows the specific type and site of access created.

Figure 3 demonstrates the effect of patient age on the type of access constructed. Younger patients underwent fistula construction more frequently than older patients. Ninety percent (90%) of patients younger than 40 years of age (10) had fistulae created. Fistula creation was 73% (37/51) among those patients younger than age 65 versus 60% (28/47) for those 65 years of age and older.

Figure 4 demonstrates the effect of obesity on the type of access constructed. Increasing BMI was associated with a lower rate of fistula placement. Most patients of normal or lean weight (BMI < 30) received fistulas (53/76, 70%) versus the cohort with a BMI > 30 (12/22, 55%). Four percent (4%) of the population was massively obese (BMI > 40) and only 1 patient out of 4 had a fistula constructed.

The rate of fistula placement was lower in diabetic patients (24/40, 60%) than in the non-diabetic cohort (41/58, 71%). The rate of graft placement among diabetics was correspondingly higher. Radiocephalic fistula construction was achieved in 42% (10/40) of diabetics versus 46% (19/41) of non-diabetics.

Surgeons opted not to create a radiocephalic fistula in 70% (69/98) patients undergoing a first upper extremity operation (Figure 5). The cephalic vein was considered too small for use in 80% (55/69) of the patients, while in 12% (8/69) of patients the cephalic vein was thrombosed or had been subjected to sufficient trauma (presumably from cannulation or phlebotomy) to preclude surgical use. Twenty-five percent of the patients preoperatively had undergone venous mapping by doppler ultrasound or venography.

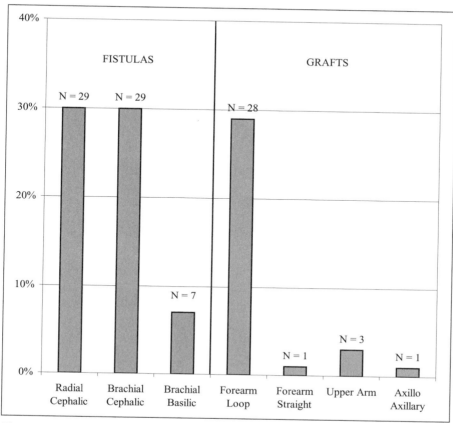

Figure 2:   Type of vascular access constructed in 98 ESRD patients
undergoing first arm access surgery

Follow-up data at six months were available for 82% (80/98) patients who underwent construction of an arm access. Eleven patients were lost to follow-up and 7
patients had died (overall mortality rate 8.8%, Figure 6). Those patients in whom a
fistula was created had a mortality rate of 9.4%; graft associated mortality was 7.4%.

Patency was defined as an access that supported hemodialysis (68/80) or, in the
pre-dialysis patient (12/80), judged suitable for cannulation. Patency at 6 months
was present in 78% of all arm access: 77% (41/53) of fistulae and 78% (21/27) of
grafts (Table 1). Patency of the radiocephalic fistula was 71% (17/24). Patency was
greater in fistula patients younger than 40 years (N=9, 100%) than in those fistula
recipients older than 65 years (19/21, 90%) and graft recipients (14/15, 93%) older
than 65 years. Fistula patency was greater in those patients of normal or lean weight
(BMI < 30, N=34/42, 81%) than in obese patients (BMI > 35, N=2/5, 40%). Graft
patency was not adversely affected by obesity, as 23 lean graft patients (BMI < 30)
had a patency rate of 68% (N=13/19) while in obese graft patients (BMI > 35) all
grafts were patent. Diabetes was associated with an 83% (19/23) patency rate for all
fistulas versus 73% (22/30) in non-diabetics. Radiocephalic fistulas were more frequently patent among diabetics (80%, 8/10) than non-diabetics (64%, 9/14).

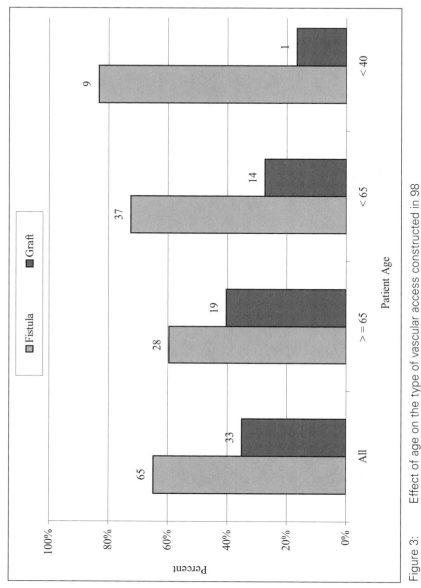

Figure 3:   Effect of age on the type of vascular access constructed in 98 patients undergoing first arm access surgery

Conclusion

The primary purpose of this Quality Improvement Project was to determine the surgical decision making influencing AV fistula construction in the ESRD population served by Network 1. A secondary purpose was to measure the frequency of wrist fistulae as the first access. In contrast to most other studies of access construction and patency, our investigation includes multiple institutions and surgeons rather than a single surgical practice.

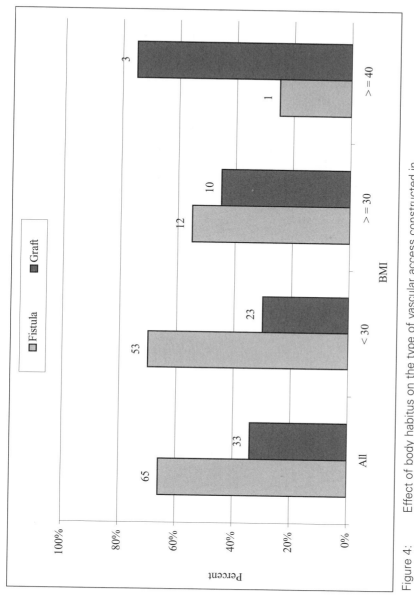

Figure 4: Effect of body habitus on the type of vascular access constructed in 98 ESRD patients undergoing first arm access surgery

In 30% (29/98) of patients, surgeons constructed a radiocephalic fistula. Review of alternative surgical choices in the other 70% of patients demonstrated that in 12% the cephalic vein at the wrist was thrombosed or traumatized from prior cannulation. This reflects the failure of vein preservation as suggested in DOQI guideline 7 and represents an area for improved quality of care in the pre-ESRD patient population. Educational materials to alert patients with chronic kidney disease, their physicians and healthcare professionals such as phlebotomists and nursing staff, may aid in long-term vein preservation. The 2% of cases in which a nephrologist or patient preferred

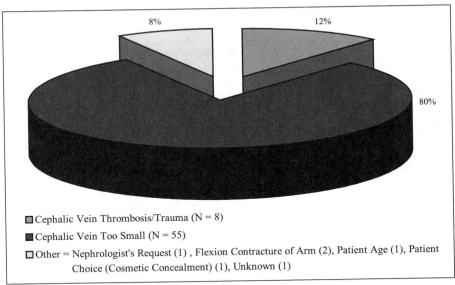

Figure 5:   Surgeon's reason for not constructing a radial cephalic fistula in 69 of 98 ESRD patients undergoing first arm access surgery

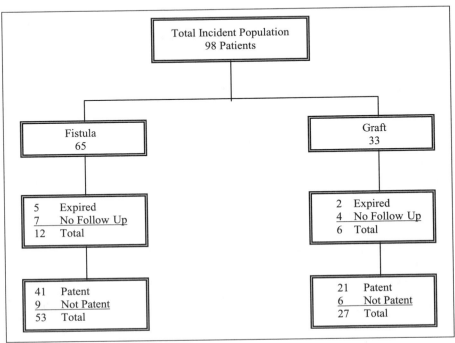

Figure 6:   Six month outcome of 98 ESRD patients evaluated for first arm access surgery

Table 1.   Six-month access patency in ESRD patients with first arm access surgery.

	Original N	6 mo. Follow-Up N	Patient at 6 mo. N	Revisions N	Patent
TOTAL	98	80	62	6	78%
FISTULA					
ALL	65	53	41	4	77%
Radio Cephalic	29	24	17	1	71%
Brachio Cephalic	29	23	19	3	83%
Brachio Basilic	7	6	5	0	83%
GRAFT					
ALL	33	27	21	2	78%
Forearm Loop	28	22	18	2	82%
Forearm Straight	1	1	1	0	100%
Upper Arm	3	3	2	0	67%
Upper Arm	1	1	0	0	0%

an alternative access site must also be considered failures to achieve adequate education regarding the benefits of an initial radial-cephalic fistula.

Eighty percent of decisions to construct alternative accesses were based on the surgeon's judgment that the cephalic vein was simply too small. While preoperative studies such as vein mapping may be performed to establish adequacy of the cephalic vein caliber and justify operative wrist exploration[4,5] the final determination of anatomic suitability remains a subjective judgment. If the surgeon uses a cephalic vein that ultimately proves to be inadequate, the fistula will thrombose or fail to mature, creating significant morbidity for the patient. This thrombosis or maturation failure also leads to prolongation of dialysis catheter use, subsequent hospitalization for additional access procedures, and increasing cost of care.[6,7]

Whether the exclusion of 80% of cephalic veins due to anatomic unsuitability was excessive is unknown. There was obviously a strong emphasis on the placement of native arteriovenous fistulae among these surgeons, as they constructed grafts in only 34% of patients. These surgeons constructed fistulae in patients irrespective of age, body habitus, or diabetic status. The primary patency rate of 77% of all fistulae suggests that appropriate access site selections were made.

DOQI guideline 35 sets no specific rate of primary AV fistula patency, thereby promoting native fistula construction. Yet, inordinately low patency rates, perhaps < 50%, should prompt consideration of inadequate surgical quality reflecting either poor surgical technique or poor judgment regarding anatomic suitability of the native vein. The primary patency rate of 71% for wrist fistulae and 77% for all fistulae in this study may serve as the initial quality indicators.

The significantly lower rate of 29% of incident patients observed to have arteriovenous fistulas in Network1 from CMS Annual CMP Report 2001 may reflect the collective failure to identify and refer pre-dialysis patients for access construction in sufficient time to avoid dependence on catheter use for the initiation of hemodialysis.[8]

Alternatively, the difference between the fistula construction rate in the six study sites and the overall Network data may reflect surgical behavior change simply through participation in a prospective study. This aspect of ESRD care is the focus of an ongoing quality improvement project.

Disclaimer

The analyses upon which this publication is based were performed under Contract Number 500-00-NW01 entitled End Stage Renal Disease Networks Organization, Network of New England, sponsored by the Centers for Medicare and Medicaid Services (CMS), Department of Health and Human Services. The content of this publication does not necessarily reflect the views or policies of the Department of Health and Human Services.

The authors assume full responsibility for the accuracy and completeness of the ideas presented. This article is a direct result of a Health Care Quality Improvement Program initiated by CMS, which has encouraged identification of quality improvement projects derived from analysis of patterns of care, and therefore require no special funding on the part of this contractor.

Acknowledgments

The Network Medical Review Board and the members of the Vascular Access Committee wish to extend their collective appreciation to all of you for your cooperation and ongoing participation in this Quality Improvement Project.

Medical Centers

Saint Francis Hospital and Medical Center, Hartford, CT
Yale New Haven Hospital, New Haven, CT
Saint Mary's Regional Medical Center, Lewiston, ME
Central Maine Medical Center, Lewiston, ME
Rhode Island Hospital, Providence, RI
Kent County Memorial Hospital, Warwick, RI
U-MASS Memorial Health Care – Hahnemann Campus, Worcester, MA
Maine Medical Center, Portland, ME

Dialysis Facilities

Gambro Healthcare Hartford, Hartford, CT
Gambro Healthcare New Haven, New Haven, CT
Lewiston-Auburn Kidney Center, Lewiston, ME

Southern Maine Dialysis Center, Portland, ME
U-MASS Memorial Health Care – Hahnemann Campus, Worcester, MA
Artificial Kidney Center of Rhode Island, East Providence, RI
Artificial Kidney Center of Tiverton, Tiverton, RI
Rhode Island Renal Institute, Warwick, RI
Rhode Island Hospital Dialysis Unit, Providence, RI

References

1. National Kidney Foundation Vascular Access Working Group. NKF-DOQI clinical practice guidelines for vascular access. New York, NY, National Kidney Foundation, *Amer J Kid Dis.* 1997; 30:S142.
2. Annual Report ESRD Clinical Performance Measures Project. Department of Health and Human Services, Centers for Medicare & Medicaid Services, Office of Clinical Standards and Quality, Center for Beneficiary Choices, Baltimore, MD, 2001.
3. ESRD Network of New England, Inc. Excerpts from The Network of New England Annual Report. New Haven, CT. ESRD Network of New England, Inc. 2000; 14-33.
4. Sands J, Young S, Miranda C. The effect of doppler flow screening studies and elective revisions on dialysis access failure. *ASAIO J.* 1992; 38:M524-M527.
5. Tordoir JHM, Hoeneveld H, Eikelboom BC, Kitslaar PJEHM. The correlation between clinical and duplex ultrasound parameters and the development of complications in the arterio-venous fistulae for hemodialysis. *Eur J Vasc Surg.* 1990; 4:179-184.
6. U.S. Renal Data System: X. The cost effectiveness of alternative types of vascular access and the economic cost of ESRD. *Amer J Kid Dis.* 1995 (suppl); 26: S140-S156.
7. Feldman HI, Kobrin S, Wasserman A. Hemodialysis vascular access morbidity. *J Am Soc Nephrol.* 1996; 7:523-535.
8. Friedman AL, Walworth C, Meehan C, Wander H, Shemin D, DeSoi W, Kitsen J, Hill C, Lambert C, Mesler D. First hemodialysis access selection varies with patient acuity. *Adv Ren Replace Ther.* 2000 (suppl); 7(4): S4-S10.

DISCUSSION

Vascular Access for Hemodialysis IX
May 6-7, 2004
Lake Buena Vista, Florida

May 6, 2004
Abstract Session 1

Dr. Candace Walworth
"First Vascular Access: The Surgeon's Viewpoint"

Question: How have you communicated the results of your data to the rest of the surgeons in New England?

Walworth: One of the problems we have found is that surgeons do not really know what their own results are, unless they have some way of tracking their own data. Now we have surgical results for almost every surgeon in New England and we are sending them maps, coded maps so we pick greater than 50% fistulas and you're not identified. You have a nice big red pin if you were getting 50% fistulas. If you weren't you would have a blue pin. So we are trying to modify surgical behavior.

Question: I think that the operative room is not the best place to examine the patient before creating a vascular access. I think it is mandatory to preserve the veins of both wrists, not only the non-dominant one.

Walworth: I do not disagree with you that the first counter between the surgeon and the patient should not take place in the operating room. But the ultimate decision takes place in the operating room. These people were all seen prior to surgery.

Question: What percentage of the patients had preoperative Doppler or venogram studies?

Walworth: Twenty five percent and this was in 1999.

Question: Did the performance of the Doppler or the venogram increase the use of fistulas or did they increase the use of forearm fistulas?

Walworth: Not in this study.

SECTION III
FACULTY PRESENTERS

10

CREATION AND MAINTENANCE OF DIALYSIS ACCESS GRAFTS: CODING REVIEW AND UPDATE

Melody W. Mulaik, MSHS, CPC, CPC-H, RCC

Coding and Reimbursement

On of the greatest challenges associated with discussing coding and billing guidelines of a diverse group of providers is that the guidelines vary from payor to payor. It is important to remember that when a third party payor is involved, the determination of reimbursement for services is the decision of the individual insurance company, based on the patient's policy and the third party payor guidelines. No presentation or paper can adequately address reimbursement issues for the hundreds of insurance payors that exist. Therefore, it is essential that each payor be contacted for their individual requirements.

Four of the key areas of concern associated with the coding and billing of creation and maintenance of dialysis grafts are the pre-surgical evaluations, new procedures, access maintenance and ensuring appropriate modifiers are appended, when necessary. When evaluating coding guidance it is important to distinguish between authoritative guidance and opinion. Only guidance provided by the insurance payors and the American Medical Association (AMA) is considered to be authoritative guidance. All other sources of information (including specialty societies, other medical groups, healthcare consultants and billing companies) provide opinion. When conflicting information is received, the source of the information should be evaluated to ensure adherence to authoritative information.

Local Coverage Decisions (LCDs), formerly known as Local Medical Review Policies (LMRPs), provide guidance and information related to the medical necessity of designated procedures. Any individual may submit information to a carrier regarding the content of an LCD. At the present time, many carriers are in the process of reviewing their LCDs, therefore this is a key opportunity to bring matters of concern to your local carrier. The medical necessity guidelines related to the pre-surgical evaluation and access maintenance vary widely between payors and there exists opportunities for improvement in coverage and corresponding reimbursement. For example, some payors will provide payment for a pre-surgical vascular ultrasound (93971) [utilizing ICD-9 code V72.83], however many payors do not address this procedure in their LCD. The absence of payor guidelines for a specific procedure does not automatically indicate that reimbursement will not be provided, however, it is very difficult to appeal for payment without written guidance from the payor.

2004 Coding Updates

The annual coding changes published in the AMA *CPT-4 Procedure Coding Guide* should be reviewed to identify the impact on new or existing procedures performed by the practice. The biggest changes for 2004 is the addition of a new DRIL code and a complete overhaul of the central venous catheter codes. A new code, 36838 [Distal revascularization and interval ligation (DRIL), upper extremity hemodialysis access (steal syndrome), is now available for use, however, it is important to review the CPT cross-references to ensure correct coding and billing practices.

The biggest coding changes for 2004 was in the central venous catheter (CVC) codes. The new procedures codes for central venous devices can be categorized as:

1. Insertion—placement of catheter through a newly established venous access
2. Repair—fixing device without replacement of either catheter or port/pump, other than pharmacologic or mechanical correction of intracatheter or pericatheter occlusion
3. Partial replacement of only the catheter component associated with a port/pump device, but not entire device
4. Complete replacement of entire device via same venous access site (complete exchange)
5. Removal of entire device

For these new codes, there is no coding distinction between venous access achieved percutaneously versus cutdown or based on catheter size. For all services except, repositioning under fluoroscopy, the appropriate CPT code describing the service may now be assigned with a frequency of two, when appropriate. If an existing central venous access device is removed and a new one placed via a separate venous access site, codes for both procedures (removal of old, if code exists, and insertion of new device) may be assigned. Also, it is important to note that the age criteria for these procedures has been changed from 2 to 5 years of age.

In addition to the numerous new central venous catheter procedure codes, two new imaging guidance codes were created in 2004 specifically for central venous catheter/device procedures.

+75998—Fluoroscopic guidance for central venous access device placement, replacement (catheter only or complete), or removal (includes fluoroscopic guidance for vascular access and catheter manipulation, any necessary contrast injections through access sites or catheter with related venography radiologic supervision and interpretation, and radiographic documentation of final catheter position) (List separately in addition to code for primary procedure)

+76937—Ultrasound guidance for vascular access requiring ultrasound evaluation of potential access sites, documentation of selected vessel patency, concurrent realtime ultrasound visualization of vascular needle entry, with permanent recording and reporting (List separately in addition to code for primary procedure)

It is important to note that the definition of 76937 requires "permanent recording". Many of the hand held ultrasound devices are not capable of capturing a permanent image which poses an operational and coding challenge. How can the use of ultrasound for central venous catheter placement be billed when no permanent record is performed? The answer is, unfortunately, not at all. The creation of these new imaging codes has negated the ability to bill for the previously utilized ultrasound guided needle localization code 76942, therefore either the definition of 76937 must be met or no charge may be created for this component of the procedure.

Percutaneous Access Maintenance

Correct code assignment for percutaneous interventions utilizes the principles of component coding. This coding methodology permits the assignment of CPT® codes that define both the surgical procedure and/or vascular access and separate codes for the radiological supervision and interpretation (S&I) portion of the service. Therefore it would be anticipated that the graft access, diagnostic imaging, thrombectomy, angioplasty and stent placement would all be coded and billed when performed and properly documented in the report.

A graft is considered to be a single vascular conduit. Coding for a declot, by any method, includes declotting the entire graft. In some situations, multiple passes of the mechanical device or the employment of several declotting methods [mechanical, balloon, lytics (pulse-spray, lyse-and-wait, short or long infusions), etc.] may be required to completely declot the graft. However, according to SIR, one graft equals one declot service and one CPT® code [36870]. Treatment of vascular stenosis is separately coded. According to SIR, the entire graft from the arterial anastomosis through the venous anastomosis, as well as the outflow vein approximately to the level of the axillary vein is considered a single vessel. All PTAs within this segment should be coded as a single venous PTA, regardless of the number of stenoses treated within the segment. Some payors may also allow for the coding of a second (separate) venous PTA performed on a stenosis identified centrally and also treated with a balloon. However, some payors (e.g., Trailblazers) has stated that the venous PTA codes may only be assigned for documented stenosis *proximal to the fistula* and that stent placements within the fistula must be assigned the unlisted code 37799. Stenosis treated at the arterial anastomosis is included in the venous PTA codes for the entire graft and would not be coded separately unless it is the only stenosis treated with PTA. Some payors consider this angioplasty as an arterial procedure and allow for the assignment of 35475+75962. Check your payor guidelines. It is appropriate to code for an additional PTA if a separate vessel from the initially treated stenotic vessel is treated, such as the subclavian vein. Modifier -59 would be used to indicate the treatment of a separate vessel.

Thombolysis of a separate vessel (e.g., embolus or thrombus) discontinuous with the occluded AVF is coded as 37201 if a separate thrombolytic infusion/pulsed spray procedure is necessary. There is no printed authoritative reference prohibiting the coding of 75820, venography of the extremity, with 75790, angiography of an arteriovenous shunt. SIR supports coding only the shunt angiography (75790) to include venous outflow all the way to the superior vena cava.

A summary description of common percutaneous intervention:

- Puncture into the graft (arterial or venous limb or arterial and venous limbs) (36145 or 36145x2)

- Declotting of graft if necessary (36870)

- PTA of vessel(s) not associated with the declot procedure (surgical and S&I components)

- Placement of stent(s) as necessary (surgical and S&I components)

- Therapeutically directed imaging of the graft (75790)

In addition to ensuring that all codes are properly assigned, it is important the modifier not be forgotten. If you are treating a patient within the global days for a particular procedure, the appropriate modifier (-78/-79) will need to be appended to ensure appropriate reimbursement.

Finally, it is important that your coding/billing operations be reviewed to ensure that charges are not inadvertently omitted or billed incorrectly. Specifically, the following questions should be raised:

- Is a charge ticket or coder utilized for CPT code assignment?

- Is there a reconciliation process to ensure all charges are captured?

- Who is responsible for modifier assignment?

- At what point in the process is the modifier assigned?

- What information is utilized for modifier assignment?

- Who is responsible for diagnosis code assignment?

- What information is utilized and what coding tools are being employed?

- How are rejects/denials being tracked?

- Who is responsible for following up on medical necessity or other coding related denials?

- What policies are in place to dictate how rejects/denials will be resolved?

In summary, ensure that your documentation is comprehensive to facilitate accurate CPT-4 and ICD-9 code assignment. Clarify any coding ambiguities with your payor and provide input if there are opportunities for improved reimbursement. Ensure that modifiers are utilized appropriately. Evaluate your current coding and billing operational processes to ensure that you have the right staff supporting your organization.

DISCUSSION

Vascular Access for Hemodialysis IX
May 6-7, 2004
Lake Buena Vista, Florida

May 6, 2004
Abstract Session II

Melody Mulaik
"Coding and Reimbursement Issues"

Question: If I do a surgical thrombectomy and follow with a fistulogram and an angioplasty as indicated. How would that be properly coded?

Mulaik: Well you have your actual surgical intervention. I'll have to look at what the code guidelines that are relevant to that. Many of times they will bundle them. Are you are talking about doing it all surgically?

Question: Doing a 36831, which is a surgical thrombectomy. Then a code for an AV fistulogram, then an opened angioplasty with the appropriate codes.

Mulaik: I'll have to look at the bundling piece for that and see whether or not they bundle. Usually the actual fistulogram itself will be included with the surgical intervention. Most times they will let you code angioplasties separate but I'm not sure if they will in that situation. I'll have to look at the bundling guidelines for that one.

Question: I am going to resume my question that I asked a while ago about the Medicare reimbursing for angioplasty. They will allow it in some situations but they will not reimburse it in a free standing surgery center. Both are independent of hospital based interventional labs, I don't understand why they will reimburse for one and not the other?

Mulaik: I can not explain the guidelines of why they will reimburse versus the other because it does not always make sense. Some of it it has to do with how the organization is designated. You said one of them is designated as an ambulatory surgery center?

Question: It is a freestanding ambulatory surgery center and we are under the guidelines of Medicare rulings. For example, they won't let us do laparoscopic gallbladders in freestanding surgery centers. They will let us do a thrombectomy, as I understand it, but the issue is angioplasty. They will not reimburse for the angioplasty, yet interventionalists are able to do it as an extension of their office. If it is a safety issue, I don't see either one is any different. I don't understand.

Mulaik: Many times when they designate where they will pay for it, it is actually based on what the perceived potential complications would be and how you could respond to that.

Comment: Exactly, my point is that the facilities are no different.

Comment: The problem is if you tried to decide on the logic of Medicare rules, you'll go crazy. They are simply wrong in doing that but it is an antiquated rule that has not been changed. Many people including myself have been trying to get them to change that but so far it has not happened.

Comment: What we should address with CMS is that if they want more fistulas, they need to give us incentives to do the cheapest way.

Question: I am very interested in your fluoroscopy code. I use fluoroscopy all of the time when I am putting in tunneled catheters or venous access ports. I will frequently get a report from the radiology department saying the fluoroscopy unit was used for one hour during this procedure and the radiologist has done nothing to help me with that. There aren't even any pictures to be taken. Are they billing for that?

Mulaik: They are not supposed to.

Levine: Can I bill for that in addition to my procedure?

Mulaik: You can bill the 75998 that you are using. The facility will capture the fluoro but the radiologist should not bill for that.

Levine: What about a surgeon myself. Can I get reimbursement?

Mulaik: If you are doing it related to the central venous catheter, yes. That is one reason why they created those codes, so they can distinguish it separately from any other types of procedures you are doing. But that is the only situation that you will be able to bill fluoro separately as a general rule.

Question: The codes that are used for selective catheterization of first and second artery branches are written from the definitions of those written predicated going from the central location peripherally. When we are working with vascular access we are going from peripherally to centrally. Should those be reversed?

Mulaik: The challenge with those is when you go in and you start non-selective, say starting in the arm, and then you go in a higher order, as in going into the SVC. That is where some of that gray area is and actually a lot of the organizations can't agree on, which is why you can't find anything in writing. When you step out, lets say outside of an AV fistula for a second, you step out and then you go more selectively that is when they start coding it. But if you go, lets say in the leg, and you start in the femoral vein, or even better, in the femoral artery and then you go to the external and then I go up to the iliac, I don't get anything additional for doing that because I have gone through what is considered a low order. But if I went down the leg to a higher order, I would get to code that. That is why with that 36145 even if you are stepping outside the fistula a little bit, a lot of times you are not going to see it coded separately. If I was just billing a 36005, which is my nonselective code for the extremity venous, I do not get to code anything extra for that. Not until I actually step out of the arm and then go some place else.

Question: You can only bill 35476 when there is a document of stenosis proximal to the fistula or graft. It may not be billed with the dilation of the venous end of the fistula, so what do we bill for the dilation of the fistula?

Mulaik: That is not addressed in their policy. That is one of those gaps in documentation.

Question: But this is 90% of our work.

Mulaik: I agree

Question: So what do we bill? Just the fistulogram?

Mulaik: According to their policy, that is the way it is written. They are saying that you should only bill the PTA if that is the location of it.

Question: If the venous graft anastomosis was 90% of the problem, you don't bill it?

Mulaik: That is what the policy states. That is one reason why I bring it up because it is a huge opportunity to address it and change it.

Comment: You should bill it and then when they deny it, you should go back to them and discuss it in length with them.

11

COVERED STENT USE IN
VASCULAR ACCESS RESCUE

Marcello A. Borzatta, M.D., F.A.C.S.
John Belville, M.D.
Mission Vascular Center
Mission Hospital Regional Medical Center,
Mission Viejo, California

Introduction

Complications associated with hemodialysis vascular access grafts, represent an important source of morbidity and mortality among chronic hemodialysis patients. Endovascular intervention utilizing thrombolytic agents, mechanical thrombectomy devices, balloon angioplasty and stent placement have proven to be as effective as surgical thrombectomy and graft revision in restoring patency of occluded dialysis grafts. However. they do not extend the life of the graft. Most dialysis access failures are not due to the graft itself, but to venous stenotic disease caused by neointimal hyperplasia. Initial balloon angioplasty techniques were employed to remedy this, but restenosis remained a problem. More recently, flexible self-expanding stents have been used. Although they appear to delay the onset of restenosis, neointimal hyperplasia occurring through the interstices and at the ends of the stent, will eventually lead to failure. The observation that the endothelial growth usually occurs within or at the ends of the stent is the basis for our premise that placing a graft lined stent may significantly extend the life of the dialysis graft by preventing neointimal growth.

Study Design

To assess the safety and effectiveness of a PTFE-lined nitinol stent graft (Viabahn, W.L.Gore& Assoc. Inc., Flagstaff, AZ) we undertook a prospective physician sponsored IDE trial. Patients presenting with arterio-venous graft failure second-ary to previously untreated venous outflow stenosis were enrolled. A registry group was also established to include all comers with failed AV grafts secondary to venous outflow lesions, regardless of the number of previous interventions.

Materials & Methods

The AV graft was cannulated in the standard fashion using an 18 gauge one-wall needle, often under ultrasound guidance. Percutaneous mechanical thrombectomy with or without pulse jet utilization of thrombolytic agents was performed. Prior to restoring inflow, a shuntogram was obtained to evaluate patency of the venous out-flow. Percutaneous transluminal angioplasty of the affected area was performed. Arterial inflow was then re-established by removing the "plug" at the arterial anas-tomosis usually using a Fogarty balloon. Once arterial flow was re-established, the area of the venous anastomosis could be properly sized and the endoprothesis selected. The Viabahn endoprothesis was then deployed across the target area, making certain that the entire segment treated with PTA would be covered. Post dilatation was performed to achieve complete apposition. A completion angiogram was obtained to image the arterial anastomosis, the entire graft and the venous out-flow. After removal of the sheath, the patients were returned to the dialysis unit.

Follow up for the trial group included venous ultrasound and plain x-ray at one, three, six, and twelve month intervals. Clinical follow up only was performed for the registry patients at the same intervals. Primary and secondary patency rates were the selected end points.

Results

Trial Patients. Eighteen endoprosthesis were deployed in sixteen patients enrolled in the FDA trial with two patients receiving two devices simultaneously to cover longer segment stenosis. Nine males and seven females with a mean age of 74 years composed this group. Endoprothesis of the following sizes were utilized: ten 8×5, four 7×5, three 9×5 and one 6×5. Patency was successfully established in all grafts. All the stent grafts were successfully placed at the target lesions. All patients were returned to hemodialysis with a functional graft. Follow up ranges to date between six and twelve months.

The primary patency rate at three, six, and twelve months was respectively 62%, 58%, and 41%. At the same intervals, the secondary patency rate was 87%, 64%, and 58%.

There were four surgical revisions for either graft infections or repeated failures. Four patients died from unrelated causes.

Registry Patients. Twenty five patients were enrolled in this group, ten males and fifteen females with a mean age of 63 years. Successful placement of the stent graft was achieved in 100% of the patients. All stent grafts were patent and functional and the patients were returned to hemodialysis at the end of the procedure. Clinical follow up ranges between six and twelve months. The primary patency rate was 54% at three months, 48% at six months and 31% at twelve months. The secondary patency rate was 94% at three months, 88% at six months, and 69% at twelve months.

There were two surgical conversions, and two deaths due to unrelated causes.

Conclusions

Arterio-venous graft rescue with stent graft implantation to treat venous outflow stenosis is a safe technique which yields encouraging preliminary results. Similar patency rates were obtained in both groups of patients. High secondary patency rates were achieved leading to the extension of the life of the access site and preservation of venous "real estate" for further access procedures. Patency of the access was re-established in all patients in an outpatient setting with immediate return to the hemodialysis unit without loss of dialysis days. Encouraging high patency rates favorably compare to historical controls but warrant further investigation.

DISCUSSION

Vascular Access for Hemodialysis IX
May 6-7, 2004
Lake Buena Vista, Florida

May 6, 2004
Abstract Session II

Dr. Marcello Borzatta
"Covered Stent Use in Vascular Access Rescue"

Question: The question that I actually have is that when I use these things and go back when they fail again, it almost is due to a development of a new stenosis. In other words, the stent is fine. That is actually not what fails. The primary patency rates are actually no better than angioplasty. So one would think that that would support not using this device. Did you find that in your study? When these failed it was not because of the stent graft, it was because of another problem at another location?

Borzatta: Most of the time the recurrence is because of a stenosis that occurs somewhere else in the device in the access graft and not necessary with the Viabahn, which is found to be completely patent. Although, we have encountered this in probably about thirty percent of the patients, that there is an edge stenosis at the distal leading edge of the device. So I say about 2/3 of the cases the device is perfectly patent and it is due to another stenosis or maybe no anatomical reason, which we encounter in about 40% of recurrent failure. They come back and there is no anatomical reason for the failure. The ones who do have an anatomical reason is about 2/3 and its somewhere else, and about 30% is at the leading edge of the device.

Question: Do you encourage or discourage cannulation through the device?

Borzatta: That is a very good question and the cannulation of the device should be discouraged because your device is usually placed right at the anastomotic level. You would not cannulate that area normally under normal circumstances anyway. Can you cannulate a Hemobahn or a Viabahn device? The company does not have an official policy on that. It has been done. It turns out actually that there is experience both with cannulating the wall graft device, which has a different construction. The Hemobahn seems to be at least conceptually easier to cannulate because you don't have continual struts, so you actually have spaces where you are going to be going through just PTFE and not the nitinol stent. If you look at the in vitro cannulation, and you can do it on your back table, the recoil of the PTFE is much greater than with the other covered stents. So can it be done, yes. Is it being encouraged, no. The company does not recommend it.

Comment/Question: This is a great technology for these of us who believe in doing local revision for the graft. Now we can do a revision by just interventional means, which allows the patient to go back to dialysis immediately without having the problem with the pain in surgery. My only concern is in many situations when these stents are placed by people who are not thinking in these terms. The deep vein might not be available in the future because the stent has already crossed that vein.

Comment: That is an excellent point but the important point to me is that you need to cover the area that you are going to be treating with your angioplasty balloon. I assume that you are treating the area that is stenotic and you should not extend your angioplasty into the native vein and therefore since you are only covering the area that you are treating with the balloon, you should not take your prosthetic device into native untouched vein. The whole idea of this is that you are going to preserve the native vein for further access sites. The only time when open surgical repair compares favorably within the interventional repair of av access graft is when you actually have done an interposition graft and you have extended your surgical reconstruction utilizing a new native vein. So the whole principle behind utilization of covered stents is that you should not extend the device into territory that you want to preserve for further access.

12

FISTULA FIRST INITIATIVE

Deborah J. Brouwer R.N., C.N.N.
Director, Therapeutic & Clinical Programs
Renal Solutions Inc.
770 Commonwealth Drive
Suite 101
Warrendale, PA 15086

The National Vascular Access Improvement Initiative (NVAII) or "Fistula First" is a United States national project to increase the number of AV fistulae for hemodialysis to reach or exceed the NKF K/DOQI Vascular Access Guideline 29.

"Primary AV fistulae should be constructed in at least 50% of all new kidney failure patients electing to receive hemodialysis as their initial form of renal replacement therapy. Ultimately, 40% of prevalent patients should have a native AV fistula."[1]

The Centers for Medicare and Medicaid Services (CMS) and the 18 ESRD Networks have adopted the NVAII as part of the scope of work for July 2003- July 2006. The ESRD Networks are nonprofit organizations that work as contractors for CMS to promote and improve the quality of care for all patients with ESRD (End Stage Renal Disease). To learn more about the role of the specific ESRD Networks visit the ESRD Forum website at www.esrdnetworks.org.

The NVAII takes the K/DOQI Vascular Access Guidelines theory and applies proven practical ideas to reach the AV Fistula goals. The Institute for Healthcare Improvement (IHI) is a not-for-profit organization that was selected by CMS to coordinate the NVAII. For more information on the IHI or the NVAII please visit the following websites: www.ihi.org and www.qualityhealthcare.org. The process to develop the NVAII started with the IHI researching the topic of hemodialysis vascular access. Numerous phone interviews were conducted with various healthcare leaders in the specific area of hemodialysis vascular access. A working group was selected to represent a cross section of the various thought leaders in vascular access. The goal for the Working Group was to provide expert assistance in developing the NVAII. The main areas included:

- Identify key opportunities for improvement
- Share practical strategies, implementation approaches and tools
- Identify important barriers to change that must be addressed to succeed

An additional duty was to review change package document and ensure that content is accurate and actionable. The Working Group Members were:

Clinicians

Larry Spergel, MD, Dialysis Management Medical Group (Chair)

Deborah Brouwer RN CNN, Director, Therapeutic & Clinical Programs, Renal Solutions, Inc.

Richard J. Gray, MD, Director, Interventional Radiology, Medstar Health

Vo Nguyen, MD, Memorial Nephrology Associates, Olympia, WA

Jack Work, MD, Interventional Nephrologist, Emory University, Renal Division

Bessie Young, MD, MPH, VA Puget Sound Health Care

Network Staff

Jeanette Cain, QI Director, The Renal Network, Inc.

Janet Crow, MBA, Administrator, Forum of ESRD Networks

Jenny Kitsen, Executive Director, ESRD Network of New England

Doug Marsh, Executive Director, Southern California Renal Disease Council

Patient Representative

Mike Zecca, Patient Representative

Providers

Mike Lazarus, MD, Chief Medical Officer and Senior VP of Clinical Quality, Fresenius Medical Care

John Sadler, MD, Pres. & CEO, Independent Dialysis Foundation

CMS

Jefferson Rowland, Government Task Leader

David Hunt, MD, Medical Officer, Quality Improvement Group, Centers for Medicare and Medicaid Services

Institute for Healthcare Improvement

Carol Beasley, Project Director

Kevin Nolan, Improvement Advisor

Rebecca Steinfield, Project Manager

The Working Group held a face to face meeting to brainstorm. The meeting resulted in the development of eleven change concepts. "A *change concept* is a *general* approach to change that has shown usefulness in developing *specific* ideas for changes that lead to improvement. *Change concepts* are intended to encourage development of *specific changes* that make sense within a particular setting."[2]

The Change Concepts are the following[2]:

1. Routine CQI review of vascular access
2. Early referral to nephrologist
3. Early referral to surgeon for "AVF only"
4. Surgeon selection
5. Full range of appropriate surgical approaches
6. Secondary AVFs in AVG patients
7. AVF placement in catheter patients
8. Cannulation training
9. Monitoring and surveillance
10. Continuing education: staff and patient
11. Outcomes feedback

The Working Group selected the eleven change concepts because the implantation of a few or all of the ideas will lead to an increase AV fistula rate for hemodialysis patients. Many of the Working Group members have personal experience with one or more of the change concepts and could testify to the impact changing practice had on a dialysis units AV fistula success rate. Unlike the K/DOQI Guidelines that outlined the goals and the rational for each guideline, the change concepts provide the how to steps for reaching the goals. The AV fistula goals have been well understood since the first publication of the NKF K/DOQI Vascular Access Guidelines, but clinical practice does not reflect achievement of the goals. The graph (figure 1) reflects the percentage of the AVF use in the various ERSD Networks for 2001. Without specific targeted efforts to increase the number of AV fistula creations in incident and prevalent ESRD patients, the goals of the K/DOQI Guidelines could take years to reach. The NVAII three year project targets the end point of more AV fistula creations for all ESRD patients.

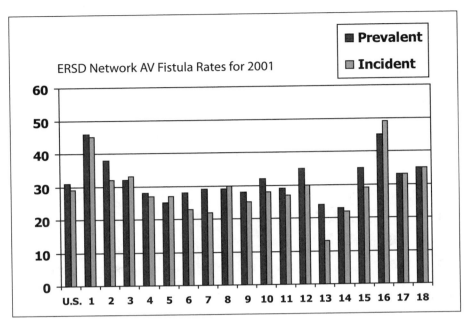

Figure 1:   2001 CPM data.

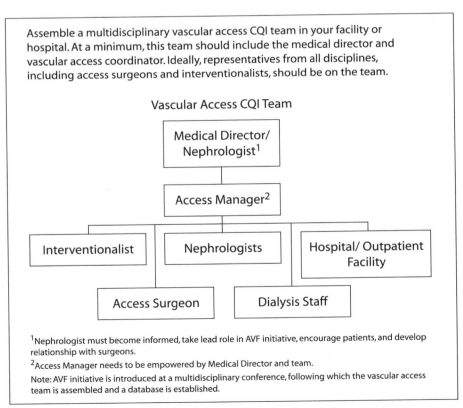

Figure 2
Source: www.qualityhealthcare.org.

The First of the Change Packet is Review Vascular Access as Part of Routine Organizational Improvement Processes.

"Dialysis facilities should incorporate vascular access into their continuous quality improvement (CQI) processes. Planning and care for vascular access spans many disciplines and settings; breakdowns in communication put patients at risk for sub-optimal treatment. In order to identify patients who will benefit from secondary arteriovenous (AV) fistula placement, facilities need processes that facilitate multidisciplinary communication, assign responsibility for vascular access information coordination, and regularly collect and use data to identify problems and opportunities for improvement."[2]

This change concept is based on clinical practices that have implemented the CQI process to improve the vascular access outcomes with in a specific clinical practice area. Several key articles explained how the use of the CQI process did result in increased AV fistula placement. The key articles are:

A multidisciplinary approach to hemodialysis access: Prospective evaluation

Allon M, Bailey R, Ballard R, et al. A multidisciplinary approach to hemodialysis access: Prospective evaluation. Kidney International. Feb 1998;53(2):473-479.

How a multidisciplinary vascular access care program enables implementation of the DOQI guidelines: Part I

Duda C, Spergel L, Holland J, Tucker T, Bander S, Bosch J. How a multidisciplinary vascular access care program enables implementation of the DOQI guidelines: Part I. Nephrology News & Issues. 2000;14(5):13-17.

Implementing a vascular access quality improvement program: Part II: Lessons learned

Duda C, Spergel L, Holland J, Tucker C, Bander S, Bosch J. Implementing a vascular access quality improvement program: Part II: Lessons learned. Nephrology News & Issues. 2000;14(6):29-32.

Multidisciplinary team approach to increasing AV fistula creation

Nguyen V, Griffith C, Treat L. A multidisciplinary team approach to increasing AV fistula creation. Nephrology News & Issues. 2003;17(7):54-57.

Change Concept #2. Establish Processes to Facilitate Timely Referral to Nephrologists

"Reach out to the primary care physician (PCP) community to educate clinicians on appropriate referral criteria."[2]

Practical ideas to reach the goal include

- Document an AV Fistula Plan

- "Document an AV fistula plan for all patients expected to require renal replacement therapy (RRT), regardless of the type of RRT being considered."[2]

- Educate Primary Care Physicians to Utilize Pre-End Stage Renal Disease/Chronic Kidney Disease Referral Criteria

"The new *Kidney Disease Outcomes Quality Initiative (K/DOQI) Chronic Kidney Disease (CKD) Guidelines* provide a clear standard for classification and management of patients with kidney disease. Primary care physicians (PCPs) should use these guidelines to evaluate, manage, and refer their patients with evidence of kidney disease. Referral to a nephrologist should be made for all patients with evidence of CKD, but certainly before the glomerular filtration rate (GFR) falls below 30 ml/minute (Stage 4 CKD) for nondiabetics or below 60 ml/minute (Stage 3 CKD) for diabetics."[2]

Ideally, the PCP's regular laboratory will convert serum creatinine measurements to GFR. If not, office staff or the PCP can easily use an *online GFR calculator* to do the conversion.[2]

Other key articles for this change concept include:

National Kidney Foundation practice guidelines for chronic kidney disease: Evaluation, classification, and stratification

Levery A, Coresh J, Balk E, et al. National Kidney Foundation practice guidelines for chronic kidney disease: Evaluation, classification, and stratification. Annals of Internal Medicine. 2003;139(2):137-149

Vascular access surgery managed by renal physicians: The choice of native arteriovenous fistulas for hemodialysis

Ravini P, Marcelli D, Malberti F. Vascular access surgery managed by renal physicians: The choice of native arteriovenous fistulas for hemodialysis. American Journal of Kidney Disease. 2002;40(6):1264-1276.

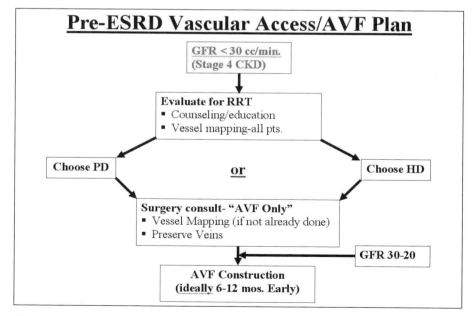

Figure 3

Assessment of a policy to reduce placement of prosthetic hemodialysis access

Gibson KD, Capt MT, Kohler TR, et al. Assessment of a policy to reduce placement of prosthetic hemodialysis access. Kidney International. 2001; 59(6):2335-2345.

Change Concept # 3 Establish Processes to Facilitate Early "AVF Only" Referral to Surgeons

"When possible, coordinate chronic kidney disease (CKD) patient care so that surgeons can evaluate patients and perform surgery with sufficient lead-time for AVF maturation. Studies show that mapping vessels can significantly increase the incidence of successful AV fistulae (e.g., *A strategy for increasing use of autogenous hemodialysis access procedures*). Establish the understanding with your surgeons that they will contact you before placing anything other than an AV fistula. Where timing is such that a temporary access must be placed (e.g., catheter), arrange for evaluation (and placement, if feasible) of an AV fistula during the initial hospitalization."[2]

The ideas behind this concept include:

- Establish Processes to Facilitate Early "AVF Only" Referral to Surgeons:

- Refer Patients for Vessel Mapping

  "Nephrologists should refer patients for vessel mapping (identification of vessel anatomy) where feasible, ideally prior to surgery referral. Doppler ultrasound or alternate technique should be used to search for suitable vessels that may be too deep to be identified on physical exam. Numerous studies have shown that vessel mapping identifies vessels suitable for an AV fistula in the majority of patients where physical exam alone classified the patient as not being a candidate for an AV fistula."[2]

Some of the Key articles:

Transition to all-autogenous hemodialysis access: The role of preoperative vein mapping

Dalman RL, Harris Jr EJ, Victor BJ, Cooga SM. Transition to all-autogenous hemodialysis access: The role of preoperative vein mapping. Annals of Vascular Surgery. 2002;16(5):624-630.

Strategy for maximizing the use of arteriovenous fistulae

Beathard GA. Strategy for maximizing the use of arteriovenous fistulae. Seminars in Dialysis. 2000;13(5):291-296.

Effect of preoperative sonographic mapping on vascular access outcomes in hemodialysis patients

Allon M, Lockhart ME, Lillo RZ, et al. Effect of preoperative sonographic mapping on vascular access outcomes in hemodialysis patients. Kidney International. 2001;60:2013-2020.

US vascular mapping before hemodialysis access placement

Robbin ML, Gallichio MH, Dieirhoi MH, Young CJ, Weber TM, Allon M. US vascular mapping before hemodialysis access placement. Radiology. 2000; 217(1):83-88.

Obese and non-obese hemodialysis patients have a similar prevalence of functioning arteriovenous fistula using pre-operative vein mapping

Vassolotti JA, Falk A, Cohl ED, Uribarri J, Teodorescu V. Obese and non-obese hemodialysis patients have a similar prevalence of functioning arteriovenous fistula using pre-operative vein mapping. Clinical Nephrology. 2002; 58(3):211-214.

A strategy for increasing use of autogenous hemodialysis access procedures: Impact of preoperative noninvasive evaluation

Silva MB, Jobson RW, Pappas PJ, et al. A strategy for increasing use of autogenous hemodialysis access procedures: Impact of preoperative noninvasive evaluation. Journal of Vascular Surgery. 1998;27:302-308.

Change Concept # 4 Select Surgeons Based on Best Outcomes.

"Collect data on the surgeons in your community to find out who has the skills and interest in placing fistulae. Choose surgeons who are willing and able to do AV fistula construction."[2]

Communicate AV Fistula Expectations to Surgeons   "Nephrologists should communicate expectations to surgeons regarding AV fistula placement and their ability to use current AV fistula surgical techniques, based on *K/DOQI Guidelines* and best practices."[2]

Refer to Surgeons Willing and Able to Meet AV Fistula Expectations "Nephrologists should refer to surgeons who are willing and able to meet AVF expectations based on *K/DOQI Guidelines* and best practices."[2]

Evaluate Surgeons on the Frequency, Quality, and Patency of Access Placements   "Data collection and outcomes tracking can be initiated and reported at the dialysis center as part of ongoing CQI processes, and may be aggregated at the ESRD Network level. Nephrologists can also potentially track the data for their patients themselves."[2]

A surgeon specific report card can help the vascular surgeon evaluate his current AV fistula placement rate for incident and prevalent ESRD patients. The dialysis units need to report back to the surgeon when the AV fistula is used successful for dialysis. The AV fistula should be reported to the surgeon as a functioning AV fistula once successful cannulations have occurred and an expectable needle gauge and blood flow rate have been achieved for routine hemodialysis. An AV fistula placed, but not yet used for dialysis needs to be evaluated at 2, 4, 6, and 8 weeks for signs of maturation. If maturation is not occurring as expected, the AV fistula should be re-evaluated for possible causes and potential treatment options to assist the AV fistula in development. If the surgeon doe not receive routine feedback on the functional status of his vascular access creations, he will be unable to truly evaluate his success rates. A successful AV fistula is a functioning vascular access used for routine hemodialysis treatments without numerous complications such as needle infiltrations.

Change Concept # 5 Use a Full Range of Appropriate Surgical Approaches.

"Surgeons who are skilled in vein transposition techniques are able to create successful AV fistulae in a substantially greater number of patients. These options require vein mapping and a surgeon's willingness to put in the additional time and effort. Make sure surgeons understand the logistics of cannulation so that they position the veins suitably and safely for cannulation."[2]

Ideas for this change concept include:

- Utilize Current Techniques for AV Fistula Placement Including Vein Transpositions

   "Surgeons should utilize current techniques for AV fistula placement including vein transpositions."[2]

Some of the key articles for this change concept include:
Aggressive treatment of early fistula failure

Beathard GA, Arnold P, Jackson J, Litchfield T. Aggressive treatment of early fistula failure. Kidney International. 2003; 64(4):1487-1494.

Durability and cumulative functional patency of transposed and nontransposed arteriovenous fistulas

Choi HM, Lal BK, Cerveira JJ, et al. Durability and cumulative functional patency of transposed and nontransposed arteriovenous fistulas. Journal of Vascular Surgery. 2003; 38(6):1206-1212.

The initial creation of native arteriovenous fistula: Surgical aspects and their impact on the practice of nephrology

Konner K. The initial creation of arteriovenous fistula: Surgical aspects and their impact on nephrology. Seminars in Dialysis. 2003; 16(4):291-298.

Arteriovenous fistula using transposed basilic vein

Butterworth PC, Doughman TM, Wheatley TJ, Nicholson ML. Arteriovenous fistula using transposed basilic vein. British Journal of Surgery. 1998; 85(12):1721-1722.

Vein transposition in the forearm for autogenous hemodialysis access

Silva MB, Hobson RW, Pappas PJ, et al. Vein transposition in the forearm for autogenous hemodialysis access. Journal of Vascular Surgery. 2002; 26(6):981-988.

The value and limitations of the arm cephalic and basilic vein for arteriovenous access

Ascher E, Hingoran A, Gunduz Y, et al. The value and limitations of the arm cephalic and basilic vein for arteriovenous access. Annals of Vascular Surgery. 2001; 15(1):89-97.

Change Concept # 6 Place Secondary AV Fistulae in Patients with AV Grafts.

"Evaluate graft patients for placement of a secondary AV fistula. In the context of the *NVAII initiative,* an AV fistula placed in a patient whose initial access was a graft is considered a "secondary" AV fistula. Staff should consider every graft patient a candidate for an AV fistula and should evaluate each patient for an AV fistula before the graft fails. In this way, a plan will be in place for providing the patient with an AV fistula when the graft begins to fail. This avoids the need for a catheter or missing an AV fistula opportunity when the graft fails and there is urgency for an immediate usable access.

Note particularly that the outflow vein from a graft is an already matured arterialized vein that could be connected and used right away (see indivual change recommendation: *Examine the Outflow Vein of All Forearm Graft Patients to Identify Suitable Veins for Secondary AV Fistula*)."[2]

Ideas for this change concept include:

- Refer to the Surgeon for Evaluation/Placement of Secondary AV Fistula Before the Graft Fails

    "Patients with an AV graft should be evaluated (including vessel mapping) for an AV fistula when the graft shows evidence of dysfunction by monitoring and surveillance. The timing of such surgical intervention to convert the outflow vein of an existing AV graft to an AV fistula, or to construct a new AV fistula in a new location, assuming suitable vessels, should be as soon as feasible but not later than following an intervention for thrombosis or clinically significant stenosis. Any delay in conversion beyond this point is likely to result in loss of the window of opportunity for an AV fistula, since further graft interventions, especially if done as an emergency, are likely to damage or utilize the outflow vein, or the graft will eventually be abandoned (usually after a failed intervention), resulting in a catheter and a new graft in a different location."[2]

- Evaluate Every AV Graft Patient for Possible Secondary AV Fistula

    Nephrologists should evaluate every arteriovenous (AV) graft patient for possible placement of a secondary AV fistula, including mapping as indicated, and document the plan in the patient's record. AV fistula evaluation of graft patients should include an updated history relevant to vascular access, physical exam with tourniquet, and vessel mapping if suitable vessels are not identified on physical exam. A secondary AV fistula plan should be documented in the chart and discussed with the patient, family, staff, and nephrologists and surgeon in anticipation of AV fistula construction on the earliest evidence of graft failure.[2]

- Examine the Outflow Vein of All Forearm Graft Patients to Identify Suitable Veins for Secondary AV Fistula

"Dialysis facility staff and/or rounding nephrologists should examine the outflow vein of all forearm graft patients during dialysis treatments (with a recommended minimum frequency of at least monthly) to identify patients who may have a suitable upper outflow vein for elective secondary AV fistula conversion in the upper arm. If such a suitable vein is found, dialysis facility staff and/or rounding nephrologists should inform the patient's nephrologist and surgeon of the need to evaluate the identified outflow vein for AV fistula conversion."[2]

Change Concept # 7 Place AV Fistulae in Patients with Catheters Where Feasible

"Higher catheter use is associated with increased infection, morbidity, mortality, and hospitalization. Evaluation and mapping of catheter patients is crucial to facilitate the

---

"SLEEVES UP" Protocol for conversion of forearm A-V graft to upper arm A-V fistula

Purpose: to identify a suitable outflow vein for conversion from an AV graft to an AV fistula, in anticipation of secondary AVF construction by the surgeon.

1. Once a month, clinic rounds to include examination of the AV graft extremity to the shoulder, by rolling *sleeves up* (or removing shirt if necessary).

2. After upper arm is exposed to the shoulder, the hand or a tourniquet is used for light compression just below the shoulder, to see if the outflow vein of the forearm graft appears suitable for immediate use as an AVF. If this appears to be the case, (often this is the case if the cephalic vein is the outflow vein), the vein is evaluated by:

- Referring patient for fistulogram (or Doppler study) to confirm that the outflow vein and draining system back to the heart is normal.

- If fistulogram is normal, the vein is "tested" by cannulating the outflow vein with the venous needle only, for 2 consecutive dialysis sessions.

- If both cannulation sessions are uneventful, the plan for surgical conversion from graft to upper arm fistula is discussed with patient, staff, nephrologists and surgeon—and documented in chart.

- Staff follows patient until AVF conversion is performed.

Figure 4:   "SLEEVES UP" Protocol for conversion of forearm A-V graft to upper arm A-V fistula

placement of AV fistulae. While catheters are necessary in some circumstances (e.g., while an AV fistula matures), the increasing prevalence of catheters in the United States is a serious health risk to patients. Strategies for reducing the number of catheters include early referral to nephrologists, monitoring and maintenance (so that accesses can be repaired before a catheter needs to be placed), and planning for a permanent access before the patient leaves the hospital."[2]

Key practical ideas include:

- Track All Catheter Patients for Early Removal of Catheters

  "Develop and implement protocols to track all catheter patients for early removal of catheters"[2]

- Evaluate All Catheter Patients for an AV Fistula

  "Regardless of prior access (e.g., AV graft), nephrologists and surgeons should evaluate all catheter patients as soon as possible for an AV fistula, including mapping as indicated."[2]

- Develop a Protocol for Catheter Indications and Removal

"Nephrologists should make every effort not to admit "catheter only" patients to the clinic. Require "catheter only" patients' nephrologists to document a plan for permanent access. Once patients arrive in the unit with a catheter only, they become part of the "catheter culture" and it becomes very difficult to counsel them to change."[2]

Change Concept # 8 Provide Cannulation Training

"Prevent fistulae from being destroyed by inexperienced staff. Discuss the basics of needle cannulation with all staff."

Key ideas include:

- Use Protocols for Initial Dialysis Treatments with New AV Fistula Patients

  "Dialysis staff should develop and use a specific protocol for initial dialysis treatments with new AV fistula patients and assign the most skilled staff to such patients."[2]

- Use Experienced Staff and Teaching Tools to Train All Appropriate Dialysis Staff on AV Fistula Cannulation

  "Identify the experienced cannulators on your staff; make sure they are available to cannulate all new fistulae and to train inexperienced staff. Identify and make available to your staff appropriate teaching tools."[2]

- Teach Self-Cannulation to Patients Who Are Interested and Able

  "Facilities should offer the option of self-cannulation to patients who are interested and able."[2]

HEMODIALYSIS ACCESS REFERRAL: EXISTING ACCESS

Date: ____/____/____   Referred to ☐ Interventional radiologist/nephrologist ☐ Surgeon
Dr._____   Phone #: _____   Fax #: _____

HEMODIALYSIS UNIT CONTACTS

Referring Nephrologist: _____ Phone #: _____ Fax #: _____
Referring Dialysis Unit : _____ Contact Person: _____ Phone #: _____ Fax #: _____

PATIENT DEMOGRAPHICS

Patient's Name _____ SS# _____ DOB ____/____/____
Address _____ City _____ State _____ Zip _____
Patient's Phone _____ Emergency Contact _____ Phone _____
Insurance _____ Phone _____

REASON FOR REFERRAL AND PROCEDURE REQUESTED

Reason _____
Procedure/Evaluation Requested _____
Desired Access _____
Date of Scheduled Procedure (If known) ____/____/____ Location: _____

CURRENT ACCESS

Type: ☐Fistula ☐Graft ☐Catheter ☐Port   Side: ☐Left ☐Right   Extremity: ☐Arm ☐Leg
Location: ☐Upper ☐Lower ☐ IJ   ☐Other
Access Insertion Date: ____/____/____ Surgeon _____ Hospital _____

Most Recent Access Blood Flow Rates/Pressures: (Check all that apply)
☐ Most recent Blood Flow Rate _____ cc/min.   ☐ Most recent Dynamic Venous Pressure _____
☐ Most recent Static Venous Pressure (SVP) _____   ☐ Most recent Arterial Pressure _____

Recent Surgical/Radiologic Interventions to Access:
1. _____ Date ___/___/___ Physician _____
2. _____ Date ___/___/___ Physician _____

Recent Access Problems/Complication - Check all that apply:
☐ Difficult cannulation   ☐ Hematoma/Infiltration   ☐ Change in bruit or thrill ☐ Pseudoaneurysm
☐ Pain in extremity   ☐ Infected Access   ☐ URR or Kt/V   ☐ Prolonged bleeding during/after dialysis
☐ Severe swelling/extremity ☐ High venous pressure   ☐ Possible Steal Syndrome   ☐ Problems with arterial flow
☐ Other (Specify) _____

SYNOPSIS OF MEDICAL HISTORY

	Yes	No
SEAFOOD OR DYE ALLERGIES * - if yes, fistulagram may be contraindicated contact Nephrologist	☐	☐
Diabetes	☐	☐
Peripheral Vascular Disease	☐	☐
History of Clotted Access	☐	☐
Anticoagulation Medicines - If yes specific medicine(s) below	☐	☐
☐Coumadin ☐Ticlid ☐ASA ☐Plavix ☐Other-list :		
Recent PT/PTT – if yes, results:	☐	☐
Recent CBC	☐	☐
Recent Chest x-ray	☐	☐
Recent EKG	☐	☐
Other pertinent medical history:		

DIALYSIS TREATMENT INFORMATION

Patient's Dialysis Schedule: M-W-F   T-Th-S   on **am / midday / pm** shift   Date of Last Dialysis___/___/___
Weight today:_____   Estimated Dry Weight: _____ Last time patient ate or drank: _____
Stat K+ drawn @ ___:___ am/pm on ___/___/___ _____meq/dl.
Transportation Service _____ Phone_____

Comments:

Figure 5

VASCULAR ACCESS DIAGRAM – FAX to Dialysis Facility and/or Nephrologist			

Patient Name:_____   Procedure Date:_____

Diagram Completed by: Surgeon (Interventional Radiologist (Interventional Nephrologist

Name (Surgeon or Interventionalist):   Phone: (   )

FAX to: (Nephrologist Name: FAX #: (   )

(Facility Name: FAX #: (   )

Procedure(s): (Check all that apply)	Access Type	Configuration	Location
SURGERY New Access Thrombectomy Revision Other- specify: _____ **INTERVENTIONAL (Endovascular)** Thrombolysis / Thrombectomy PTA Stent Catheter insertion or revision Diagnostic Fistulogram only Other- specify: _____	A/V Graft A/V Fistula Port device Central venous Catheter If new catheter, priming volume: _____ml Cuffed Non-cuffed **Graft Material** **(if applicable)** PTFE Other – specify: _____	**Graft (if applicable)** Loop Straight Curved **Fistula Construction** **(if applicable)** Radio-cephalic Brachio-cephalic Transposed Type: _____ _____ Other – specify: _____	Right Left Forearm Upper arm Leg/Thigh Other—specify: _____ Subclavian Internal Jugular Femoral Other – specify: _____

Figure 5 (Continued)

Key reference include:

Cannulation camp: Basic needle cannulation training for dialysis staff

Brouwer J. Cannulation camp: Basic needle cannulation training for dialysis staff. Dialysis and Transplantation. 1995;24(11):606-612.

The care and feeding of the AV fistula…the road to improvement? Part 2 Brouwer, DJ, Nephrology News and Issues 19 (7):pp 2003

Back to basics: The arteriovenous Graft: How to use it effectively in the dialysis unit. Brouwer DJ, Peterson P, Nephrology News and Issues 16 (12): pp. 41-49, 2002

Directing care for the vascular access: first steps. Brouwer DJ. Nephrology News and Issues 16 (6): pp., 2002

Constant site (buttonhole) method of needle insertion for hemodialysis

Twardowski Z. Constant site (buttonhole) method of needle insertion for hemodialysis. Dialysis & Transplantation. 1995;24(10):559-576.

A perfect AV fistula can be surgically created, but if the dialysis unit staff does not have a basic understanding of the AV fistula cannulation, the fistula can fail. Cannulation of a new AV fistula is very different than the routine cannulation of a mature AV fistula or of an AV graft. The dialysis units should have a specific new AV fistula cannulation policy and procedure that outlines the best cannulation practice to protect the new AV fistula from harm.

The best person to cannulate an AV fistula is the patient. Many hemodialysis patients can easily be taught to perform self cannulation in just a few training sessions. Educating patients to self cannulate solves many of the current dialysis unit problems associated with cannulation. Patients often request specific dialysis staff to perform their cannulation and this can cause staff issues and tension in the unit. If a short period of time such as 10 minutes per dialysis session over a two week period, the patient can easily master the skills required to self cannulate. The patient can then gain some independence and control of their own therapy. Most empowered patients become more compliant with dialysis therapy and become a partner in their own care with the entire ESRD Healthcare Team.

The buttonhole cannulation technique (constant-site AV fistula cannulation technique) allows patients to perform self cannulation. The use of the sharp AV fistula needle for six cannulations in the exact same site and at the exact same angle creates a tunnel track in the skin and tissue just like a pieced earring. The vessel wall forms a flap that displaces as the needle enters the vessel. After six cannultaions, the needle is changed to a Medisystems ButtonHole™ Needle Set with Anti-Stick Dull bevel for Constant-Site AV fistula access. The dull needle bevel is painless to insert into the buttonhole cannulation sites. Patients experience a pain free cannulation with the ButtonHole™ needles. The buttonhole cannulation technique has been used for many years with standard AV fistula needles. The technique is gaining popularity because the advance of the dull needle bevel is a smooth, well defined buttonhole needle track. The sharp needles created small nicks within the needle track walls and caused bleeding as new tissue could be cut with each cannulation. The dull needle bevel can not cut new tissue and thus will not alter the original buttonhole needle track or vessel flap. The dull bevel also helps to greatly reduce the risk of infiltrations once the needle is inside the vessel because the dull bevel can not puncture the vessel wall. Dialysis staff can be easily trained to perform the buttonhole cannulation techniques. The buttonhole technique is supported by the NVAII project and training for the buttonhole technique is part of the NVAII at the ESRD Network level. A full description and training tools are available from Medisystems at their web site www.medisystems.com.

Change Concept # 9 Establish Processes for Monitoring and Maintenance to Ensure Adequate Access Function

"The health care team should establish a process for monitoring and maintenance of AV fistulae to ensure adequate access function. It is extremely important to catch problems with fistulae early. Problems must be caught within 24 hours or the fistula will fail and be irreparable. There is a 20 to 30 percent failure rate for early fistulae."[2]

Practical ideas for this change concept include:

- Establish Processes for Monitoring and Maintenance to Ensure Adequate Access Function

  "The health care team should establish a process for monitoring and maintenance of AV fistulae to ensure adequate access function. It is extremely important to catch problems with fistulae early. Problems must be caught within 24 hours or the fistula will fail and be irreparable. There is a 20 to 30 percent failure rate for early fistulae."[2]

- Conduct a Post-Operative Physical Evaluation of AV Fistulae at Four Weeks

"Nephrologists and surgeons should conduct post-operative physical evaluations of AV fistulae at four weeks to detect early signs of failure and refer for
diagnostic study and remedial intervention as indicated."[2]

**Adopt Standard Procedures for Monitoring, Surveillance, and Timely
Referral for the Failing AV Fistula**   The K/DOQI has established recommendations and *guidelines for monitoring and surveillance:*

- Monitoring, which K/DOQI defines as physical examination techniques to
  detect access dysfunction, has been shown in many studies to be able to identify the majority of patients with AV fistula dysfunction.

- Surveillance involves the use of a variety of tests to detect access dysfunction.
  Intra-access blood flow measurement over time is the best surveillance method
  available for assessing AV fistula function and detecting dysfunction.

Two other methods offer significant value for AV fistula surveillance:

1. Pre-pump arterial pressure, which is measured on almost all dialysis machines,
   indicates the ease or difficulty with which the blood pump is able to draw
   blood from the access (inflow). A significant restriction of inflow will cause an
   excessively negative pre-pump arterial pressure. Since most causes of AV fistula dysfunction are inflow problems, an excessively negative pre-pump arterial pressure is often the earliest indication of such a problem.
2. Access recirculation measurement. An AV fistula may remain patent but not
   provide enough blood flow to meet the prescribed blood pump flow rate,
   resulting in underdialysis. If there is any question about adequacy of blood
   flow for dialysis, or if there is difficulty dialyzing the patient at the prescribed
   pump rate, a recirculation study will determine if the AV fistula blood flow is
   not sufficient to meet the prescribed blood pump flow rate.

Note: While physicians commonly use venous pressure measurement to detect
access dysfunction, it is of very limited value in AV fistula surveillance. This is
because most of the flow-limiting problems in AV fistulae are on the arterial of the
venous needle (and often the arterial needle as well) and therefore are not detectable
by pressure measurements made at the venous (or arterial) needle, which can only
detect an outflow obstruction downstream of the measuring needle(s). In addition,
the fistula has tributaries that can dissipate pressure in the presence of an outflow
obstruction. Finally, access pressure measurements are not likely to identify centrally located venous obstructions.[2] The K/DOQI Guidelines and full references can be
found on the National Kidney Foundation web site at www.kidney.org under
Practice Guidelines.

Change Concept # 10 Educate Caregivers and Patients

"To make good decisions about their care, dialysis patients and their caregivers need
support and resources, including information about the value of fistulae over other
access types, protecting their veins, and advocating for themselves with their health
care team."[2]

Practical ideas for this change concept include:

- Educate Patients to Improve Quality of Care and Outcomes

  "Facilities should educate patients on practices that can improve the quality of their care and their outcomes (e.g., prepping puncture sites, applying proper pressure at needle sites without clamps).

- Patients should be taught, where feasible, to manage their puncture sites without the use of clamps. This is especially important for self-care and home dialysis. Emphasizing patient education and self-care (e.g., prepping cannulation sites, patient or family member holding pressure, etc.) is beneficial for patients and can actually reduce the workload for the staff (reducing dependence on routine use of clamps).[2]

- Develop Routine In-Servicing and Education Programs in Vascular Access for Facility Staff

  'Facilities should provide routine in-servicing and education programs for all staff to communicate the value of fistulae over other access types and best treatment practices for patients with fistulae."

- Provide Continuing Education for All Caregivers

  "Provide continuing education for all caregivers to include periodic in-services by nephrologists, surgeons, and interventionalists."[2]

A major role of the ERSD Networks in the NVAII is to provide education about the eleven change concepts to all members for the ESRD Healthcare Team. The current ERSD Healthcare team that is responsible for the care plans of every dialysis patient currently includes the patient, nephrologist, dialysis nurse, renal social worker, renal dietitian, and a representative of the renal transplant team. I would suggest the vascular access surgeon is a key missing member of the care plan team. Every patient should have a vascular access plan as part of their on going care plan. Everyone on the ESRD Healthcare Team should know the next vascular access location should the current vascular access show signs and symptoms of failure. The current vascular access status should be documented as part of the routine care plan with the future plan clearly documented for easy reference. This way the entire ESRD Healthcare Team knows what should be done if the current vascular access requires any interventions and the plan should be clearly communicated to any specialist that will perform interventions on the vascular access. This way a patient with a failing lower arm AV graft can easily have the failing AV graft surgically converted to an upper arm AV fistula as the upper arm vein would be identified with the "sleeve up" program and clearly documented on the care plan.

The Final Change Concept # 11 Provide Outcomes Feedback to Guide Practice

Facilities can start by measuring performance on a monthly basis by access type — catheter, AV graft, and AV fistula — since access type is the major determinant of outcomes and directly affects dialysis delivery and adequacy. It is also important to focus specifically on native AV fistula outcomes and performance, including tracking the monthly AV fistula placement and failure rate in incident as well as prevalent patients.

The National Vascular Access Improvement Initiative (NVAII) has developed a data collection tool (Vascular Access Tracking Tool (VATT) and Instructions) that can help facilities measure and track AV fistula rates (and all access types) in incident and prevalent patients. This data tool permits simple tracking of not only AV fistulae that are in use but also AV fistulae that have been placed and are awaiting maturation.

Performance outcomes for specialists (surgeons, nephrologists, and interventionalists) should also be tracked and reported to everyone on the team on a regular basis:

- For surgeons, track the AV fistula placement rate (compared to *K/DOQI standards*) as well as success and patency rates.

- For nephrologists, track the distribution of access types their patients receive, with a focus on the AV fistula rate and the percentage of new patients starting dialysis with only a catheter.

- For interventionalists, measure the success rate of interventions and track patency rates for their procedures.

Key article for this change concept:

Increasing AV fistula creation: The Akron experience

Spuhler C, Schwarze K, Sands J. Increasing AV fistula creation: The Akron experience. Nephrology News & Issues. 2002;16(6):44-49.

The NVAII or Fistula First is an important project to change the current United States practice patterns from AV graft and hemodialysis catheter placement to the gold standard of an AV fistula placement. All members of the ERSD Healthcare Team, including the vascular access surgeon, interventional radiologist or interventional nephrologist need to understand the eleven change concepts. Implementation of the change concepts will retire the team effort, but will help to move the current clinical practice towards AV fistula placement as the vascular access of choice for new and current hemodialysis patients.

References

1. National Kidney Foundation. K/DOQI Clinical Practice Guidelines for Vascular Access, 2000. Am J Kidney Dis 37:S137-S181, 2001 (suppl 1) www.kidney.org
2. Department of Health and Human Services, Centers for Medicare and Medicaid Services, Office of Clinical Standards and Quality, End Stage Renal Disease Program. 2003. Fistula First: The National Vascular Access Improvement Initiative. Baltimore, MD

Web Sites for Additional Information

www.kidney.org Official web site for the National Kidney Foundation with full listing of all the NKF K/DOQI Guidelines

www.ihi.org and www.qualityhealthcare.org Web sites for the Institute for Healthcare Improvement

SECTION IV
ABSTRACT PRESENTERS

13

CURRENT HEMODIALYSIS AS A RISK FACTOR FOR PATENCY OF THE ARTERIO-VENOUS FISTULA

Brian W. Haag, MD, FACS
Ann S. Ewbank, MD
Colin L. Terry, M.S.

Introduction

Achieving successful long-term hemodialysis access is a well-known problem for many patients who are diagnosed with end stage renal disease (ESRD) each year. The population of patients who depend upon hemodialysis has been steadily increasing and currently includes an estimated 310,000 patients in the United States.[1] Of these patients, many will be hospitalized for difficulty in maintaining dialysis access patency. In fact, it has been estimated that dialysis patients are hospitalized 3 days out of every 3 months, and their perceived overall life satisfaction is significantly lower than normal control patients or transplant recipients.[2] Therefore, in determining the type of vascular access for each patient, the physician's goal should be that which provides the longest period of primary patency with minimal complications. The National Kidney Foundation Dialysis Outcomes Quality Initiative (DOQI) has confirmed that arterio-venous fistulas (AVF) provide patients with the best chance for prolonged uninterrupted hemodialysis access.[3] This initiative recommends construction of AVF in at least 50% of incident patients, which should eventually lead to 40% prevalence among patients at a steady state. Historically some centers in the United States have aggressively pursued the AVF, while with the advent of Doppler ultrasound, others are increasing their utilization of previously missed veins.

In order to determine which population of patients would most benefit from an AVF, as well as establish risk factors, we conducted a retrospective review of patients from a single vascular surgery practice who underwent construction of a new AVF. This population of patients included both those previously on hemodialysis as well as those patients with chronic renal insufficiency for which surgery was performed electively in preparation for hemodialysis.

Methods

We retrospectively reviewed data from 245 patients who had native AVF placement at Methodist Hospital performed between March 1997 and November 2001. The data was collected by review of pre-operative office notes and operative records. Follow up was assessed through examination of post-operative office records, and communication with the dialysis units. Attention was directed toward etiology of renal failure and other basic patient demographics including age, gender, and whether or not they were currently being dialyzed. Fistulas were differentiated between forearm (radiocephalic) and upper arm (brachiocephalic). Primary and secondary patency including the required revisions for each access failure was recorded. At the end of this study, patient status was categorized by: those with a functioning fistula, new AVF, conversion to PTFE graft, hemodialysis by way of a venous catheter, patients on peritoneal dialysis, patients with a kidney transplant, and death.

Results

Two hundred forty-five patients had native AVF placement during the period between March 1997 and November 2001. The majority of the renal disease in the study group was due to diabetic nephropathy (46.5%). Hypertension accounted for the second largest group (29.4%). Other etiologies included glomerulonephritis as well as urologic issues and are listed in Table I.

Demographic data for the series are summarized in Table II. This included 166 males (67.8%) and 79 females (32.2%). The mean age was 54.7 years. The fistula type in this population of patients included 136 brachiocephalic (55.5%) and 107 radiocephalic (43.7%). There were 2 basilic vein transpositions at the time of this study. Of those studied 68 (27.8%) were on dialysis at the time the fistula was performed.

Table I.   Etiology of Renal Failure (N=245).

Disease	Number (Percent)
Diabetes Mellitus	114 (46.5%)
Hypertension	72 (29.4%)
Glomerulonephritis	32 (13.1%)
Urologic	9 (3.7%)
Other	18 (7.4%)

Table II.   Patient Demographics (N=245).

Age	54.7 (16.0)
Gender	
Male	166 (67.8%)
Female	79 (32.2%)
Fistula Type	
Radiocephalic	107 (43.7%)
Brachiocephalic	136 (55.5%)
Basilic Vein Transposition	2 (0.8%)
Current hemodialysis	68 (27.8%)

Primary and secondary patency rates are summarized in figure 1. At 6 months the primary patency was 62.4% and the secondary patency was 70.2%. At 1 year the primary patency had dropped to 46.2% with the secondary patency being 52.3%. At 3 years the primary patency was 24% with the secondary patency being 32.0%. Thirty-four patients (13.9%) required at least one revision.

The reason for the first failure is summarized in table III. The majority of failed AVF simply thrombosed in the early post-operative period. Thirty-five patients (24.7%) maintained patency, but their AVF were non-maturing and unable to be used for dialysis.

At the end of the study, 105 patients (42.9%) were still using their AVF. Sixty-four (26.1%) were converted to a PTFE graft. These results are summarized in Table IV. It should also be noted in Table IV that 24 patients (9.8%) underwent creation

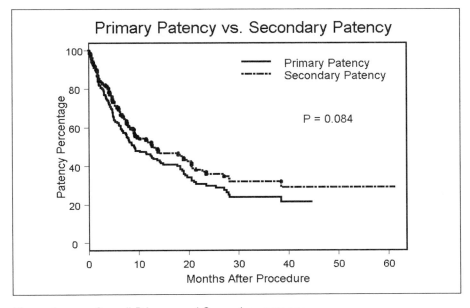

Figure 1:   Overall Primary and Secondary patency

Table III.   Etiology of First "Failure" (N=142).

Complication	Number (Percent)
Thrombosis	74 (52.1%)
Non-Maturing	35 (24.7%)
Stenosis	22 (15.5%)
Pseudoaneurysm	11 (7.8%)

Table IV.   Outcome of Arterio-Venous Fistula (N=245).

Outcome	Number (Percent)
Still Using AVF	105 (42.9%)
New AVF	24 (9.8%)
Converted to PTFE Graft	64 (26.1%)
Permacath	19 (7.8%)
Transplant	21 (8.6%)
CAPD	6 (2.5%)
Death	6 (2.5%)

of a new AVF. Twenty patients (83.3%) of this subgroup were still using their AVF. This is demonstrated in Table V.

The demographics for patients receiving "2nd chance" fistulas are summarized in table VI. As can be seen, the majority of these "2nd chance" patients had an upper AVF placed following failure in the forearm. Seven (29.2%) of these patients had prior hemodialysis compared to 27.8% of the original group. The most significant

Table V.   Outcome of "2nd Chance" AVF (N=24).

Outcome	Number (Percent)
Still Using 2nd Fistula	20 (83.3%)
New (3rd) AV Fistula	4 (16.7%)

Table VI.   Patient Demographics for 2nd AVF (N=24).

Age	49.5 (16.2%)
Gender	
Male	19 (79.2%)
Female	5 (20.8%)
Diabetic	10 (41.7%)
2nd Fistula Type	
Radiocephalic	3 (12.5%)
Brachiocephalic	21 (87.5%)
Current hemodialysis	7 (29.2%)

difference was the location of the AVF, more patients receiving a brachio-cephalic AVF than the original group.

Gender did not impact patency rates. Males did slightly better than females, but the difference did not prove to be statistically significant (P=0.870). This is illustrated in figure 2.

Although younger patients generally showed greater patency rates, no statistical significance (P=0.335) could be seen as shown in figure 3.

Fistula patency was greater for the non-diabetic past one year. However, it was not statistically significant (P=0.651) shown in figure 4.

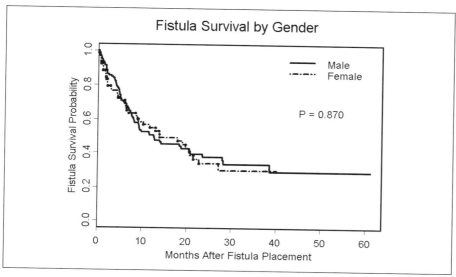

Figure 2:   Fistula survival by gender

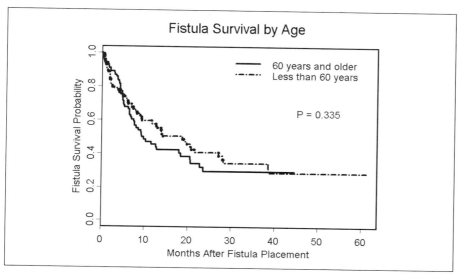

Figure 3:   Fistula survival by age

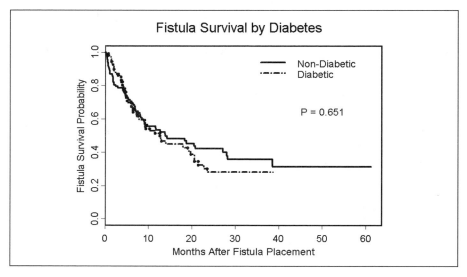

Figure 4:   Fistula survival by diabetes

Fistula type was a significant factor influencing patency rates. Upper arm (brachiocephalic) AVF had a greater survival (76.3%) in comparison with forearm (radiocephalic) AVF (59.1%) beginning at 6 months. At the end of 3 years, 35.9% of upper arm fistulas were still patent and functioning versus 23.2% for the forearm type. This can be seen in figure 5.

The most interesting finding of this study was AVF survival when looked at with respect to whether the patient was on dialysis at the time of AVF placement. Figure 6 illustrates that prior hemodialysis is a significant risk factor, P<0.001.

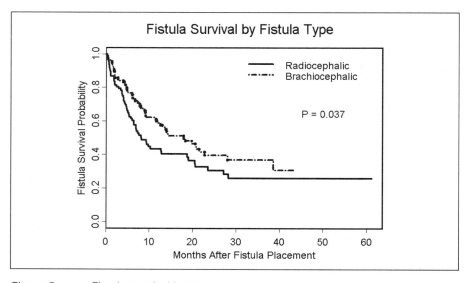

Figure 5:   Fistula survival by type

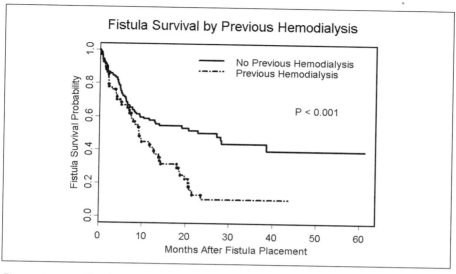

Figure 6:   Fistula survival by previous hemodialysis

Discussion

In 1997, The National Kidney Foundation Dialysis Outcomes Quality Initiative (DOQI) published guidelines proposing that AVF be constructed in at least 50% of incident patients. Additionally, another DOQI goal was to achieve a prevalence rate of 40% AVF in all hemodialysis patients.[3] Despite this, the Dialysis Outcomes and Practice Pattern Study (DOPPS) reported that AVF accounted for only 24% of all access procedures in the United States, compared with 80% in Europe.[4] There is no question that since the publication of DOQI guidelines, both access surgeons and nephrologists have made efforts to increase the number of AVF for hemodialysis patients.

While DOQI was very specific as to the success rate for PTFE grafts, there are no corresponding rates suggested for AVF. Likely the intent was to encourage the creation of AVF without being "penalized" for failure. However, this raises the question of what is an acceptable maturation rate and what can be done pre-operatively to minimize the number of unsuccessful attempts at fistula creation.

Pre-operative assessment with duplex ultrasound (US) scanning has been used as a means to identify veins not apparent by clinical examination thereby leading to increased AVF construction rates. Using routine pre-operative duplex ultrasound, Silva et al increased the rate of AVF from 14% to 63% in their practice.[5] Using a selective protocol of duplex ultrasound and venography, Patel et al increased AVF creation from 61% to 73%. Unfortunately, this aggressive approach resulted in a lower maturation rate.[6]

In this study, routine duplex US was not included in the initial pre-operative assessment. If physical examination resulted in identification of a suitable vein, an AVF was placed. Patients with a cephalic vein of 3.5 mm or larger were the best candidates for AVF placement and demonstrated optimal maturation rates. Decreased dialysis usage rates were found in patients with a cephalic vein diameter of 2.0 to 2.5 mm. Duplex US was used prior to AVF placement selectively, primarily in obese and younger patients who had potential for central venous stenosis or vein inadequacy.

Regarding primary and secondary patency, one can see a smaller difference in our series than generally seen for PTFE grafts. This is because the options for revision are more limited with an AVF. One of the biggest challenges that the access surgeon faces is turning a non-maturing or thrombosed AVF into an access that the dialysis unit can reliably use.

Even the non-maturing (non-salvageable) forearm AVF can be converted to a functioning AVF when shifted to the upper arm. When an upper arm fistula is placed in the setting of a non-maturing forearm fistula, a success rate in excess of 80% can be achieved. While this can be explained in some measure simply because of larger vessels in the upper arm, increased venous flow from the immature AVF undoubtedly plays a role by dilating the vein. Even if an AVF cannot be created, it is easier to perform a forearm PTFE loop graft into a dilated antecubital vein proximal to non-maturing AVF.

The finding that hemodialysis is such a strong risk factor for AVF survival reinforces long held suspicions. While others have shown that current hemodialysis decreases the rate of AVF creation,[7-9] this study now demonstrates that it can diminish patency rates as well. It should be noted that the majority of hemodialysis patients in this study had only a permacath in place. Few had prior AVF or graft attempts. Therefore, the differences relating to hemodialysis cannot be explained by anatomic limitations relating to prior access procedures.

Having said this, it is likely that other technical and anatomic issues do account for some of the differences in AVF patency. The dialysis patient has clearly had extensive interaction with the medical community. He has likely had multiple intravenous lines, multiple phlebotomies, and perhaps multiple central lines. He may have even spent time in an intensive care unit. At a minimum, he has been in an interventional radiology department or surgery suite.

Other factors that may play a role in the difference in AVF survival relate to hemodynamic aspects of dialysis. Certainly, hypotension would be at the top of the list. Hemoconcentration of the blood and other fluid shifts that decrease access blood flow would also compromise the new AVF at a time when outflow stenosis is not an issue.[10]

A thorough discussion of coagulation and hemodialysis access thrombosis is beyond the scope of this paper, but deserves mention. Surgeons tend to focus on the known qualitative platelet abnormalities, which lead to an increased bleeding tendency. This might seem paradoxical given the findings of this study. However, hypercoagulability can be one of the reasons for access failure. Platelet and coagulation factor activation may explain the hypercoagulable state.[11] It is possible that these factors are different, more problematic, and severe in the patient on hemodialysis than those with chronic renal failure.

In conclusion, the quest to fulfill DOQI standards has lead many centers to increase the rate of AVF formation. This well-intentioned goal has unfortunately led some groups to recognize unintended consequences and pitfalls. We believe that the best results can be achieved with a vein of at least 3.5 mm in diameter. In the event a forearm AVF fails, excellent results can be obtained with an upper arm AVF. Age, diabetes, and gender did not prove to be significant risk factors in this study. Given the significant differences in AVF survival between the two groups as noted in this study, creation of the AVF before initiation of dialysis is critical.

We thank Crystal Lott for secretarial assistance with preparation of this manuscript.

References

1. US Renal Data System 1999 annual report. Bethesda, MD: National Institutes of Health, National Institute of Diabetes and Digestive and Kidney Diseases; 1999.
2. Simmons RG, Abress L. Quality-of-life issues for end-stage disease patients. *Am J Kid Dis.* 1990; 15:201-8.
3. The Vascular Access Work Group. NKF-DOQI clinical practice guidelines for vascular access. National Kidney Foundation-Dialysis Quality Initiative. *Am J Kid Dis.* 1997; 30(suppl 3): S150-91.
4. Pisoni RL, Young EW, Dykstra DM, Greenwood RN, Hecking E, Gillespie B, et al. Vascular access use in Europe and the United States: results from the DOPPS. *Kidney Int.* 2002; 61:305-16.
5. Silva MB Jr, Hobson RW II, Pappas PJ, Jamil Z, Araki CT, Goldberg MC, et al. A strategy for increasing the use of autogenous hemodialysis access procedures: impact of perioperative noninvasive evaluation. *J Vasc Surg.* 1998; 27:302-7.
6. Patel ST, Hughes J, Mills JL. Failure of Arteriovenous fistula maturation: An unintended consequence of exceeding DOQI guidelines for hemodialysis access. *J Vasc Surg.* 2003; 38:439-45.
7. Allon M, Robbin MC. Increasing arteriovenous fistulas in hemodialysis patients: problems and solutions. *Kidney International.* 2002; 62:1109-24.
8. Astor BC, Eustace JA, Powe NR, Klog MJ, Fink NE, Coresh J. Timing of nephrologist referral and arteriovenous access use: The CHOICE study. *Am J Kid Dis.* 2001;38(3):494-501.
9. Arora P, Obrador GI, Pulhazer R, Kausz A, Meyer K, et al. Prevalence, predictors, and consequences of late nephrology referral at a tertiary care center. *J Am Soc Nephrol.* 1999; 10:1281-6.
10. Windus DW. Permanent vascular access: a nephrologists view. *Am J Kid Dis.* 1993; 21:457-71.
11. Smits J, Linden J, Blankestijn P, Rabelink T. Coagulation and hemodialysis access thrombosis. *Nephrol Dial Transplant.* (2002) 15:1755-60.

DISCUSSION

Vascular Access for Hemodialysis IX
May 6–7, 2004
Lake Buena Vista, Florida

May 6, 2004
Abstract Session II

Dr. Brian Haag
"Prior Hemodialysis as a Risk Factor for the Autogenous AV-Fistula"

Question: In regards to your comment about AV access, one thing has been mentioned and I'd like to hear some about interventional radiologists and radiologists in general is the use of the PICC line. Nothing is going to destroy an upperarm fistula more than a PICC line, which now has become very popular and residents order them all the time thinking nothing of it.

Haag: I agree and about the only thing I can say is often times in our institution PICC lines are done in probably the brachial or basilic veins so from my perspective first time around being leaning heavily on the cephalic vein I'm not as worried. But your point is well taken. PICC lines have taken over the hospitals.

Question: My question is also about PICC lines. It is almost a standing order now when the patient gets admitted along with his diet order, that they get a PICC line. I am wondering if we are burning our bridges with upperarm veins?

Haag: I think the centers that do a lot of basilic vein transpositions will have to answer to that. I do not know if Tom is still here or not but I know his group does about 39% BVTs and I think they would have to answer that. Again, great point.

Question: PICC line placements are actually contraindicated in our renal patients and there is a big note in the angio suite "do not place PICC line in patients with ESRD". It takes a while to educate the house staff and your residents and fellows when you are working with them. But you actually must keep the PICC lines out of all the veins because PICC lines damages most of the vein going up. The vascular surgeon that I was working with will tell you when she goes in to put in the fistula and she opens it up, she'll see little pieces of fiber and strands and junk inside, so you can not put these in. What do you do when you have a patient with complicated medical history and they need access? What we do is to place the mini tunnelled distant catheters or you can use a home catheter. It is an IJ catheter and Cook makes a 25 cm catheter with a little cuff and it is only six french and you get a single and double lumen. So any patient that needed long term antibiotics for six weeks or whatever reason, will get a mini IJ catheter going down because we thought that smaller was better. In fact, in some patients that had tunneled dialysis catheters we also put in these little mini tunneled catheters and we would give them access that way.

Comment: That is a good point but two years ago when we presented our results from Michigan on our basilic vein transposition and one of the findings from that study was the single most important negative predictor for success was an ipsilateral central line of any kind. So even the short cannula that you are describing might not be a good thing.

14

THE BENEFIT OF MICROSURGERY IN CHILDREN FOR CREATION OF ARTERIOVENOUS FISTULAS IN RENAL AND NON-RENAL DISEASES

Pierre BOURQUELOT*MD., Fabien RAYNAUD** MD., Nicola PIROZZI*** MD.
* Clinique Jouvenet, Angioaccess Department, 6 square Jouvenet, 75016, Paris, France, Tel 33 1 42 15 42 15, Fax 33 1 42 15 40 11, pbourquelot@magic.fr
** Clinique des Ceseaux, Clermont-Ferrand, France
*** Casa di Cura Nova Itor, Roma, Italy

Introduction

In children, the first reports on hemodialysis angioaccess[1-3] indicated a 50% immediate failure due to small size vessels, often reduced by spasm provoked by arterial dissection. The first vascular microanastomosis on 1 mm diameter vessels was described in 1960 by Jacobson and Suarez. In 2004 it is of paramount importance for every surgeon and nephrologist to recognize that microsurgery can have a dramatic benefit when applied to arteriovenous fistula (AVF) creation in children with ESRD. For long term non-ESRD therapy in children requiring repeated blood access, the microsurgical creation of an AVF is also a safe and durable alternative to peripheral venipuncture and central venous catheter (CVC).

Methods

The condition of the vein is assessed by careful preoperative clinical examination. A duplex scan is necessary if there is any doubt of size or quality and venous angiography is mandatory in cases of a previous central venous catheter. A prophylactic broad spectrum antibiotic is prescribed.

The equipment needed includes: ophthalmologic scissors, microsurgical needle holders, disposable ophthalmologic scalpel, Dumont forceps, single and double microsurgical clamps, heparinised saline, surgical microscope with two facing binoculars, and Ethilonâ 9 to 10/0 (BV 70 and BV 50) sutures.

The rule for "no-touch" microsurgical suturing is that forceps must never grasp the intima. The thinnest possible needles are used. Intraluminal saline injection is prohibited. Preventive hemostasis using a pneumatic tourniquet[4] makes extensive arterial dissection for clamping unnecessary and therefore arterial spasm induced by arterial dissection is avoided. When hemostasis is incomplete, atraumatic microclamps are placed on the artery after minimal dissection. Anticoagulation is mandatory in hypercoagulation conditions (nephrotic syndrome mainly).

Results and Discussion

In 1981[5] , we published our results for AVF microsurgery in children under 10 kg. In 1990[6] we reported 380 children receiving microsurgery for AVF. The percentage of autologous AVFs vs. grafts was 93% and creation of distal AVF was possible in 78% of the children. The immediate patency rate was 96% and the 24 month patency rate was 85% in distal radial-cephalic AVF, 72% in brachial-basilic AVF, 47% in brachial-cephalic AVF and only 5% in AV bridge-grafts. Sixty per cent of the distal fistulas were patent after 4 years (Fig.1).

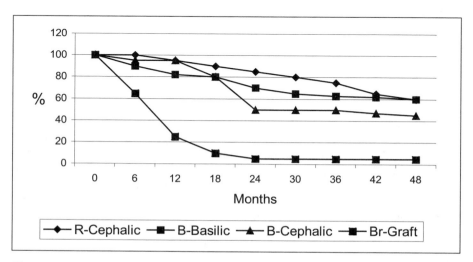

Figure 1:   AVF in ESRD children. Long-term patency.

The benefits of microsurgery for children were re-emphasised by a Canadian team[7] in 1984, by a Spanish team in 1993[8] and by an Italian team in 1998[9].

In a cross-sectional survey of the three pediatric nephrology departments in Paris on 1 February 2003 we observed that 70% of ESRD children were being hemodialyzed via an autologous fistula, 24% via a CVC, while 6% were on peritoneal dialysis. This compares favorably with the annual publication of the North American Pediatric Renal Transplant Cooperative Study in 1996[10] reporting that between January 1992 and January 1996, two-thirds of children and adolescents on dialysis were maintained on peritoneal dialysis, despite an overall peritonitis rate of 1 episode every 13 patient months, and that the majority of hemodialysis accesses were percutaneous catheters, with the subclavian vein the most common site.

In 2001 we retrospectively reviewed 69 AVFs in a young (mean age 20 years) and difficult cohort of 64 non-renal chronic disease patients requiring a permanent angioaccess for repeated transfusions, perfusions, aphereses or drug injections. The disease processes were sickle cell anemia (n=19), parenteral nutrition (n=16), mucoviscidosis (n=9), hemophilia (n=6), hypercholesterolemia (n=5), hemochromatosis (n=3), and miscellaneous conditions (n=6). Although there had been no previous venous preservation strategy, it was possible with microsurgery to create distal AVF in 68% of cases; and insertion of a graft was necessary in only 4%. Long-term patency rate was around 60% after 10 years (Fig.2).

Without microsurgery limited-quality arteriovenous fistulas are frequently observed in children. Proximal fistulas and grafts are easier to construct in children, but they have high complication rates and they will destroy proximal veins, threatening the long term survival of the patient. Lumdsen[11] reported in 1994 on 61 angioaccesses in children without microsurgery; mean age was 11 years and only 25% were simple AVF and 30% of them failed to mature. The mean functional patency was 6.2 months; 75% of the accesses were grafts, mostly in the upper arm or in the thigh, with mean patency of 10 months. Sheth[12] in 2002, reported on 52 arteriovenous angioaccesses in 13-year-old (mean-age) children. The percentage of autologous AVF was low (46%) and the percentage of primary failures (failed to mature) was high (33%). Curiously, these 2 authors demonstrated no interest in microsurgery and made no reference to any of the previous publications concerning

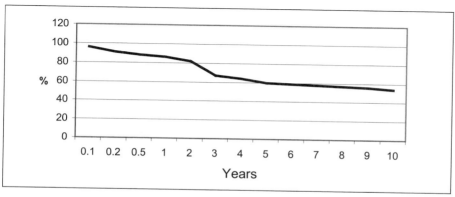

Figure 2:   AVF in non-ESRD young patients. Long-term patency.

Table 1.   Arteriovenous angioaccess in children—Major publications since 1990.

	Bourquelot France	Sanabia Spain	Lumsden USA	Bagolan Italy	Sheth USA
Year of publication	1990	1993	1994	1998	2002
Microsurgery	yes	yes	no	yes	no
Number of accesses	434	86	61	112	52
Failed to mature AVF	10%	10%	30%	5%	33%
% Grafts	7%	14%	76%	0%	54%

microsurgical creation of AVF in children. Furthermore, Sheth stated incorrectly that "the literature contains very little data regarding the success of permanent vascular access in pediatric patients".

In fact, the 3 European surgical teams who used microsurgery for angioaccess in children (Table 1) reported only 5% to 10% percentage of fistulas failing to mature and a 0 to 14% percentage of grafts versus AVFs. These results compare favorably with those of the 2 American teams not using microsurgery; 30 and 33% of their AVF failed to mature and 76% to 54% were grafts.

Conclusion

Children must have a microsurgically created distal radial to cephalic AVF created several months (3 months) before use. In children less than 10 kg, the interval should be longer. When a distal AVF is not possible, a proximal AVF is indicated, The cephalic vein is used first, then the basilic vein.

Grafts, which are still recommended by a few authors[13], must be avoided at all costs in children[14] in view of the rapidity with which they become complicated by stenosis of the venous anastomosis.

Microsurgery is mandatory for creation of arteriovenous fistulas. It is the best form of angioaccess in children treated by hemodialysis or requiring repeated access to blood in various non-renal diseases.

References

1. Sicard GA, Merrell RC, Etheredge EE, et al. Subcutaneous arteriovenous dialysis fistulas in pediatric patients. *Trans Am Soc Artif Intern Organs.* 1978;24:695-698.
2. Broyer M LC, Gagnadoux M, Cukier J, et al. "Bypass" et fistule artério-veineuse en vue de l'hémodialyse chronique chez l'enfant. *Arch Fr Pediatr.* 1973;30:145-161.
3. Gagnadoux M F, Pascal P, Bourquelot P, et al. M. L'abord vasculaire chez l'enfant traité par hémodialyse chronique. *Néphrologie.* 1978;12:935-944.

4. Bourquelot PD. Preventive haemostasis with an inflatable tourniquet for microsurgical distal arteriovenous fistulas for haemodialysis. *Microsurgery.* 1993;14(7):462-463.

5. Bourquelot P, Wolfeler L, Lamy L Microsurgery for haemodialysis distal arteriovenous fistulae in children weighing less than 10kg. *Proc Eur Dial Transplant Assoc.* 1981;18:537-541.

6. Bourquelot P, Cussenot O, Corbi P, et al. Microsurgical creation and follow-up of arteriovenous fistulae for chronic haemodialysis in children. *Pediatr Nephrol.* 1990;4(2):156-159.

7. Yazbeck S, O'Regan S. Microsurgery for Brescia-Cimino fistula construction in pediatric patients. *Nephron.* 1984;38(3):209-212.

8. Sanabia J, Polo JR, Morales MD, et al. A. Microsurgery in gaining paediatric vascular access for haemodialysis. *Microsurgery.* 1993;14(4):276-279.

9. Bagolan P, Spagnoli A, Ciprandi G, et al. A ten-year experience of Brescia-Cimino arteriovenous fistula in children: technical evolution and refinements. *J Vasc Surg.* 1998;27(4):640-644.

10. Lerner GR, Warady BA, Sullivan EK, et al. Chronic dialysis in children and adolescents. The 1996 annual report of the North American Pediatric Renal Transplant Cooperative Study. *Pediatr Nephrol.* 1999;13(5):404-417.

11. Lumsden AB, MacDonald MJ, Allen RC, et al. TF. Hemodialysis access in the pediatric patient population. *Am J Surg.* 1994;168(2):197-201.

12. Sheth RD, Brandt ML, Brewer ED, et al. Permanent hemodialysis vascular access survival in children and adolescents with end-stage renal disease. *Kidney Int.* 2002;62(5):1864-1869.

13. Brittinger WD, Walker G, Twittenhoff WD, et al. N. Vascular access for hemodialysis in children. *Pediatr Nephrol.* 1997;11(1):87-95.

14. Bourquelot P, Gagnadoux MF. Vascular access for hemodialysis in children. *Pediatr Nephrol.* 1997;11(5):659-660.

DISCUSSION

Vascular Access for Hemodialysis IX
May 6-7, 2004
Lake Buena Vista, Florida

May 6, 2004
Abstract Session II

Dr. Pierre Bourquelot
"Microsurgery in Children for Creation of Arteriovenous Fistulas in Renal and Non-Renal Diseases"

Question: Your results with the non-ESRD children were very remarkable. Do you anticoagulate those children?

Bourquelot: Never, only for children having nephrotic syndrome with a hyperco-agulable state.

Comment: So you are really saying that you think that most of the failures from autologous fistulas at the wrist are technical in nature? Do you think that it is purely a technical issue?

Bourquelot: Yes I do think it is especially true in children because some of them have never been punctured so they have nicer vessels and it is very small. So you have to have a very good technique to make the anastomosis and this is very useful to use microsurgery. Actually I use microsurgery in others and I do not have all that problem you noticed before with women. It is more difficult to do an AV fistula in women but with the microscope, there is no difference.

Question: What role has the tourniquet had in the preparation of the vein and the stripping of peri-venous tissue? What part of the microsurgery and what proportion is the lack of clamping?

Bourquelot: I think the use of a tourniquet is very important. Not only for the vein but also it avoids any dissection of the artery. You just have to open the artery, you don't have to dissect it and ligate the branches and place clamps. So it's a very respectful technique.

Comment: I just finished reporting a series of 47 children and I use the operating microscope for only three and my two year patency rate was 100%. There are major differences between our series, which highlight the difference between Americans and Europeans series. First of all , the average age of my children was 14 years and the average age of European children was five. It is absolutely remarkable. We use so much peritoneal dialysis and transplant patients in the United States. Secondly, only one third of my accesses were radiocephalic. I had a large number of upperarm basilic vein transplants and brachial cephalics and I think the major difference is that I would only construct the fistula based on vein size. For me, I did not care how old the child was, I wanted to have a minimal vein size of 2.5 millimeters and I use an operating microscope only when the radial artery was minuscule. I am dealing with a small artery and not so much the small vein because my vein was always an adequate size. Your results are just phenomenal.

Question: Can you explain why the survival of the brachial fistula is worse than radial fistula in your time table?

Bourquelot: In the long term, the distal radial artery fistula has much better results than proximal AV fistula. I have patients with a fistula constructed 25 years ago and they are still functioning. The flow is lower in distal artery AV fistula. This is probably one of the explanations for why the long-term results are much better.

15

CIMINO AND BRACHIAL-CEPHALIC FISTULA RECOMMENDATIONS FOR CONSTRUCTION, MAINTENANCE, AND TREATMENT OF COMPLICATIONS

Stephen L. Hill, M.D., F.A.C.S.
Antonio T. Donato, M.D, F.A.C.S.

Corresponding author:
Stephen L. Hill, M. D., F.A.C.S.
1125 South Jefferson Street
Roanoke, Virginia 24016
Phone-540-982-1141
Fax-540-982-5802
e-mail: stoverhill@aol.com

Introduction

Chronic renal failure is permanent in most patients and thus dialysis access can be a chronic problem with significant morbidity and mortality. It has been shown in numerous studies that a successful autogenous dialysis access offers the best chance for long term dialysis with a minimum of complications.[1,2,3,4,5] The ability to provide consistent, reliable hemodialysis access is of paramount importance and therefore a planned approach to the patient with renal failure is vital. The planning becomes particularly important if the goal is to provide an autogenous fistula since there are only a limited number of veins available and they must be protected from intravenous lines and blood drawing. There has been a resurgence of interest in the construction of autogenous dialysis access mainly due to The National Kidney Foundation Dialysis Outcomes Quality Initiative in 1997 that stated that all hemodialysis centers should strive to have fifty per cent of their patients with an autogenous access.[6] In order to achieve this goal we soon realized that there were many changes we would have to institute in the workup of patients with renal failure.

Methods

We reviewed all of the autogenous hemodialysis accesses performed in a two man surgical group over a twenty-year period. The fact that there were only two surgeons who provided all the dialysis accesses we felt provided consistency in the evaluation, work up and surgical technique. We noted the types of access and the changes that occurred through the years. All complications including infection, thrombosis, steal syndrome, and aneurysm formation were carefully tabulated. In addition, the different types of fistulae, as well as their success rate were recorded. We made note of the many changes that have occurred over the twenty-year period and made recommendations concerning certain procedures we followed in the later years to significantly increase our percentage of successful autogenous fistulae.

Results

There were a total of 366 patients who had 1,120 procedures performed to provide hemodialysis access over the twenty-year period. In this group there were 123 patients who had 128 attempts at autogenous hemodialysis access. There were an additional 21 procedures performed to preserve and maintain patency in these patients. During this same time period there were 314 prosthetic grafts placed in 213 patients, requiring a total of 516 operative procedures to achieve and maintain patency in the prosthetic group.

In this study we used only two types of autogenous fistula including the well-known Cimino fistula and transposition of the upper arm cephalic vein over the brachial artery. We have found, through the years, that these two are the best types of autogenous fistula to perform for hemodialysis access. They are simple to construct, require limited dissection, have only one anastomosis, and are superficial in location (Figure 1).

There were 52 Cimino fistulae placed in fifty patients over the twenty-year period. There were 22 (42%) that were either immediate failures or never adequately matured for successful hemodialysis. There were 30 Cimino fistulae (58%) which had long-term patency and were used for hemodialysis. Their average primary patency was 60.7 months with a cumulative average patency of 70.4 months. There were eight patients who died during the study with a functioning fistula and their average patency at the time of their death was 20.5 months. There were 15 patients with an intact Cimino fistula at the end of the study and their average patency was 108.3 months. Therefore in this study, 82% of the patients with a Cimino fistula had

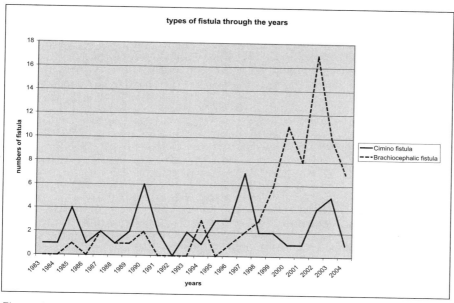

Figure 1:

a functioning fistula at the time of their death or the end of the study. The remaining 18% were changed over to a brachiocephalic fistula, prosthetic graft, tunneled dialysis catheter, or switched to peritoneal dialysis. (See Table 1)

In assessing the overall success of Cimino fistulae, the statistics reveal that 42% (22/52) of all attempts were patent at 12 months and 33% (17/52) were patent at 24 months. If it is analyzed further to include only those fistulae which were successful then the numbers are even better where 82% (22/28) were functioning at 12 months and 60.7% (17/28) were still patent and functioning at 24 months.

There were 12 fistulae that required revision and/or thrombectomy to maintain and prolong patency. The operative procedure was successful in six cases (50%) prolonging the life of the fistula an average of 30.3 months (range 14 – 240 months). In virtually all of these cases a vein patch angioplasty was used to repair a stenosis, in addition to the thrombectomy if there was a thrombosis. Some of the fistulae were too deep for adequate dialysis and the arterialized vein had to be raised to a more superficial location.

Other complications associated with autogenous fistulae are the steal syndrome and infection. There was one patient who experienced a steal syndrome with a Cimino fistula (3.6%) and there were no infections found in patients with a Cimino fistula in this study.

In reviewing the patients with a brachiocephalic fistula there were a total of 73 patients who had attempts at 76 fistulae. There were 17 failures (22%) and there were 59 brachiocephalic fistulae (78%) that were used for dialysis. The average primary patency for brachiocephalic fistula was 17.3 months with an average cumulative patency of 21 months. There were 16 (22%) patients who died during the study with a functioning brachiocephalic fistula and their average patency at the time of

Table 1.

	CIMINO FISTULA	BRACHIALCEPHALIC FISTULA
PATIENTS	50	73
ATTEMPTED FISTULA	52	76
SUCCESS	30 (58%)	59 (78%)
FAILURE	22 (42%)	17 (22%)
TRANSPLANT	1	2
LONG TERM OCCLUSIONS	6	9
DEATH	8	16
END OF STUDY	15	32
PRIMARY PATENCY (MONTHS)	60.7	17.3
CUMULATIVE PATENCY (MONTHS)	70.4	21
REVISONS	12	9
	6 SUCCESSFUL	6 SUCCESSFUL
	50%	66%
ADDED MONTHS	30.3	24.2
RANGE (MONTHS)	14-240	8-118

their death was 16.3 months. There were 32 (44%) patients at the end of the study with a functioning brachiocephalic fistula and their average patency at the end of the study was 23.3 months. Two patients with functioning brachiocephalic fistulae received a transplant and their average patency at the time of the transplant was 26 months. Therefore in this study a total of 50 patients (68%) had a functioning brachiocephalic fistula at the time of their death, transplant, or the end of the study. In the functioning brachiocephalic fistulae 36 fistulae (47%) were patent after 12 months and 24 fistulae (32%) were patent after 24 months.

There were nine brachiocephalic fistulas which required revision/repair to maintain patency. The operative procedure was successful in six cases (66%) prolonging the life of the fistula an average of 24.2 months (range 8 – 118 months).Here , as in the Cimino fistula group, some of the brachiocephalic fistulae were too deep for adequate dialysis and the fistula had to be raised to a more superficial location.

In the group of patients who received brachiocephalic fistulae there were five infections (6.5%), two of which were treated and the graft was salvaged. The steal syndrome occurred in two patients with brachiocephalic fistula and one fistula was able to be salvaged by revising the anastomosis. In reviewing the 3 patients (3.5%) who manifested signs and symptoms of the steal syndrome all were insulin dependent diabetics and two out of the three were female.

Many of the brachiocephalic fistulae developed aneurysmal dilatation from repetitive sticks in the same location. In contradistinction to prosthetic grafts with aneurysmal dilatation which often become infected or always require operative replacement, the vast majority of autogenous fistulae continue to function.[7, 8] In only two patients (2.3%) did aneurysm formation preclude dialysis and necessitate operative intervention. In one brachiocephalic fistula we were able to repair the problem while the other one had aneurysmal dilatation due to infection and had to be ligated.

Beginning in 1996, the percentage of autogenous fistulae for dialysis access began to significantly increase (Figure 2). In dividing this study into three periods (1983-1990; 1991-1997; 1998-2004) there were significant changes and increases in the number of autogenous fistula through the periods. In the first period (1983-1990) the percentage of autogenous dialysis access was only 15.6% of the total accesses performed for hemodialysis access. In the second period (1991-1998) it slightly increased to 19%; in the final period the percentage of autogenous accesses as a function of the total number of hemodialysis access increased significantly to 55%. (Figure 3)

Discussion

The use of an autogenous fistula for hemodialysis access has long been advocated as the best long-term conduit for dialysis.[1, 2] However, as medical technology progressed, there was an extended period where new prosthetic grafts were challenging this long held belief. This was partially due to the fact that many individuals did not have a usable cephalic vein at the wrist by the time they had come to dialysis. This,

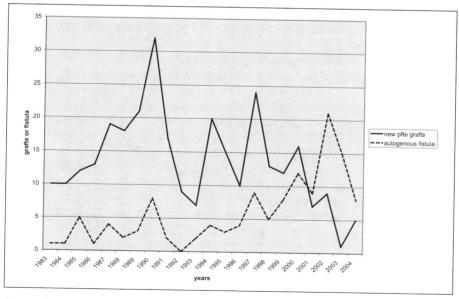

Figure 2:

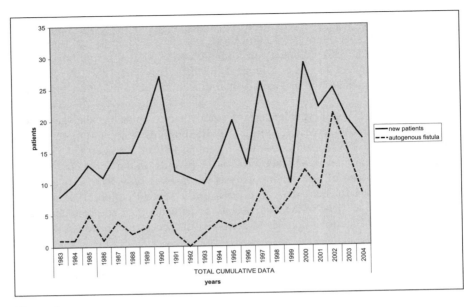

Figure 3:

in conjunction with the development of ePFTE and other prosthetic grafts which claimed to have as good a patency rate as vein, caused a trend in many areas of the country to where a prosthetic graft was used almost exclusively for dialysis access.[9, 10, 11] It was easy, could be used for dialysis almost immediately, and did not require a six to eight week maturation period. The construction of an autogenous fistula was technically more demanding and another means for dialysis would have to be available while the fistula matured, since most patients required immediate and continuing dialysis.

There were several developments that caused a change in this trend. The vascular laboratory which had became prominent in the early 1980's expanded its capabilities to the field of hemodialysis access; this then afforded surgeons the ability to evaluate and use veins that heretofore had not been available.[12, 13, 14] The upper arm cephalic vein is a perfect example; it is almost as superficial in the upper arm as down at the wrist and is often spared the multiple needle sticks and intravenous lines seen in the cephalic vein at the wrist. In addition, the vascular laboratory can be used to evaluate other veins in the arm such as the basilic vein for a possible basilic vein transposition or the deep veins in the upper arm in preparation for use with a prosthetic graft for dialysis. It is also extremely helpful in defining the arterial anatomy of the arm prior to placement of a fistula or dialysis graft. In some individuals there is a high bifurcation of the brachial artery or significant arterial disease in a radial or brachial artery which might prevent the construction of a functioning dialysis access. We have also begun to use the vascular laboratory to evaluate the internal jugular veins and subclavian veins in preparation for a tunneled dialysis catheter. Many of the patients requiring dialysis have had other major disease processes which may have required central lines and thus there may be occlusions or stenoses which could preclude cannulation and/or effective hemodialysis.[15] In addition, since many of our patients go directly to dialysis after placement of the tunneled dialysis catheters, the internal jugular veins are marked by the vascular laboratory in an effort to prevent errant sticks, hematoma, or arterial puncture.

The development of tunneled dialysis catheters that could be used for months has also encouraged the trend toward more autogenous fistula construction. Now a patient can be referred for immediate dialysis and a tunneled catheter is placed thus allowing time for construction and maturation of a fistula. Other institutions have used the tunneled dialysis catheters in a similar fashion to increase their rate of autogenous fistula.[13] We have found, however, this, too, is not without significant risks. There are significant complications which can occur with these catheters such as occlusion of the central veins giving rise to extensive edema and morbidity. If this occurs in a patient who has a functioning graft/fistula in the affected extremity the edema can be massive and the dialysis access will be put at risk for thrombosis due to low flows and outflow obstruction.

The third change which brought emphasis back to the use of autogenous fistulae for hemodialysis access was the National Kidney Foundation Dialysis Outcomes Quality Initiative in 1997. They made a list of recommendations and guidelines for dialysis access which they felt should be strived for in all hemodialysis centers to lower costs and improve care. One of their main tenets was that an attempt should be made in most patients to place an autogenous fistula such that over time at least 40% of all renal failure patients would have an autogenous fistula.[6] This was a dramatic departure from what was occurring in many major centers across the nation where most forms of hemodialysis access was provided by a prosthetic graft.[9, 10, 11]

One other factor that influenced the change in emphasis towards the formation of an autogenous fistula is one that is affecting all of medicine and that is patients are living longer.[16, 17] While the chronic renal failure population clearly does not live as long as the rest of the population, they are living longer than in years past. This can be a major problem with dialysis access. The prosthetic grafts clearly, and undeniably in most patients, have a significantly shorter patency rate and this taken in conjunction with a longer life expectancy can lead to major problems with vascular access after a few years and several failed accesses.

We have noticed all these changes and incorporated them into our practice. It is the use of the vascular laboratory in conjunction with the effective tunneled dialysis catheters that have significantly increased our autogenous fistula construction through the years.

In light of the fact that many patients do not have an adequate cephalic vein at the wrist, the next best source for an autogenous fistula appeared to be the cephalic vein in the upper arm.[1] It was here that the vascular laboratory assisted in finding and evaluating these veins and thus increasing our ability to provide an autogenous hemodialysis access to many patients. Several authors have shown excellent patency rates and longevity in brachiocephalic fistulae.[8, 13] The Cimino and the brachiocephalic fistulae appear to be the easiest to construct and offered the best hope of conforming to the National Kidney Foundation Dialysis Outcomes Quality Initiative Guidelines.

Unfortunately, the autogenous fistula is not a panacea. It comes with its own group of problems and complications that must be addressed in order to have good patency rates and a minimum of complications.

The cephalic vein in the upper arm must be at least 2.0 mm in size and extend almost down to the antecubital space to be adequate for transposition over to the brachial artery. The surgery is technically more demanding and the orientation of the vein in the tunnel needs to be exact and superficial. It often cannot be used for at least six to eight weeks and then the first several weeks are difficult due to hematoma and extravasation. In the elderly (greater than sixty years old) the veins are often very thin walled and bleed excessively after the first several treatments. Other authors have noticed a similar problem in older patients with autogenous accesses.[18, 19] We have made it a policy to leave the tunneled dialysis catheter in place for at least one month after the autogenous fistula has been used to allow for these mishaps.

As is already known, the cephalic vein at the wrist is often not available to the surgeons for vascular access due to intravenous lines and needle sticks. In many cases, even when it is patent it is unusable due to a thrombus further up the cephalic vein. Oftentimes when patent, at surgery it is found to be sclerotic or too thin walled and cannot or will not mature with time. In some cases the radial artery is the culprit, it is too small, or in diabetics, is calcified and thus cannot vasodilate and increase the flow to provide adequate arterial inflow for a dialysis fistula. It is for all of the above reasons that the success rate for a Cimeno fistula hovers around fifty percent, at best.[1, 20, 21]

Despite all of these drawbacks the autogenous fistula still offers the best patency rates, longevity, and least complications.[20, 22, 23] Those patients who require chronic hemodialysis oftentimes have a multitude of other problems and complications which are costly and life threatening; in addition, their basic disease process makes them prone to poor healing, infectious complications, and peripheral vascular disease. The successful construction of an autogenous fistula affords them one less major morbidity with which to deal.

Bibliography

1. Hakaim AG, Nalbandian M, Scott T. Superior maturation and patency of primary brachiocephalic and transposed basilic vein transposition arteriovenous fistulae in patients with diabetes. *J Vasc Surg.* 1998;27: 154-7.
2. Ad Hoc Committee on Reporting Standards, Society for Vascular Surgery/North American Chapter, International Society for Cardiovascular Surgery. Suggested standards for reports dealing with lower extremity ischemia. *J Vasc Surg.* 1986;4:80-94.
3. United States Renal Data System. URDS 1995 annual data report. The National Institutes of Health, National Institue of diabetes and Digestive and Kidney Diseases. *Am J Kidney Dis.* 1998;32 (suppl 1): S2-162.
4. Brotman DN, Fandos L,Faust GR, et al. Hemodialysis graft salvage. *J Am Coll Surg.* 1994; 178: 431-4.
5. Bitar G, Yang S, Badosa F. Ballon versus patch angioplasty as an adjuvant treatment to surgical thrombectomy of hemodialysis grafts. *Am J. Surg.* 1997; 174: 140-2.
6. National Kidney Foundation. K/DOKI Clinical Practice Guidelines for Vascular Access 2000. *Am J Kidney Dis.* 2001; 37 (supp 1): s137-8
7. Kherlakian GM, Roedersheimer LR, Arbaugh,JJ. Comparison of autogenous fistula for hemodialysis *Amer J Surg.* 1986;152: 238-240.

8. Nazzal MMS, Neglen P, Naseem J., et al. The Brachiocephalic fistula : a successful secondary vascular access procedure.*VASA.* 1990; 19:326-329.

9. United States Renal Data System. URDS 1999 Annual Data Report. The National Institutes of Health, National Institute of Diabetes and Digestive and Kidney Diseases. *Am J Kidney Dis.* 1999;34; 59-19

10. United States Renal Data System.URDS 1995 annual data report. The National Institutes of Health,National Institue of Diabetes and Digestive and Kidney Diseases. *Am J Kidney Dis.* 1995; 26: S140-56.

11. Chertow GM. Grafts vs fistulas for hemodialysis patients. Equal access for all? *JAMA.* 1996;276:1343-1344.

12. Malovrh M. Approach to patients with end stage renal disease who need an arteriovenous fistula. *Nephrol Dial Transplant.* 2003;18 (Suppl 5)v 50-52

13. Huber TS, Seeger J. Approach to patients with "complex" hemodialysis access problems. *Seminars in Dialysis.* 2003;16: 22-29.

14. Silva MB Jr. Hobson RW, Pappas PJ, et al. A strategy for increasing use of autogenous hemodialysis access procedures; impact of preoperative non-invasive evaluation. *J Vasc Surg.* 1998; 27:302-307

15. Surratt RS, Picus D, Hicks ME. The importance of preoperative evaluation of the subclavian vein in dialysis access planning. *AJR Am J Roentgenol* 1991 ; 156: 623-625.

16. Rettig RA. The social contract and treatment of permanent kidney failure *JAMA.* 1996;275 :1123-112

17. McClellan WM, Flanders DA, Gutman RA. Variable mortality rates among dialysis treatment centers. *Ann Intern Med* 1992; 117: 332-336.

18. Staramos DN, Lazarides MK, Tzilalis VD, et al. Patency of autologous and prosthetic arteriovenous fistulas in elder patients. *Eur J Surg.* 2000; 166: 777-781.

19. Shina MJ, Neumayer MN, Healy DA, et al. Influence of age on venous physiologic parameters. *J Vasc Surg.* 1993; 18: 749-752.

20. Konner K. Vascular Access in the 21st Century. *J Nephrol.* 2002; 15 (suppl 5) : S28-S32.

21. Murphy GJ. Nicholson, ML. Autogenous elbow fistulas: The effect of diabetes mellitus on maturation, patency and complication rates. *Eur J Vasc Surg.* 2002; 23: 452-457.

22. Ascher E, Gade P, Hingorani A, et al. Changes in the practice of angioaccess surgery: Impact of dialysis outcome and quality initiative recommendations. *J Vasc Surg.* 2000;31:84-92

23. Golledge J, Smith CJ, Emery J, et al. Outcome of primary radiocephalic fistula for haemodialysis. *Br J Surg.* 1998;86:211-216

DISCUSSION

Vascular Access for Hemodialysis IX
May 6-7, 2004
Lake Buena Vista, Florida

May 7, 2004
Abstract Session III

Dr. Stephen Hill
"Cimino and Brachial-Cephalic Fistulae – Recommendations for Construction, Maintenance, and Treatment of Complications"

Question: Could you tell me what the primary unassisted patency of the Brescia-Cimino fistula was in your hands?

Hill: The primary patency in our hands was about 65% and as I said that usually lasted for a year or two. Then we had to treat stenosis, sometime with a vein patch angioplasty.

Question: I often found that the veins in the upperarm are better than the veins in the forearm. My problem has been that when I do my anastomosis there is only a very short segment of vein that is superficial enough to be used for dialysis in the upperarm. I was wondering if anyone does a procedure where you can do a side to side anastomosis, pass the valve cutter down into the forearm to try to get your retrograde flow for your fistula so maybe more of the superficial veins in the forearm can be used for dialysis access instead?
I am not sure if it has been done or not but for several patients I thought that would be nice if I could get the flow to go the opposite direction.

Comment: I have not done that. The way I have dealt with it was to elevate a segment of the vein by making a fairly long incision along the side of the cephalic vein and creating a tunnel. Sometimes you can try to do it through one incision but by making a tunnel you have raised that portion of the cephalic vein so it is available and further up the arm. So you have about a three to four inch area. In some patients, particularly the people who are slightly obese, you sometimes have to go back and raise that. I have had that happen on only two occasions.

Comment: I have done it to and I think it is a good idea to do. Actually I am surprised about the way the blood figures out how to get back to the heart. You cannot necessarily predict that. I don't think there is anything wrong with that.

Hill: The advantage of doing that is that I make a tunnel, which then raises that vein and it is higher up for you. Then you use that tunnel that you have and it gives you at least a two or three inch superficial vein. So that is why I do it that way through one incision. But then, often times it is sometimes deeper and harder for them to cannulate.

16

CLINICAL EVALUATION COMPARED WITH TRANSONIC MEASUREMENTS FOR SURVEILLANCE OF HEMODIALYSIS ACCESS

Earl Schuman, M.D.
Patti Heinl, RN
Carolyn Barkley, RN
1130 NW 22nd St.
Portland, Or 97210
Office number
Fax number
schumane@earthlink.net

Assessment of hemodialysis access was historically done by the dialysis staff examining the graft or fistula and possibly measuring venous and arterial pressures. These efforts were not well organized and did not seem to impact the outcome of the access. Over the last 15 years, more organized attempts were made at evaluation with a focus to prevent access thrombosis.[1,2,3] These included specific measurements of venous resistance under controlled circumstances.[4,5] This progressed to flow measurements[6,7] and use of ultrasound[2,8,9,10] for screening purposes. All of these evaluations were non-invasive. Transonic flow assessment provides quantitative data and is the most common mode used to evaluate access. Final assessment of the access was by angiography, which also allowed for simultaneous treatment. But some feel that many of these newer assessments are inaccurate,[11,12] of questionable value,[13] and costly.

To see if there was an alternative to these newer surveillance techniques, we undertook a prospective cohort study to determine if an organized clinical assessment could provide an outcome similar to transonic measurements. An evaluation tool was developed with input and cooperation from the dialysis staff.

Methods

The group A cohort were patients from a dialysis unit that performed bimonthly transonic assessments by one trained nurse. This individual had 2 years experience with Transonics before the initiation of this study. The group B cohort was a unit in a separate dialysis system that had been trialing ultrasound assessments on a quarterly basis and was willing to undertake clinical evaluation based on the tool developed. There were 100 patients in each cohort at the beginning of the study.

All patients were enrolled in September 2002 and followed for 1 year or until an end point was reached. End points included access abandonment, death, transplant or lost to follow-up. Data was entered concurrently on data entry sheets and later entered into an Excel spreadsheet. Source documents were used by the entering dialysis unit and applicable data transmitted to the surgeon's office by a consult form (Fig 1). Both units followed urea reduction ratios (URR) and kinetic modeling (Kt/V) in addition to the evaluations under investigation. No other surveillance studies were utilized in this population for the duration of the study.

The clinical assessment tool was utilized by the dialysis staff for each hemodialysis treatment (Fig. 2). This tool and the consult form were developed by the nurse coordinators with input from dialysis and office staff. At each session the patient's access was evaluated and the data entered on the form. The graft or fistula was visually assessed for signs of infection, pseudoaneurysms, ecchymosis, bleeding or changes in overall access appearance. The staff then listened to the access at 2-3 locations (arterial anastomosis, mid-access and venous anastomosis). They listen for a change in the bruit, pulse rate or a high pitched sound that is new for that access. Finally, the access is palpated to check for new aneurysmal formations, quality of the thrill or pulse and topography of the graft or fistula (dips and curves). If changes in the examination persist for 3 dialysis treatments, the patient is referred to the surgeon's office. Determination is then made to obtain an angiogram, surgically revise, or observe further.

Transonic assessments were done every 2 months. Data was transmitted to the surgeon's office and patients with flows less than 600cc/min. were evaluated by angiography. For either cohort a decreasing URR or Kt/V would prompt an angiogram.

Outcome measures included primary patency (from enrollment to access thrombosis), total primary patency (from access creation to thrombosis), secondary patency (from enrollment to access abandonment or end of study) , total secondary patency (access creation to abandonment or end of study), number of angiograms, thrombectomies, revisions and total procedures per access (calculated from the start of study to completion or an end point).

Results

There were 176 patients available for evaluation, 90 in the Transonic group and 86 in the clinical evaluation cohort. The average age was 62 years (Transonic-58 and

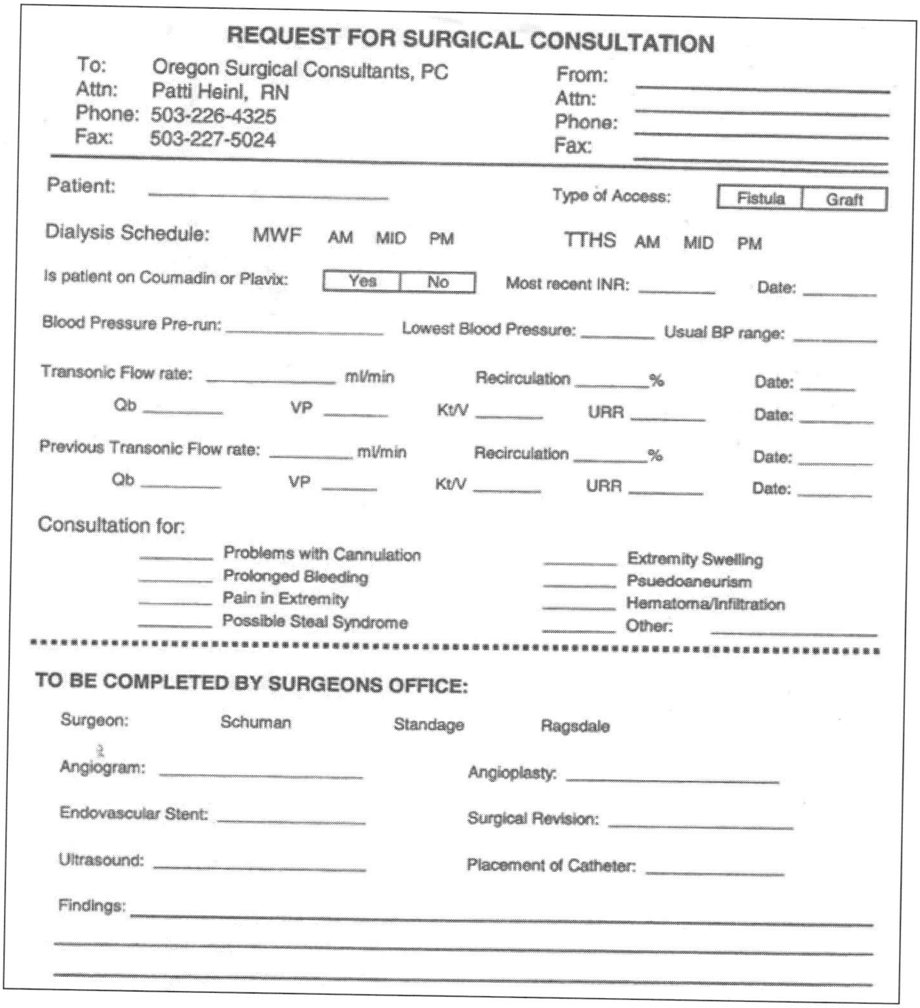

REQUEST FOR SURGICAL CONSULTATION

To: Oregon Surgical Consultants, PC
Attn: Patti Heinl, RN
Phone: 503-226-4325
Fax: 503-227-5024

From: ______
Attn: ______
Phone: ______
Fax: ______

Patient: ______ Type of Access: Fistula | Graft

Dialysis Schedule: MWF AM MID PM TTHS AM MID PM

Is patient on Coumadin or Plavix: Yes | No Most recent INR: ______ Date: ______

Blood Pressure Pre-run: ______ Lowest Blood Pressure: ______ Usual BP range: ______

Transonic Flow rate: ______ ml/min Recirculation ______% Date: ______
Qb ______ VP ______ Kt/V ______ URR ______ Date: ______

Previous Transonic Flow rate: ______ ml/min Recirculation ______% Date: ______
Qb ______ VP ______ Kt/V ______ URR ______ Date: ______

Consultation for:

______ Problems with Cannulation
______ Prolonged Bleeding
______ Pain in Extremity
______ Possible Steal Syndrome
______ Extremity Swelling
______ Psuedoaneurism
______ Hematoma/Infiltration
______ Other: ______

TO BE COMPLETED BY SURGEONS OFFICE:

Surgeon: Schuman Standage Ragsdale

Angiogram: ______ Angioplasty: ______

Endovascular Stent: ______ Surgical Revision: ______

Ultrasound: ______ Placement of Catheter: ______

Findings: ______

Figure 1: Consult form.

clinical –65). Diabetes was the cause of renal failure in 37% of the Transonic patients and 50% of the clinical patients. The access was a fistula in 111 patients and grafts in 65 patients. There was a similar incidence of fistula use in both cohorts with 61% in Transonics group and 65% in the clinical group. The age of the access prior to enrollment was slightly longer in the clinical group (878 days vs. 813 days). Of the 30 patients lost to the study before completion, 23 died, 3 were transplanted, 2 had their access abandoned and 2 were lost to follow-up.

Primary patency averaged 346 days in the clinical group and 349 days in the Transonics cohort. This patency was similar in the graft patients (287 days transonics and 288 days for clinical group) with a small difference in the fistula group (390 days in clinical group and 416 in the transonic group).

Average number of procedures to maintain patency was 1.56 per access in the clinical group and 2.09 in the Transonics group. This difference was significant (p=.014). The remainder of the data is shown in Table 1.

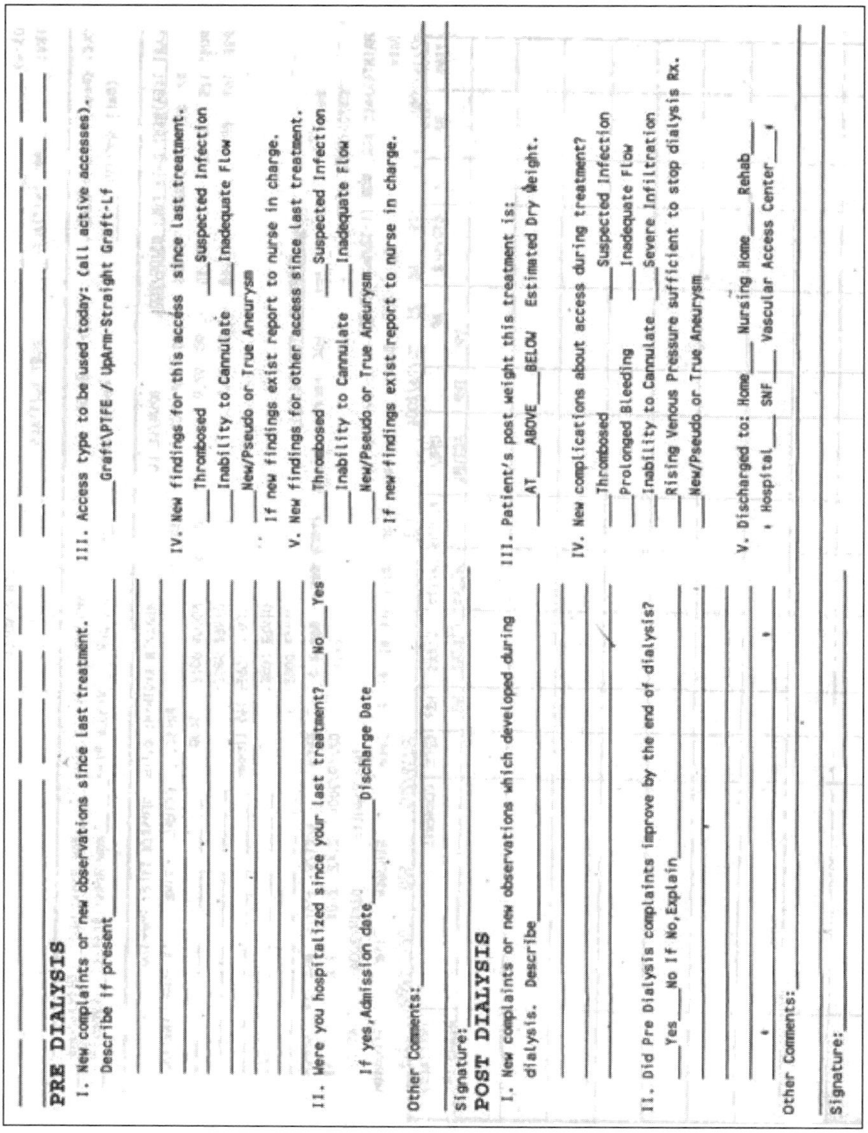

PRE DIALYSIS

I. New complaints or new observations since last treatment.
Describe if present____________________

II. Were you hospitalized since your last treatment?___No___Yes

If yes,Admission date__________Discharge Date__________

III. Access type to be used today: (all active accesses).
____Graft\PTFE / UpArm-Straight Graft-Lf

IV. New findings for this access since last treatment.
___Thrombosed ___Suspected Infection
___Inability to Cannulate ___Inadequate Flow
___New/Pseudo or True Aneurysm
If new findings exist report to nurse in charge.

V. New findings for other access since last treatment.
___Thrombosed ___Suspected Infection
___Inability to Cannulate ___Inadequate Flow
___New/Pseudo or True Aneurysm
If new findings exist report to nurse in charge.

Other Comments:____________________

Signature:____________________

POST DIALYSIS

I. New complaints or new observations which developed during dialysis. Describe____________________

II. Did Pre Dialysis complaints improve by the end of dialysis?
___Yes___No If No,Explain____________________

III. Patient's post weight this treatment is:
___AT___ABOVE___BELOW Estimated Dry Weight.

IV. New complications about access during treatment?
___Thrombosed ___Suspected Infection
___Prolonged Bleeding ___Inadequate Flow
___Inability to Cannulate ___Severe Infiltration
___Rising Venous Pressure sufficient to stop dialysis Rx.
___New/Pseudo or True Aneurysm

V. Discharged to: Home___ Nursing Home___ Rehab___
Hospital___ SNF___ Vascular Access Center___

Other Comments:____________________

Signature:____________________

Figure 2: Data collection tool.

Table 1.

	Transonic	Clinical
Primary patency	365 days	354 days
Total primary patency	1162 days	1199 days
Total secondary patency	1197 days	1270 days
Total procedures	2/ patient	1.56/ patient
Average thrombectomy	.38/ patient	.317/ patient

Discussion

About fifteen years ago many investigators proposed that an organized surveillance program for hemodialysis access could improve longevity of the access and decrease the number of thrombectomies needed to keep the access functional. Previous surveillance was sporadic and was limited to watching the venous and arterial resistance on the dialysis machine, looking for abnormalities in the physical appearance of the access, or obvious signs of recirculation. Newer methods were developed to assess access function, including Doppler dilution flow measurement, color flow ultrasound, static and dynamic pressure ratios and determinations of dialysis adequacy as a surrogate of access function. The Transonic flow measurement has become the most widely used method and is readily available. Although it is recommended that these measurements be taken monthly,[6,14] this frequency is difficult to attain in the current setting as this study is not reimbursed for the majority of patients. Also, some have questioned the accuracy of these measurements and their high variability from one Transonic session to the next[15]. Still others have noted that many grafts clot despite active surveillance programs[13,14]. Clearly, the ideal approach is yet to be found.

A definite benefit demonstrated by surveillance studies is that an organized program is superior to a sporadic one, as in the past. We decided to study whether an organized clinical assessment program could detect abnormalities as well as an organized Transonic program. Although no formal cost analysis was done, we do know that the training, equipment costs and time to perform assessment were all greater with the Transonic evaluation. The assessment form (fig.2) both directed the dialysis personnel in their exam and simplified the recording of the exam, saving time and money. Although most clinical assessments were completed in 1-3 minutes, there is a learning curve and initial exams could take a little longer. Cooperation and collaboration with dialysis personnel are critical to the success of a clinical program.

The similarity in patency rates between the two arms may have a variety of factors involved. Although the Transonic program has been well validated for access surveillance, the clinical evaluation of the access many times a week gives an excellent surveillance overview of that access to the dialysis personnel. Also, a downward trend in the parameters followed can signal a significant stenosis which can then be treated. This is validated by the significantly lower procedure rate and lower thrombectomy rate in the clinical group.

One should recognize a note of caution. The quality and dedication of those doing the assessment may vary from one dialysis unit to the next, and our study compared only 2 units. These data may not transfer to other dialysis units. It requires the efforts of all involved, including physicians, dialysis personnel and patients, to make this approach successful.

These intermediate results suggest that an organized program of clinical surveillance can be as successful as transonics measurements in avoiding thrombosis and maintaining adequate patency rates for dialysis grafts and fistulas. There may be an advantage in clinical assessment reducing the total number of procedures done and reducing costs. Further evaluations will be needed for a definitive statement on the validity of a clinical assessment program as the primary surveillance mode for dialysis access.

Bibliography

1. Safa AA, Valji K, Roberts AC, et al. Detection and treatment of dysfunctional hemodialysis access grafts: effect of a surveillance program on graft patency and the incidence of thrombosis. *Radiology.* 1996; 199:653-657.
2. Sands JJ, Ferrell LM, Perry MA. The role of color flow Doppler ultrasound in dialysis access. *Semin Nephrol.* 2002; 22:195-201.
3. Gallego Beuter JJ, Hernandez Lezana A, Herrero Calvo J, et al. Early detection and treatment of hemodialysis access dysfunction. *Cardiovasc Intervent Radiol.* 2000; 23:40-46.
4. Besarab A, Lubkowski T, Frinak S, et al. Detecting vascular access dysfunction. *Asaio J.* 1997; 43:M539-543.
5. Frinak S, Zasuwa G, Dunfee T, et al. Dynamic venous access pressure ratio test for hemodialysis access monitoring. *Am J Kidney Dis.* 2002; 40:760-768.
6. Krivitski NM, Gantela S. Access flow measurement as a predictor of hemodialysis graft thrombosis: making clinical decisions. *Semin Dial.* 2001; 14:181-185.
7. May RE, Himmelfarb J, Yenicesu M, et al. Predictive measures of vascular access thrombosis: a prospective study. *Kidney Int.* 1997; 52:1656-1662.
8. Robbin ML, Oser RF, Allon M, et al. Hemodialysis access graft stenosis: US detection. *Radiology.* 1998; 208:655-661.
9. Dumars MC, Thompson WE, Bluth EI, et al. Management of suspected hemodialysis graft dysfunction: usefulness of diagnostic US. *Radiology.* 2002; 222:103-107.
10. DeVita MV, Ky AJ, Fried KO, et al. Assessment of sonographic venous peak systolic velocity in detecting hemodialysis arteriovenous graft stenosis. *Am J Kidney Dis.* 2000; 36:797-803.
11. Agharazii M, Clouatre Y, Nolin L, et al. Variation of intra-access flow early and late into hemodialysis. *Asaio J.* 2000; 46:452-455.
12. Daugirdas JT, Schneditz D, Leehey DJ. Effect of access recirculation on the modeled urea distribution volume. *Am J Kidney Dis.* 1996; 27:512-518.
13. Work J. Does vascular access monitoring work? *Adv Ren Replace Ther* 2002; 9:85-90
14. Arbabzadeh M, Mepani B, Murray BM. Why do grafts clot despite access blood flow surveillance? *Cardiovasc Intervent Radiol.* 2002; 25:501-505.
15. Wang E, Schneditz D, Levin NW. Predictive value of access blood flow and stenosis in detection of graft failure. *Clin Nephrol.* 2000; 54:393-399.

DISCUSSION

Vascular Access for Hemodialysis IX
May 6-7, 2004
Lake Buena Vista, Florida

May 6, 2004
Abstract Session II

Dr. Earl Schuman
"Clinical Evaluation Compared with Transonic Measurements for Surveillance of Hemodialysis Access"

Question: Are you planning to or have you already separated the graft patients from the fistula patients?

Schuman: Yes, they have been separated and you can see the majority 60-65% were native fistulas. There was similar outcomes in both groups, with the grafts there were no significant difference in any category.

Question: I question the methodology. You can't be half pregnant. If you use surveillance then you use it first monthly and second, with two thresholds. As soon as you use only one threshold to doing by monthly you decrease two or three times the power of surveillance. It is very clear on thrombotic events. Thirty eight percent from both events per patient per year is two times more than it should be if you look at different publications. You should use surveillance as a tool like a DOQI guideline. If you kind of do half of a surveillance, then you don't know what it could be. If you do four times surveillance, decrease thrombosis rate to levels that you usually see in the literature, and then compare. This is a major problem.

Schuman: We heard this morning, though, is that the most common may not be the right way, but one of the most common ways of using this is bimonthly. The common use is not necessarily the right way.

Comment: But you use the major threshold because you may have just missed half of the patients and decreased the success. You have 38 per patient per year thrombotic event. If you look at the literature, it is much less common with people who use normal document guidelines.

Question: What was this graft inflow based on? Large artery like the brachial mostly or radial artery? The reason for that is the brachial artery based grafts tend to have high flows and in the presence of high flows, the clinical picture may not be very different from Transonics. But if you have vessels based on a low flow system, there is probably a difference between accurate flow measurements and clinical exam.

Schuman: If I understand your question correctly, the grafts average 900-1000 ccs of flow. Off hand I cannot tell you what the fistulas were averaging. Most of the grafts were brachial based.

Question/Comment: Brachial artery based systems are generally high. Usually close to a liter. In that situation clinical findings may be okay. With lower flows, which one sees in radial artery based access graft or a fistula, their flows are within 600-800 range. In those situations, clinical exam can be sometime misleading.

Schuman: I appreciate that and the majority of these, both grafts and fistulas, were brachial based. But I will look at that more closely.

17

PROSPECTIVE, NON-RANDOMIZED, MULTICENTER EVALUATION OF THE MESENTERIC VEIN BIOPROSTHETIC GRAFT FOR HEMODIALYSIS ACCESS IN PATIENTS WITH PRIOR FAILED PROSTHETIC GRAFTS

Howard E. Katzman, MD[1]; Marc H. Glickman, MD[2];
A. Frederick Schild, MD[3]; Roy M. Fujitani, MD[4];
Jeffrey H. Lawson, MD, PhD[5]

Institutions:
Cedars Medical Center, Miami, Florida
Vascular & Transplant Specialists, Eastern Virginia Medical School, Norfolk, Virginia.
University of Miami School of Medicine, Miami, Florida
University of California Irvine Medical Center, Irvine, California
Duke University Medical School, Durham, North Carolina

Contact Information for All Authors:
Howard E. Katzman, MD
Surgical Group of Miami
1321 N.W. 14th St., Suite #306
Miami, FL 33125
Phone: 305-324-4840
Fax: 305-545-9562
Email: hkatzman4@adelphia.net

Marc H. Glickman, MD
Vascular & Transplant Specialists
880 Kempsville Road, Suite 1000
Norfolk, VA 23502
Phone: 757-466-6513
Fax: 757-466-8698
Email: mglickman@vascularandtransplant.com

Frederick A. Schild, MD
University of Miami
1611 N.W. 12th Ave.
Jackson Memorial Hosp. East Tower #3016
Miami, FL 33136
Phone: 305-585-5286
Fax: 305-585-3794
Email: fschild@med.miami.edu

Roy Fujitani, MD
Chief, Division of Vascular Surgery
UCI Medical Center 101 The City Drive, South
Bldg. 53, R. 122
Orange, CA 92868
Phone: 714-456-5452
Fax: 714-456-6070
Email: rmfujita@uci.edu

Jeffrey H. Lawson, MD, PhD
Duke Univ. Medical Center
RM 479 MSRB Research Dr., Box 2622
Durham, NC 27710
Phone: 919-681-6432
Fax: 919-681-1094
Email: lawso006@mc.duke.edu

Support:

All authors received reimbursement from Hancock Jaffe Laboratories, Inc., for costs of conducting the clinical investigation for the MVB graft. None of the authors have a direct financial relationship with Hancock Jaffe Laboratories or a financial interest in the Mesenteric Vein Bioprosthetic graft.

Introduction

The United States Renal Data System reports that more than 300,000 Americans underwent hemodialysis for the treatment of end-stage renal disease (ESRD) in 2002. For each of these patients adequate hemo-access for dialysis is essential for survival. Access to the patient's blood can either come in the form of a catheter, native arteriovenous fistula or prosthetic graft. The importance of establishing and maintaining vascular access for dialysis patients was recognized by the National Kidney Foundation in its development of the Dialysis Outcomes Quality Initiative (DOQI) guidelines, which were published in 1997 and amended in 2000. The DOQI guidelines recommend that all newly created vascular access sites be considered for the creation of an autologous arteriovenous fistula[1], however, fewer than 50% of patients in most dialysis populations in the United States have functional autologous arteriovenous fistula.[2] From these data it is apparent that both the number of new "incident" patients as well as "prevalent" patients will continue to increase requiring stable forms of vascular access.

An alternative to the autologous arteriovenous fistula is the placement of a synthetic vascular graft prosthesis which have lower patency rates and a higher overall complication rate.[3,4,5,6]

The search to modify existing options and develop new graft materials with the goal of improving the clinical outcome for hemodialysis patients continues to receive attention.[7] Based on the supposition that natural tissue could best mimic the compliance of native vascular tissue, avoiding the disruption of blood flow patterns and associated turbulence caused by more rigid synthetic materials, a number of biological alternatives have been offered including human umbilical vein and bovine carotid artery. Although biologic in nature, the structure of these materials does not allow for a bioprosthesis capable of providing compliance similar to native vascular tissue. Furthermore, there have been reports of degeneration.[8,9] Cryopreserved human vein is another alternative with mixed reports of both success and failure in the literature.[10,11]

A new Mesenteric Vein Bioprosthesis (MVB) is evaluated for use in patients who require chronic access to the vascular system for hemodialysis. The utilization of the bovine mesenteric vein allows the production of a bioprosthesis with a high elastin content and moderate wall thickness. Following harvesting of the bovine mesenteric vein, it is treated with a patented process of glutaraldehyde crosslinking and gamma radiation that renders the graft resistant to host rejection and degradation while maintaining viscoelastic compliance similar to saphenous vein (Figures 1 and 2). Secondary patency for the mesenteric vein has been reported to be significantly higher than PTFE at 12 months.[12] In this manuscript, we report the results of a large, prospective, non-randomized, mulitcenter trial that was conducted to evaluate the safety and effectiveness of the MVB in hemodialysis patients with one or more failed synthetic prosthesis.

Methods

Between October 1999 and February 2002, 183 patients were enrolled in a study to evaluate the Mesenteric Vein Bioprosthesis (MVB) as an access conduit. This study

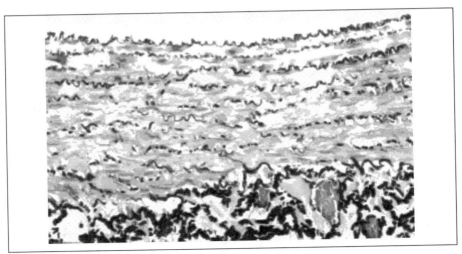

Figure 1:   Photomicrograph of the Mesenteric Vein Bioprosthesis.
Photomicrograph of MVB in cross section, oriented with graft
lumen at top of diagram demonstrates the complete internal elastic
membrane at the luminal surface and the media containing collagen
and numerous elastic fibers appearing as wavy fibers in the radially
oriented tunica media and as dark staining transverse sections in
the longitudinally oriented media at bottom of picture (X100, stained
with Verhoeff's elastica).

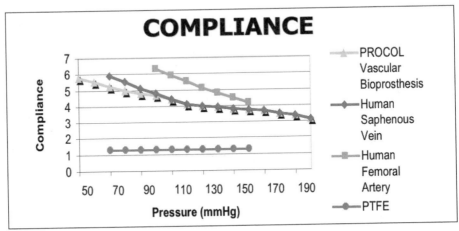

Figure 2:   Compliance of the Mesenteric Vein Bioprosthesis compared to
human saphenous vein, human femoral artery and ePTFE conduits
under pulsatile flow conditions.

was conducted at six participating sites under an Investigational Device Exemption approved by the Food and Drug Administration. The protocol was approved at each site by the individual Institutional Review Board prior to initiating the study. All subjects gave informed consent. Criteria for patient inclusion in the study were; a history of a prior failed synthetic graft(s), in addition to any native fistula or catheter-based access, and the absence of systemic septic disease or preexisting localized infection at the time of implant. Enrollment at the participating investigational sites was: Cedars Medical Center, Miami, Florida (37 MVB); Duke University Medical Center, Durham, North Carolina (62 MVB); University of California Medical Center, Irvine, California, (18 MVB): University of Miami School of Medicine, Miami, Florida (20 MVB); Vascular and Transplant Specialist, Eastern Virginia Medical School, Norfolk, Virginia, (44 MVB), California University at Long Beach (2 MVB). All MVB subjects (n=183) received a 6-mm bioprosthesis (ProCol® graft, Hancock Jaffe Laboratories, Inc., Irvine, CA).

Concomitant Control Patients   As a point of reference, concomitant control patients were selected consecutively from patients with grafts implanted at the same sites by surgeons who were not active clinical investigators during the same period of the trial (n=93). Concomitant control patients received a synthetic graft which were in all but three cases straight 6-mm or 4-7 mm tapered ePTFE grafts, by manufacturers including: Gore-Tex (Flagstaff, AZ), Impra/Bard (Tempe, AZ), and Boston Scientific (Natick, MA). Three patients receiving synthetic grafts manufactured from silicone (n=1) or polyetherurethaneurea (n=2) were also included in the concomitant control cohort. This group of patients was in no way intended to represent true randomized controls but rather to serve as a benchmark of synthetic graft patency over the same time period as the MBV graft implantation study.

Internal Control Patients   As a second point of reference, patient histories for all MVB patients were reviewed. When accurate dates of both implant and abandonment of the patient's most recent prior synthetic graft were available (n = 128), the data was captured as an internal control (INT) and compared to secondary patency for the MVB cohort. Accurate historical data on 55 patients in the MBV group could not be obtained with respect to implantation of the prior synthetic graft, therefore, those patients were not included in the internal control analysis.

Patient demographics, prior graft history, and co-morbidities were captured and recorded. Comparisons between graft types used Fisher's exact test or the 2-sample *t*-test. There were no limitations on implant position or graft configuration. Access in the MVB group was not initiated until at least 14 days post implant.

Follow-up examinations were performed 6 weeks, 6 months, and 12 months postoperatively and at six-month intervals thereafter by a combination of the implanting surgeon, nephrologist or dialysis clinic nurse in charge. For some concomitant control patients data was gathered by review of patient records.

Graft patency rates were generated using the Kaplan-Meier survival curve analysis, and groups were compared using the log-rank test. All patients were included in the intent to treat group for analysis with censoring at the time of death, lost to follow-up, or withdrawal. Definitions for primary and secondary patency were taken from the recommended standards for reports dealing with arteriovenous hemodialysis accesses.[13]

Complications, graft interventions, total number of events, the linearized rate (events/graft year), and the number of grafts with events were computed. Linearized rates were compared using Cox's approximate F-Test. Mean cumulative failure analysis was used to predict the total number of thromboses in the two groups over time. All reported P-values are two-tailed. Statistical analyses were performed using SAS® (version 8.2, Cary, NC).

Results

Population   Between October 1999 and February 2002, a total of 183 patients received the MVB and 93 concomitant control patients received an ePTFE graft for vascular access at six investigational sites. All patients had at least one prior failed synthetic graft and generally, previously failed autologous fistulas and histories of multiple catheter placements. Patient characteristics were comparable between the two groups (Table I). Prior graft history, comorbidites and graft configurations are noted in Table II. The history of prior failed synthetic grafts and the higher percentages of female and African American patients were consistent with a high-risk population. Multivariate analysis found no significant difference in the results related to any of the captured variables with the exception of graft placement in the thigh where secondary patency rates favored the MVB.

Follow-up   Data was collected per the study protocol for up to 30 months postoperatively for total follow-up of 280 years, 188 years for MVB and 92 years for the ePTFE control group. Mean follow-up was 1.0 year for the MVB group and 0.9 years for the ePTFE group. During the study there were a total of 26 deaths in the

Table I.   Patient Characteristics.

Patient Characteristic	MVB	ePTFE	P Value
Total patients (n)	183	93	
Sex			1.000
Male	40.4% (74/183)	40.9% (38/93)	
Female	59.6% (109/183)	59.1% (55/93)	
Ethnicity			0.221
African American	71.3% (129/181)	75.00% (69/92)	
Hispanic	11.0% (20/181)	4.35% (4/92)	
White	17.7% (32/181)	20.65% (19/92)	
Asian	<1% (1/181)	0	
Unreported	<1% (1/181)	0	
Age			<0.001
Mean years (± SD)	50.9 (±14.7)	58.1 (±15.1)	
Range (y)	17-86	25-93	

Table II.   Medical and vascular access history.

Patient Characteristic	MVB	ePTFE
Total patients (n)	183	93
Prior synthetic grafts		
Mean grafts (± SD)	2.1 (±1.13)	1.6 (±0.94)
Range	1-6	1-5
Co-morbidities		
Hypertension	85.8% (157/183)	90.2% (83/92)
Diabetes	44.8% (82/183)	54.3% (50/92)
Graft Placement		
Forearm loop	8.2% (15/183)	12.9% (12/93)
Forearm straight	9.3% (17/183)	1.1% (1/93)
Upper arm loop	19.1% (35/183)	16.1% (15/93)
Upper arm straight	39.9% (73/183)	35.5% (33/93)
Thigh loop	21.9% (40/183)	26.9% (25/93)
Chest	1.6% (3/183)	7.5% (7/93)
Virginal limb (no prior synthetic graft)	44.4% (80/180)	43.0% (40/93)

MVB cohort and 6 in the ePTFE group, none of which were related to the use of the graft. Two patients could not be contacted and were lost to follow-up in the MVB group and 4 ePTFE patients were lost. Ten patients were censored for patency analysis when a transplant was received (n=2), further dialysis was refused (n=5), or an alternate method of dialysis was requested (n=3).

Patency   Efficacy was determined by primary and secondary patency of the MVB compared to the ePTFE control cohort and when available, the patient's own prior prosthesis (for secondary patency only). Primary patency was defined as any event that caused a loss of graft patency or required an intervention to the lumen of the graft. Primary patency at 12 months was 35.6% for MVB vs. 28.4% for ePTFE (Fig. 3). Secondary patency was the cumulative graft survival time from graft placement until the graft was considered no longer salvageable and deemed abandoned. Secondary patency for the MVB (n=183) was compared to patency rates for both the ePTFE control cohort (n=93) and patient's prior synthetic graft or internal control cohort (n=128). Secondary patency rates at 12 and 24 months were 65.6% and 60.3% for MVB compared to 55.5% and 42.9% for ePTFE (P=.036). The difference was even more significant (P<.0001) when MVB was compared to the patient's own prior synthetic graft which had secondary patency rates at 12 and 24 months of only 33.6% and 18.0% (Fig. 4). This comparison is particularly meaningful because the patient's own hemostatic and vascular physiology is eliminated as a variable.

Interventions   The improved patency experienced with the MVB cohort was achieved with a lower incidence of interventions. The rate of interventions per year was 0.97 with MVB compared to 1.37 interventions/y for ePTFE (Table III). The

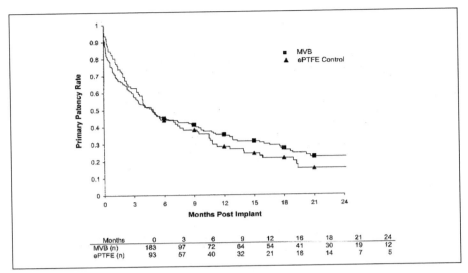

Months	0	3	6	9	12	16	18	21	24
MVB (n)	183	97	72	64	54	41	30	19	12
ePTFE (n)	93	57	40	32	21	18	14	7	5

Figure 3:   Primary patency by Kaplan-Meier Analysis for Mesenteric Vein Bioprosthesis (MVB) and ePTFE concomitant control. P=.5249 (log-rank). Standard error by Greenwood's algorithm for MVB and ePTFE at 12 months is 0.036 and 0.049 and at 24 months 0.036 and 0.045.

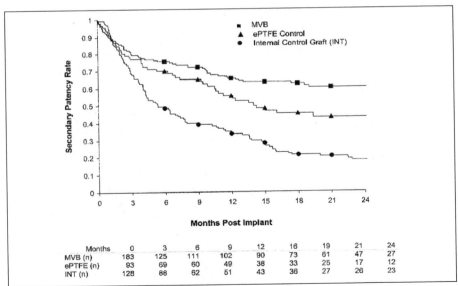

Months	0	3	6	9	12	16	19	21	24
MVB (n)	183	125	111	102	90	73	61	47	27
ePTFE (n)	93	69	60	49	38	33	25	17	12
INT (n)	128	88	62	51	43	36	27	26	23

Figure 4:   Secondary patency rates by Kaplan-Meier Analysis for Mesenteric Vein Bioprosthesis (MVB), ePTFE concomitant control, and Internal Control Graft (patient's most recent graft prior to receiving MVB). P=.036 (MVB vs ePTFE control) and P < .0001 (MVB vs Internal Control Graft) by log-rank test. Standard error by Greenwood's algorithm for MVB, ePTFE and Internal Control Graft (INT) graft at 12 months is 0.038, 0.042, and 0.055 and at 24 months 0.041, 0.034, and 0.058.

Table III.   Graft interventions to maintain or restore patency.

Event	MVB (n=183 grafts)			ePTFE (n=93 grafts)				RR†
								(95% Two-tailed
	n events	n grafts	rate‡ event/y	n events	n grafts	rate‡ event/y	P value*	Confidence Limits)
Total interventions (1.12–1.79)	183	108	0.97	126	55	1.37	.003	1.41
Revision	23	19	0.12	11	10	0.12		
Angioplasty	20	28	0.15	8	7	0.07		
Thrombectomy	49	41	0.26	23	19	0.25		
Thrombectomy/ Angioplasty	32	25	0.17	50	29	0.55		
Revision/ Thrombectomy	42	35	0.22	31	25	0.45		

*Cox F-Test: to compare total number of events
† Relative risk (RR) computed as ePTFE / MVB
‡ Total graft years for calculation of linearized rate is 188.16 (MVB), 91.68 (ePTFE)

number of grafts requiring intervention was similar in both study groups (59%) but due to the need for repeat procedures the incidence of intervention was greater in the ePTFE group and relative risk for an intervention to be performed in the ePTFE control cohort was 1.4 fold greater than in the MVB cohort (95% CL 1.1-1.8). Despite the increased number of interventions in the ePTFE control cohort the resultant secondary patency at 24 months was 42.9% with ePTFE compared to 60.3% attained with the MVB.

Complications   No unexpected or catastrophic complications were experienced in either group. Similar types of complications were reported for MVB and ePTFE including those noted in Table IV with comparisons of the rates of occurrence. There was no difference in the incidence of events of bleeding, steal, and swelling of the extremity. Prolonged bleeding due to increased venous resistance, a frank hole in the graft, and hemorrhage caused by an ulcer over the graft, which was repaired by revision, were reported as bleeding events in the ePTFE control cohort. Bleeding events in the MVB group included prolonged bleeding related to hypertension (n=1) and anticoagulation therapy (n=1), both of which were repaired, and one large hematoma of undetermined cause. Cannulation trauma occurred at a similar rate in both groups. Pseudoaneurysm formation in the MVB group was related directly to needle stick events in seven of ten instances. No events of seroma, unique to synthetic materials, were reported with MVB.

The risk of thrombosis was 1.8 times greater in the ePTFE group. The incidence of thrombosis in the MVB group at 0.78 events/year was significantly lower than the 1.36 events/year experienced in the ePTFE control group (P<.001). Graft infection was also less frequent in the MVB group at 0.05 events/yr compared to 0.20 events/yr for the ePTFE group (P<.001) making the relative risk of infection 3.7 fold greater with ePTFE than with MVB (95% CL 1.7-8.3). All but one of the graft

Table IV.   Complications.

Event	MVB (n=183 grafts)			ePTFE (n=93 grafts)				RR†
	n events	n grafts	rate‡ event/y	n events	n grafts	rate‡ event/y	P value*	(95% Two-tailed Confidence Limits)
Bleeding	3	3	0.016	4	2	0.044	.177	2.75 (0.62-12.50)
Dilatation	6	6	0.032	0	0	N/A	.052	N/A
Infection	10	8	0.053	18	15	0.196	<.001	3.70 (1.72-8.33)
Dialysis cannulation trauma	12	12	0.064	7	5	0.076	.688	1.19 (0.45-2.94)
Pseudoaneurysm	10	8	0.053	6	4	0.065	.669	1.23 (0.43-3.33)
Seroma	0	0	N/A	6	4	0.065	<.001	N/A
Steal	3	3	0.016	2	2	0.022	.696	1.37 (0.21-7.69)
Swelling of limb	20	12	0.106	9	4	0.098	.861	0.93 (0.41-1.96)
Thrombosis	146	100	0.776	125	59	1.364	<.001	1.72 (1.39-2.22)
Total Events	210	123	1.12	177	74	1.93	<0.001	1.72 (1.41-2.12)

*Cox F-Test: to compare total number of events
† Relative risk (RR) computed as ePTFE / MVB
‡ Total graft years for calculation of linearized rate is 188.16 (MVB), 91.68 (ePTFE)

infections experienced with the MVB developed initially from a wound infection following either the implant procedure or an intervention.

Rates of infection, thrombosis and seroma were all significantly lower with the MVB. The linearized rate of all events was significantly lower in the MVB cohort with a rate of 1.1 events/graft year compared to a rate of 1.9 events/graft year in the ePTFE group (P<.001).

Abandonment   Grafts were abandoned with greater frequency in the ePTFE group (P=.027). A total of 33% of MVB grafts (n=61) were abandoned at a rate of 0.32 grafts/year compared to 0.52 grafts/year in the ePTFE group with 49% of ePTFE (n=46) grafts abandoned. The primary causes for abandonment were thrombosis and infection with the risk of abandonment due to thrombosis 2.3 fold greater (95% CL 1.3-4.0) and of infection 4.5 fold greater (95% CL 1.6-14.3) in the ePTFE group. Eight MVB grafts, or 4 % of all grafts implanted, were explanted due to infection (n=5), dilatation (n=2) or thrombosis (n=1), and eleven infected ePTFE grafts, representing 12% of the population, were explanted.

Discussion

The primary and secondary patency rates reported for most synthetic vascular graft studies are based on incident patient populations or database registries. Many of the studies have different definitions for patient inclusion and patency. In some cases, only accessed patients are considered and all other patients are excluded from the analysis. In this study all patients were included in the analysis.

The expected patency rates achieved in this study should be lower than the published rates for incident populations with widely varying results. In one study, the authors' reported that the presence of a previous failed access graft created a 1.8 fold risk increase of primary access failure, a 2.6 fold risk increase of secondary access failure and a 1.8 fold risk increase in the incidence of access revision.[14] The only significant risk factor for failure of a subsequent ePTFE graft was a history of a previous unsalvageable ePTFE graft. Odds ratio for primary patency failure were 1.4, 1.9 and 2.6 and for secondary patency failure was 1.6, 2.7 and 4.4 for one, two, and three prior failed grafts, respectively.[15] These two authors reported secondary patency rates at 12 months of 58% and 59% for a combined population of over 300 patients with primarily ePTFE grafts. Although these studies included patients without a history of prior unsalvageable prostheses, the results are consistent with the 55% reported for the ePTFE control group in this study. A high percentage of female subjects and grafts implanted in the upper arm and thigh, further identify the study population with factors associated with a high risk of graft failure.[16,17] The 34% secondary patency rate at 12 months for the internal control cohort confirms that 70% of the MVB population had a dismal history of unsuccessful hemodialysis access survival.

Despite the challenging access histories and high risk nature of the population, the MVB provided 66% secondary patency at one year approaching the 70% patency recommended by the DOQI as a target for access grafts in all patients. When results obtained with MVB are compared to the prior graft experience from the same patient population the improvement is highly significant at 24 months (P<.0001). This improved secondary patency not only allows the preservation and use of a critical access site for an extended period of time, but additional benefits are realized in the form of reduced costs to maintain the access and less disruption to the patient's personal lifestyle.

Complication rates by category were comparable to or lower for MVB than ePTFE and the overall frequency of both complications and interventions were significantly lower for MVB. Infection and thrombosis are among the most frequent causes of graft failure and the most significant differences between the two groups were observed in these categories (P<.001). The Dialysis Outcomes Quality Initiative advises that the rate of infection should not exceed 10% in dialysis access grafts1. A large retrospective review of 850 patients at a single institution reported that 10.2 % of the population underwent removal of access grafts or fistula for infection[18]. In our study, graft infection was 4.44 times more likely with ePTFE and infection was reported in 16% of ePTFE and 4% of MVB grafts. Twelve percent of ePTFE grafts and 4% of MVB grafts were explanted as a result of infection.

Thrombosis occurred in a similar percentage of grafts in each group, however, rethrombosis was less frequent with MVB and the rate of all thrombotic events in the MVB group was nearly half that of the ePTFE control group (0.78 events/year MVB vs 1.36 events/year ePTFE). The lower rate of thrombosis and correspondingly reduced number of interventions required to maintain superior graft patency is a distinct benefit to the MVB patient. The lower overall complication rate with MVB in this study resulted in a lower number of grafts abandoned (33% MVB vs 49% ePTFE) and offered another option to the patient with a history of unsalvageable synthetic accesses.

One of the shortcomings of this study was the fact that the MVB group was not directly "randomized" to a direct control group. This was initially by intent, whereby when the study was initiated it was intended to be a safety study of the graft, where patients were only asked to participate if they had already failed a prior ePTFE graft. Both the concomitant control patients and the internal control patients were intended to only serve as points of reference for the progress of the MVB study. In spite of the limitations of the control group design, both groups are consistent with other reports of ePTFE graft failure rates. Furthermore, regardless of the control group, the MVB graft appears to be a safe alternative to ePTFE grafts in patients who have a history of prior ePTFE graft failure. These data further support the initiation of a true direct randomized control study of MVB graft with ePTFE to ascertain its true utility as an access conduit.

Conclusions

The data established that in this high-risk patient population with one or more previously failed prosthetic access graft(s) demonstrates that MVB primary patency rates are equal to ePTFE. There is a statistically significant benefit to the patient with the MVB in secondary patency rates. Secondary patency results achieved with the MVB approached the National Kidney Foundation-Dialysis Outcomes Quality Initiative goal of 70% at 12 months. The MVB graft offers these patients fewer thrombotic events, fewer infectious events, and an overall reduction in the number of interventions to maintain a permanent access site. Finally, these conclusions and the data reported support the principle that the MVB graft may be a suitable alternative graft for patients with a history of prior failed synthetic grafts.

Acknowledgments

Coinvestigators:

Bradley H. Collins, MD
Martin E. Fogle, MD
John L. Gray, MD
Richard L. Hurwitz, MD
C. Scott McEnroe, MD
Rasesh M. Shah, MD
Gordon K. Stokes, MD

Clinical Coordinators:

Janice Devlin, RN
Kellie Lynn, RN
Marilyn Nolan, RN

Statistical Analysis

William N. Anderson, PhD

References

1. DOQI III. NKF-K/DOQI Clinical Practice Guidelines for Vascular Access: update 2000 *Am J Kidney Dis.* 2001; 37(1 Suppl 1).S137-81.
2. Owen LV, Keagy BA, Marston WA. Management of the thrombosed dialysis-access graft. In: *Advances in Vascular Surgery.* St. Louis MO: Mosby, Inc; 2000; 131-146.
3. Ascher E, Gade P, Hingorani A, et al. Changes in the practice of angioaccess surgery; impact of dialysis outcome and quality initiative recommendations *J Vasc Surg.* 2000; 31(1).84-92.
4. Berman SS, Gentile AT. Impact of secondary procedures in autogenous arteriovenous fistula maturation and maintenance *J Vasc Surg.* 2001; 34(5).866-871.
5. Gibson KD, Caps MT, Kohler TR,et al. Assessment of a policy to reduce placement of prosthetic hemodialysis access *Kidney Int.* 2001; 59(6).2335-2345.
6. Gray R. Regarding "prospective randomized comparison of surgical versus endovascular management of thrombosed dialysis access grafts" *J Vasc Surg.* 1998; 27(2).392-393.
7. Xue L, Greisler, HP. Biomaterials in the development and future of vascular grafts *J Vasc Surg.* 2003; 37(2).472-480.
8. Dardik H, Ibrahim IM, Sussman B, Kahyn M, Sanshez M, Klausner S, et al. Biodegradation and aneurysm formation in umbilical vein grafts. Observations and a realistic strategy *Ann Surg.* 1984; 199(1).61-68.
9. VanderWerf BA, Kumar SS, Rattazzi LC, Perez G, Katzman HE, Schild AF. Long-term follow-up of bovine graft arteriovenous fistulas *Proc Clin Dial Transplant Forum.* 1976; 6.85-88.
10. Matsuura JH, Johansen KH, Rosenthal D, Clark MD, Clarke KA, Kirby LB. Cryopreserved femoral vein grafts for difficult hemodialysis access *Ann Vasc Surg.* 2000; 14(1).50-55.
11. Bolton WD, Cull CL, Taylor SM, Carsten CG 3rd, Snyder BA, Sullivan TM, Youkey JR, Langan EM 3rd, Gray BH. The use of cryopreserved femoral vein grafts for hemodialysis access in patients at high risk for infection: a word of caution *J Vasc Surg.* 2002; 36(3).464-468.
12. Bacchini G, Del Vecchio L, Andrulli S, Pontoriero G, Locatelli F. Survival of prosthetic grafts of different materials after impairment of a native arteriovenous fistula in hemodialysis patients *ASAIO J.* 2001; 47(1).30-33.
13. Sidaway, Anton, et al. Recommended standards for reports dealing with arteriovenous hemodialysis access *J Vasc Surg.* 2002; 35(3).603-610.
14. Gibson KD, Gillen DL, Caps MT, Kohler TR, Sherrard DJ, Stehman-Breen CO. Vascular access survival and incidence of revisions: A comparison of prosthetic grafts, simple autogenous fistulas, and venous transposition fistulas from the United States Renal Data System Dialysis Morbidity and Mortality Study *J Vasc Surg.* 2001; 34(4).694-700.
15. Hodges TC, Fillinger MF, Zwolak RM, Walsh DB, Bech F, Cronenwett JL. Longitudinal comparison of dialysis access methods: risk factors for failure *J Vasc Surg.* 1997; 26(6).1009-1019.
16. Tashjian DB, Lipkowitz GS, Madden RL, et al. Safety and efficacy of femoral-based hemodialysis access grafts *J Vasc Surg.* 2002; 35(4).691-693.

17. Rayner HC, Pisoni RL, Gillespie BW, et al. Creation, cannulation and survival of arteriovenous fistulae: Data from the Dialysis Outcomes and Practice Patterns Study *Kidney Int.* 2003; 63(1).323-330.
18. Schild AF, Simon S, Prieto J, Raines J. Single-center review of infections associated with 1,574 consecutive vascular access procedures *Vasc Endovascular Surg.* 2003; 37(1).27-31.

DISCUSSION

Vascular Access for Hemodialysis IX
May 6-7, 2004
Lake Buena Vista, Florida

May 6, 2004
Abstract Session II

Dr. Howard Katzman
"Development and Maintenance of Hemodialysis Access in Patients with Prior Failed Synthetic Grafts: Impact of ProCol Bioprosthetic Vein Graft"

Question: Can you comment on the mechanism of failure of your grafts? Do they tend to fail from obstructive lesions within the conduit or is it venous anastomotic hyperplasia?

Katzman: A degree of hyperplasia is much much less in these. On many of the failed grafts when we had to do percutaneous salvage the clot was very easy to dissolve or distract. There was no hyperplasia that we could identify. These were usually technical reasons and one of them is that the vein tends to elongate. You need to stretch it when you implant it to avoid kinking on the stretching of the graft material. But your question is a good one in that we have not seen a lot of hyperplasia in this particular anastomosis.

Question: I don't discount any of your data here but I'm wondering how are you using PTFE versus the mesenteric vein? Are you paralleling a failed graft, are you going to the upper extremity, are you going to the opposite extremity, or are you going to the leg? Is there any way you can compare that you used your mesenteric vein in the same position that you use PTFE?

Katzman: The answer to that is that we are using a mesenteric vein exactly as you would use a PTFE. In a loop, in a straight configuration, forearm, upperarm, and in a few cases in a thigh setting.

Question: I understand that but if you have lost a straight forearm AVG, do you parallel that and or are you paralleling a mesenteric vein to a PTFE? Are you going to the upperarm?

Katzman: No you go to a different site. That is correct and certainly you point out a significant question. You know I have submitted this paper for review and the reviewers always come back with the same questions regarding the control groups and the fact that the comparison is probably not as it should be. In order to answer that, another trial is being conducted to compare primary implants, so that we don't need to look at failed prior prosthesis and compare those two groups. It will take a controlled prospective randomized trial to try to answer those questions.

18

RENEWED INTEREST IN BOVINE HETEROGRAFT FOR VASCULAR ACCESS; A COMPARISON BETWEEN POLYTETRAFLUOROETHYLENE AND BOVINE

Casandra A Anderson M.D., Chad J Richardson M.D.,
Arthur L Ney M.D., Richard T Zera M.D., PhD.,
Brent Nykamp M.D., Greg Ausmus M.D., Mark D. Odland M.D.

Hennepin County Medical Center, Minneapolis, MN 55415

Corresponding Author:
Casandra A Anderson
HCMC
701 Park Ave. Mail Code 813B
Minneapolis, MN 55415
Telephone: 612-873-2810
Fax: 612-904-4297
Email: casandra.a.anderson@co.hennepin.mn.us

Introduction

Recent emphasis has been placed on practice guidelines to improve health care in patients maintained on chronic hemodialysis.[1] Recommendations have advocated the use of native arteriovenous fistulas (AVF) over graft placement. Although the Brescia-Cimino[2] and brachiocephalic AVF[3, 4] have been shown in most studies to have superior patency rates as compared to prosthetic grafts, their use is limited in patients who have inadequate vessels. In 1972, Chivitz et al[5] described the use of the modified interposed bovine heterograft in the construction of an AVF. Following this, the use of PTFE in creation of AVF was described by several authors.[6,7] Since this time it has been debated which material is better suited for vascular access in patients requiring chronic hemodialysis. At our institution, between 1972 and 1986[8, 9] bovine heterograft was placed in the majority of patients who required graft placement. This trend shifted to the use of PTFE for the next decade, however presently the preferred material is again bovine. This study retrospectively reviews our last 15 years of experience with vascular access graft placement. Patency, complications, and interventions required to maintain dialysis access were evaluated and compared between the two graft materials.

Materials and Methods

Subjects   From 7/6/89 to 7/30/03, 245 bovine heterografts ("Artegraft", North Brunswick, NJ) and 446 polytetrafluoroethylene (PTFE) grafts were placed in 538 patients for hemodialysis access. All patients were referred to a single institution where arteriovenous graft placement was performed primarily by renal transplant surgeons. Data was obtained from a prospectively collected clinical database as well as from chart review.

There were 283 females and 255 males, mean age 63 years (range 20-95). The most common underlying cause of renal failure was diabetes mellitus (table 1). The number of patients with diabetes mellitus was equally distributed between the two

Table 1.   Underlying cause of renal failure.

Disease	No. of patients
Diabetes Mellitus	172
Diabetes Mellitus & Hypertension	88
Hypertension	99
Glomerulonephritis	47
Polycystic kidney disease	19
Obstructive nephropathy	16
HIV nephropathy	9
Lupus	9
Other	79

groups. The majority of grafts were placed in the forearm, (548) usually in a looped fashion. Upper arm grafts were created in 112 cases and thigh grafts in 31 cases. Most procedures were done with conscious sedation and regional anesthetic. Preoperative antibiotics were routinely administered. A broad loop was created to avoid kinking, and tunneling was facilitated by a distal incision. An ace wrap bandage was applied for the first 24 hours postoperatively, while patients were observed overnight in the hospital. Dialysis was initiated 3-4 weeks after graft placement.

Distribution of graft material used over the fifteen year study period is illustrated in figure 1. Total follow-up time was 850 years for PTFE and 271 years for bovine grafts. Average follow-up time for individual grafts was 13.2 months (range: .1-164) for bovine, and 22.0 months (range: .1-121) for PTFE (p=<.001).

Analysis   Primary and secondary patency rates were calculated using life table analysis. Primary patency was defined as a widely patent graft which required no additional intervention after placement. Secondary patency was defined as restoration of graft patency after occlusion. The Log-Rank test was used for comparison of patency rates between bovine and PTFE grafts. The X^2 correlation was used to assess associations between qualitative variables using the Fisher's exact p-value and the student t-test was used for evaluating quantitative variables. The Cox F-test was used to compare event rates between the two groups.

Results

Patency   Primary patency (figure 2) for PTFE and bovine grafts at 1 and 3 years was 36% (95% CI: 31.0-41.0) and 13% (95% CI: 8.79-17.21), and 34% (95% CI: 26.6-41.3) and 17% (95% CI: 8.2-25.7) respectively (p=.049). Secondary patency

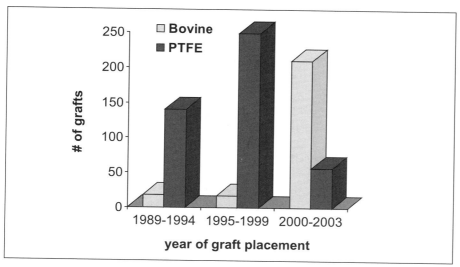

Figure 1:   Time distribution of graft material used in AV graft placement

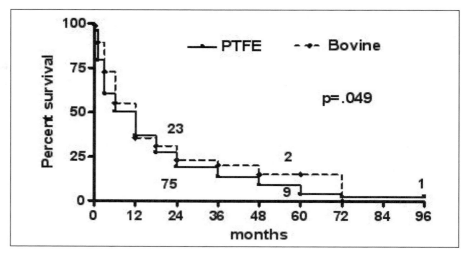

Figure 2:   Comparative primary patency rates for Bovine and PTFE heterografts followed up to 8 years. Numbers on graph represent grafts at risk.

(figure 3) for PTFE and bovine grafts at 1 and 3 years was 82% (95% CI: 78.0-86.0) and 64% (95% CI: 58.4-69.6), and 86% (95% CI: 80.8-91.3) and 62% (95% CI: 50.3-73.7) respectively, (p=.06). Because of the time distribution in which the grafts were placed, the average follow-up time per graft was statistically different between the two groups. A separate analysis was performed on a subgroup of patients who had grafts placed between 2000-2003. In this subgroup the average follow-up time per graft was 10.7 months (range: .1-36) for bovine and 12.0 months (range: .1-45) for PTFE (p=.40). When comparing patency rates in this subgroup (figures 4 and 5),

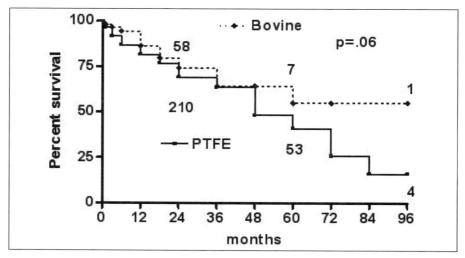

Figure 3:   Comparative secondary patency rates for Bovine and PTFE heterografts followed up to 8 years. Numbers on graph represent grafts at risk.

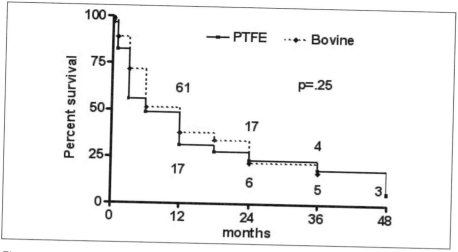

Figure 4:   Comparative primary patency for Bovine and PTFE heterografts placed between 2003–2004 followed up to 4 years. Numbers on graph represent grafts at risk.

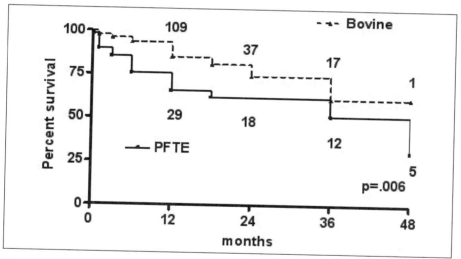

Figure 5:   Comparative secondary patency for Bovine and PTFE heterografts placed between 2003–2004 followed up to 4 years. Numbers on graph represent grafts at risk.

secondary patency was statistically higher for bovine grafts, 73% (95% CI: 63.02-82.98) at 2 years versus 59% (95% CI: 43.6-74.3) for PTFE grafts (p=.006).

Complications   Table 2 is a list of complications. Steal syndrome occurred in 4.1% of patients with bovine grafts compared to 5.2% with PTFE grafts. Twenty-seven (5.0%) episodes occurred in forearm grafts and 9 (5.3%) in upper arm configurations. Nine grafts required ligation and 24 were revised with banding. Steal syndrome was

Table 2.   Comparison of complications between Bovine and PTFE grafts.

	Bovine	PTFE	p-value
Steal	10 (4.1%)	23 (5.2%)	.58
Pseudoaneursym	10 (4.1%)	29 (6.5%)	.23
Infection	12 (4.9%)	46 (10%)	.01
Occlusion	40 (16.3)	151(33.9%)	<.0001

associated with significant complications in 5 patients. Two patients with upper arm grafts and 1 with a forearm graft required amputations. Additionally, two patients with forearm grafts had early occlusion (<30days) following banding.

Aneurysms that required intervention occurred more frequently in patients with PTFE grafts (6.5% vs. 4.1%), but this difference was not statistically significant. Overall, 8 grafts were ligated and 31 were salvaged with revision. Four bovine grafts required ligation and 6 were revised, 5 with bovine and 1 with PTFE. Similarly, 4 PTFE grafts were ligated and 25 were revised, 21 with PTFE and 4 with bovine. Mean time to aneurysm repair or ligation was not significantly different between the two groups, 38.5 months for bovine versus 31 months for PTFE.

There were statistically more infectious complications with PTFE grafts than bovine, 10% versus 4.9% respectively (p=.01). All 12 of the infected bovine grafts required removal. Four of the PTFE grafts had limited disease and were able to be treated with antibiotics and local wound care. Additionally, 1 graft was able to be salvaged with removal of the infected portion followed by a delayed revision. The remaining 41 PTFE grafts required removal. Mean time to infection was 653 days for bovine grafts and 548 days for PTFE grafts (p=.67).

One hundred ninety-one grafts occluded and patency was unable to be restored, 16% of bovine grafts compared to 34% of PTFE grafts (p=<.001). To maintain patency, 452 interventions were performed in bovine grafts as compared to 1927 interventions in PTFE grafts. Interventions include surgical thrombectomy, interventional stenting and angioplasty, and graft repair for venous stenosis, pseudoaneursyms and infections. Bovine grafts required significantly fewer interventions per graft life (1.8 vs. 4.3, p=<.001) and per year (1.7 vs. 2.3, p=<.001) as compared to PTFE grafts. When evaluating the subset of patients with grafts placed from 2000-2003, similar results were found. Bovine grafts required fewer interventions per graft life (1.5 vs. 2.6, p=.008) and per year (1.7 vs. 2.7, p=<.001), (1.5 and 1.7) than PTFE grafts. .

Discussion

Radiocephalic AVF is the preferred choice of primary vascular access in patients requiring chronic hemodialysis. Secondary patency for radiocephalic AVF at 3 and 5 years range from 64-72% and 37-72% respectively[10]. According to the DOQI guidelines[1], the next recommended AVF is a brachiocephalic fistula which has reported secondary patency rates of 50-70% and 34-53% at 3 and 5 years respectively[10]. In our patient population, approximately 50% of patients present with previously failed dialysis access and few have adequate vessels for the formation of a radiocephalic fistula. To preserve sites for future access placement, typically our practice is to create a forearm graft before an upper arm fistula. Secondary patency rates of 62% and 50% at 3 and 5 years respectively were obtained when using bovine heterograft in this series. These patency rates compare favorably to the secondary patency rates for grafts suggested by the DOQI guidelines as well as to patency rates for brachiocephalic AVF. Other published series have also reported comparable 3 year patency rates for bovine heterografts ranging from 59 to 80%.[8, 11-13]

Some authors have suggested that PTFE grafts may have better secondary patency,[7, 9-10] withstand infection, and have fewer aneurysmal complications[11, 14] as compared to bovine heterografts. These conclusions were not consistent with the findings in our retrospective series. Infection rates associated with PTFE grafts have been reported at 8-19%.[3-4, 15] In our experience the incidence of infection with the used of PTFE was 10%, while using bovine heterograft the incidence decreased to 4.9%. Aneurysmal complications occurred equally in both PTFE and bovine heterografts and patency was maintained in the majority of these grafts with revision.

When comparing grafts with similar follow-up, secondary patency was significantly higher for bovine than PTFE grafts, 73% versus 59% at 2 years. Bacchini et al[16] published similar results, reporting secondary patency of 50% for PTFE grafts at 12 months and 82% for bovine grafts at 19 months.

Bovine heterografts also required fewer interventions per year to maintain patency, 1.7 vs. 2.3. The DOQI guidelines suggest that thrombosis rate per year should not exceed .5/year. Our intervention rate per year is higher because it includes not only interventions for thrombosis but also for stenosis and revisions for infections and pseuodaneursyms. This aggressive approach to maintaining graft function has afforded us a 12-16% greater secondary patency than that suggested by the DOQI guidelines.

Conclusions

To our knowledge, there are no published prospective randomized trials comparing the use of bovine versus PTFE for vascular access in hemodialysis patients. Bacchini et al described starting such a trial in his 2001 article which retrospectively showed improved graft survival with bovine heterograft. In our series, we found secondary graft patency was significantly improved with the use of bovine heterografts, in a subgroup of patients with similar follow up. Overall, bovine grafts required fewer interventions to maintain patency. Additionally, bovine heterografts had a decreased incidence of infection and were not associated with an increase in aneurysmal complications. This data would suggest bovine carotid heterograft may be the preferred material for hemodialysis vascular access grafts when native fistulas are unable to be created or have failed. However, a prospective study is needed to verify these results.

References

1. NKF-DOQI *Clinical Practice Guidelines for Vascular Access.* New York, National Kidney Foundation, 1997.
2. Brescia NJ, Cimino JE, Appel K, Hurwich BJ. Chronic hemodialysis using venipuncture and surgically created arteriovenous fistula. *N Engl J Med* 1966; 275: 1089-1092
3. Kherlakian GM, Roedersheimer LR, Arbaugh JJ, et al Comparison of autogeneous fistula versus expanded polytetrafluoroethylene graft fistula for angioaccess in hemodialysis. *Am J Surg* 1986; 152: 238-43.
4. Palder SB, Kirkman RL, Whittemore AD, et al. Vascular access for hemodialysis: patency rates and results of revision. *Ann Surg* 1985; 202: 235-9.
5. Chivitz JL, Yokoyama T, Bower R, et al. Self sealing prosthesis for arteriovenous fistula in man. *Trans Am Soc Artif Intern Organs* 18: 452, 1972.
6. Johnson JM, Baker LD, Williams T. Expanded polytetrafluoroethylene: a subcutaneous conduit for hemodialysis. *Dial and Transpl* April 1976.
7. Volder JG, Kirkham RL, Kolff WJ. A-V shunts created in new ways. *Trans Am Soc Artif Inern Organs* 1973; 19: 38-42.
8. Andersen RC, Ney AL, Odland MD, et al. Minnesota Medicine 1988; 71: 608-613.
9. Merickel JH, Andersen RC, Knutson R, et al. Bovine carotid artery shunts in vascular access surgery. *Arch Surg* 1974; 109: 245-250.
10. Murphy GJ, White SA, Nicholson ML. Vascular access for haemodialysis. *Brit J Surg* 2000; 87(10):1300-1315.
11. Bulter HG, Baker LD, Johnson JM. Vascular access for chronic hemodialysis: PTFE versus bovine heterograft. *Am J Surg* 1977; 134:791-793.
12. Brems J, Castaneda M, Garvin PJ. A five-year experience with bovine heterograft for vascular access. *Arch Surg* 1986; 121:941-944.
13. Nordling J, Lynggaard F, Poulsen LR, et al. Experience with bovine heterografts and Impra grafts for vascular access in chronic haemodialysis. *Scand J Urol Nephrol* 1982; 16: 69-72.
14. Winsett OE, Wolma FJ. Complications of vascular access for hemodialysis. *Southern Med J* 1985; 78: 513-517.
15. Enzler MA, Rajmon T, Lachat M, Largiader F. Long-term function of vascular access for hemodialysis. *Clin Transplant* 1996; 10:511-15.
16. Bacchini G, Sel Vecchio L, Andrulli S, et al. Survival of prosthetic grafts of different materials after impairment of a native arteriovenous fistula in hemodialysis patients. *ASAIO* 2001; 47(1): 30-33.

DISCUSSION

Vascular Access for Hemodialysis IX
May 6-7, 2004
Lake Buena Vista, Florida

May 6, 2004
Abstract Session II

Dr. Casandra Anderson
"Renewed Interest in Bovine Heterograft for Vascular Access, A Comparison Between Polytetrafluoroethylene and Bovine"

Question: I was wondering in the Bovine graft patients, did you have any patients who had previously failed PTFE and compare how the Bovine graft acted in that patient who had a previously failed PTFE?

Anderson: We did not specifically look at that but over half of our patients had more than one graft at the time of presentation. But we did not separately analyze those.

19

INITIAL EXPERIENCE WITH AN INTRAWALL, RADIALLY SUPPORTED EXPANDED POLYTETRAFLUOROETHYLENE GRAFT FOR VASCULAR ACCESS

Louis C. Thibodeaux, MD, FACS,[a] and Alvaro A. Reyes, MD[b]

From [a]General and Vascular Surgical Specialists, Inc.; and [b]Nephrology and Hypertension, Inc., Cincinnati, Ohio

Address correspondence to
Louis C. Thibodeaux, MD,
FACS,
5564 Cheviot Road,
Cincinnati, OH 45247;
telephone: 513-385-1919; fax: 513-385-6208;
e-mail: cajunlou@aol.com.

Introduction

Expanded polytetrafluoroethylene (ePTFE) grafts are the most commonly used prostheses for vascular access for hemodialysis in patients with end-stage renal disease (ESRD) in whom creation or use of a native arteriovenous (AV) fistula is not feasible. Several types of ePTFE prostheses are available, including grafts made of "stretch" and standard ePTFE material and grafts that have an external-ring or spiral support system. Stretch ePTFE grafts have been found to have higher patency rates than standard grafts.[1-3] Externally placed rings have been observed to minimize graft kinking and compression, which may be a special concern with grafts that cross joints.[4-7] Although external support systems are useful, some surgeons have found the rings or spiral to interfere with cutting and suturing of the graft, especially during revision. Recently, a stretch ePTFE access graft with a support system located within the wall of the graft became available (Gore-Tex® Intering Vascular Graft, W.L. Gore & Associates, Inc., Flagstaff, AZ; Figure 1).[6,8] The intrawall support system in an Intering graft consists of radially arranged segments of ePTFE material. The luminal surface of the graft is smooth. Placement of the support system within the wall of the graft was intended to provide kink and compression resistance in a prosthesis with a low profile, as well as to facilitate cutting of the graft at desired angles and suturing it with minimal resistance.

We began to use the Intering graft in 2002. Here, we retrospectively review our initial experience with the patency and handling of the prosthesis in a series of 86 patients.

Methods

Beginning in June 2002, a 4-6 mm tapered Intering graft was implanted in 86 consecutive private-practice patients (44 men and 42 women; mean age, 67 years) with ESRD due primarily to diabetes mellitus (76 patients), hypertension (76 patients), or both, and in whom a native AV fistula had failed or could not be created. Patients

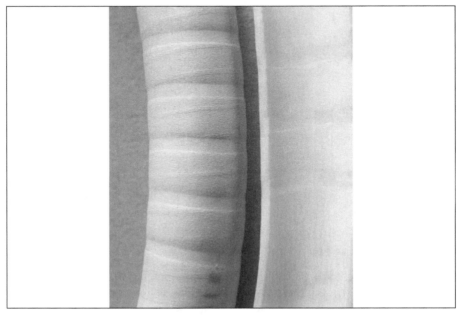

Figure 1:   Photograph of Intering stretch graft for vascular access for hemodialysis showing its full-length intrawall radial support system and smooth lumen. The graft is available in two tapered forms (4-6 mm and 4-7 mm by 45 cm) and one nontapered form (6 mm by 40 cm).

were excluded from receiving grafts only if they had open skin lesions at potential implantation sites, other skin conditions (such as scleroderma) that would increase their risk of graft infection, or vessels deemed too small for graft implantation after a preoperative ultrasound assessment. Intering grafts are available in both tapered (4-6 mm and 4-7 mm) and nontapered configurations. Although whether tapering improves the overall performance of a graft is controversial,[8-11] use of tapered grafts has been found to decrease arterial steal and high-output failure substantially,[11] especially in patients with diabetes and poor vascular resistance. Because most of the patients in this series were older, had atherosclerosis or diabetes (or both), and smaller vessels, minimization of arterial steal was an important consideration; thus, we used tapered Intering grafts exclusively.

For the implantation procedure, an axillary block was used in 35 patients, local anesthesia or sedation in 37, and general anesthesia in 14. Implantation sites were the forearm in 63 patients, the upper arm in 4, and the thigh in 11; the remaining 8 patients were given a jump graft for revision of the venous anastomosis of an access graft previously implanted by another surgeon. A loop configuration was used in 73 patients and a straight configuration in 5. In 17 patients, surgical U-clip Anastomotic Devices (Coalescent Surgical, Inc., Sunnyvale, CA) were used instead of sutures at the graft-vein anastomosis.

Postoperatively, all patients were followed closely by the same surgeon (LCT) and nephrologist (AAR) for up to a year. Follow-up assessments included clinical examinations, venous pressure readings during dialysis, and ultrasonographic evaluations that included Doppler flow measurements. Primary patency rates based on time to first thrombosis, with or without stenosis, were calculated by using survival analysis. Log-rank tests were used to compare subgroups of patients (for example, men compared with women and patients with and without hypertension or diabetes). A P value of less than 0.5 was considered to represent a significant difference.

Results

During implantation, the Intering graft was easy to cut and suture anywhere along the length of its radial support. No kinking or problems in angulating the anastomosis occurred. Intraoperatively, the thrill appeared somewhat less palpable than that with standard stretch grafts. We found that the best outcomes were achieved if use of cellulose-based hemostatic agents and forcible irrigation of the graft were avoided. Cannulation was performed immediately after implantation surgery in 4 patients, within 2 weeks of the procedure in 2 patients, and after a standard graft-maturation period in the remaining 80 patients. There were no adverse effects associated with early cannulation.

The mean observation (follow-up) time among the 86 patients in the series was 7.0 months (range, 1 to 14 months). Fifteen patients were followed for at least 1 year. As shown in Figure 2, the primary patency rate at 6 months was 76% (95% confidence interval [CI], 66% to 86%), and that at 1 year was 73% (95% CI, 63% to 84%). During the observation period, stenosis (venous intimal hyperplasia) developed in 12 patients and thrombosis in 13. Thrombectomy was successful in restoring patency in all 25 cases. Eleven of the patients with stenosis were given a jump graft; one underwent percutaneous transluminal angioplasty.

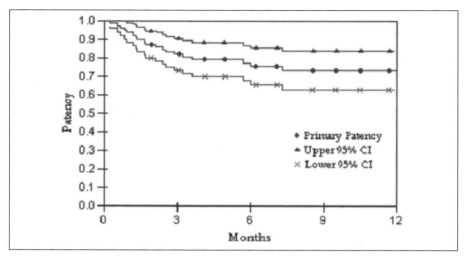

Figure 2:   Results of survival analysis showing primary patency of Intering expanded polytetrafluoroethylene stretch graft in 86 patients. CI denotes confidence interval.

Subgroup analyses using log-rank tests found no significant differences in patency related to patient age or sex; concomitant hypertension, hyperlipidemia, diabetes, congestive heart failure, peripheral vascular disease, or smoking; type of anesthesia used during graft implantation; implantation site; or type of graft configuration (loop compared with straight).

Five infections developed in patients in the series (infection rate, 6%), including one due to methicillin-resistant *Staphylococcus aureus*. All infected grafts were removed and replaced with new Intering grafts placed in a newly created tissue tunnel. Arterial steal developed in two patients. There were no pseudoaneurysms, seromas, or episodes of excessive redness or swelling in the absence of infection. Hematoma formation was minimal. The Intering grafts did not seem to "sweat" as standard grafts do. The staff in our dialysis unit observed no differences between the Intering grafts and standard stretch grafts with respect to palpation, cannulation, and hemostasis during dialysis sessions.

Conclusions

The primary patency rates achieved with the Intering graft in our series were similar to those in previously reported series in which patients were given a stretch ePTFE graft for vascular access. Davidson[12] had a rate of 76% at 1 year for 420 grafts. In the series of Derenoncourt,[1] primary patency rates for 118 stretch grafts from graft insertion to clotting were 93% at 6 months and 79% at 1 year; these results were significantly better ($P = 0.0004$) than those obtained with 192 non-stretch (standard) ePTFE grafts in the same series. Hakaim and Scott[13] had 6-month and 1-year primary patency rates of 88% and 71%, respectively, for 79 stretch grafts, 48 of which were subjected to early cannulation (performed 24 to 72 hours after implantation surgery). In the only previously published evaluation of use of the Intering graft, Davidson and Munschauer[6] reported an assisted 1-year patency rate of 64% and a clot-free survival rate of 37% for 11 jump grafts (used for revision) that crossed the antecubital fossa.

Our experience suggests that, compared with externally supported stretch ePTFE grafts, the Intering graft offers easier surgical manipulation without a decrease in patency. They may also allow routine early cannulation, perhaps as soon as immediately after surgery. Larger, longer studies are needed to determine whether the graft has superior long-term patency or other advantages. We believe that its lower profile (a reduction of about 24% in cross-sectional area compared with an externally ringed graft with the same luminal diameter) may be found to be associated with an increase in patient comfort and opportunities for early cannulation and a decrease in seromas and, possibly, infections. It is also possible that the intrawall radial support system of the Intering graft may provide some resistance to the development of thrombosis resulting from the compression applied to a vascular access graft after removal of the cannulation needle.

References

1. Derenoncourt FJ. PTFE for A-V access: six years of experience with 310 reinforced and stretch grafts. In: Henry ML, Ferguson RM, eds. *Vascular Access for Hemodialysis—IV.* Chicago, IL: WL Gore & Associates and Precept Press; 1995; 286-291.

2. Tordoir JH, Hofstra L, Bergmans DC. Stretch versus standard expanded PTFE grafts for hemodialysis access. In: Henry ML, Ferguson RM, eds. *Vascular Access for Hemodialysis—IV.* Chicago, IL: WL Gore & Associates and Precept Press; 1995; 277-285.

3. Colonna JO II, Swanson SJ, Shaver TR. Successful early use of the stretch PTFE graft. In: Henry ML, Ferguson RM, eds. *Vascular Access for Hemodialysis—IV.* Chicago, IL: WL Gore & Associates and Precept Press; 1995; 273-276.

4. Mukherjee D. Rescue of failed forearm arteriovenous access grafts using an externally supported polytetrafluoroethylene graft. *Am J Surg.* 1993; 166.306-307.

5. Barone GW, Hudec WA, Webb JW. Antecubital jump revisions for salvaging hemodialysis grafts. *Vasc Surg.* 2000; 34.11-15.

6. Davidson IJ, Munschauer CE. Preliminary experience with a new intrawall radially supported expanded PTFE graft. In: Henry ML, ed. *Vascular Access for Hemodialysis—VIII.* Arlington Heights, IL: WL Gore & Associates and Access Medical Press; 2002; 95-101.

7. Kao CL, Chang JP. Fully ringed polytetrafluoroethylene graft for vascular access in hemodialysis. *Asian Cardiovasc Thorac Ann.* 2003; 11.171-173.

8. Scher LA, Katzman HE. Alternative graft materials for hemodialysis access. *Semin Vasc Surg.* 2004; 17.19-24.

9. Dammers R, Planken RN, Pouls KP, et al. Evaluation of 4-mm to 7-mm versus 6-mm prosthetic brachial-antecubital forearm loop access for hemodialysis: results of a randomized multicenter clinical trial. *J Vasc Surg.* 2002; 37.143-148.

10. Hiranaka T. Tapered and straight grafts for hemodialysis access: a prospective, randomized comparison study. In: Henry ML, ed. *Vascular Access for Hemodialysis—VII.* Chicago, IL: WL Gore & Associates and Precept Press; 2001; 219-224.

11. Bell DD, Rosental JJ. Arteriovenous graft life in chronic hemodialysis: a need for prolongation. *Arch Surg.* 1988; 123.1169-1172.

12. Davidson IJ. PTFE bridge grafts. In: Davidson IJ, ed. *On Call in Vascular Access: Surgical and Radiologic Procedures.* Austin, TX: RG Landes; 1996; 37-76.

13. Hakaim AG, Scott TE. Durability of early prosthetic dialysis graft cannulation: results of a prospective, nonrandomized clinical trial. *J Vasc Surg.* 1997; 25.1002-1006.

DISCUSSION

Vascular Access for Hemodialysis IX
May 6-7, 2004
Lake Buena Vista, Florida

May 6, 2004
Abstract Session II

Dr. Louis Thibodeaux
"Initial Experience with an Intrawall, Radially Supported ePTFE Graft for Vascular Access"

Question: Do you cross the elbow joint with this graft?

Thibodeaux: That is a good question. Initially we were very cautious to do it. In some incidences you don't have a choice and it works very well. I have not had any trouble with kinking or bending of the graft.

20

CONVERSION OF FAILED NATIVE VEIN FISTULAS TO PTFE GRAFTS YIELDS 90% ACCESS FUNCTION AT ONE YEAR

Ingemar JA Davidson, MD, PhD, FACS, Karen Brava, RN,
Carolyn Munschauer, BS, Donna Nichols, RVT,
William H Frawley, PhD

University of Texas Southwestern Medical Center and Parkland
Memorial Hospital
5323 Harry Hines Blvd. Suite E7.108
Dallas TX 75390-9031

Corresponding author:
Ingemar Davidson, MD
5323 Harry Hines Blvd
UT Southwestern Med Ctr
Suite E7.108
Dallas, TX, 75390-9031
Phone 214.648.4823
FAX 214.648.4784
Email Ingemar.Davidson@UTSouthwestern.edu

In recent years much emphasis has been placed on native vein fistulas (AVF) over PTFE for hemodialysis access. With increasing AVFs placed a larger number of malfunctioning or not usable for hemodialysis access is likely to occur. Despite an aging ESRD population with diabetes and obesity in more than half of cases, AVFs represent 53% of all access placed for hemodialysis by the authors. This is partly achieved by using a two-staged procedure, with an initial radio-cephalic AVF at the wrist followed by a PTFE graft to the now enlarged vein. This strategy will preserve access sites and yield better outcome than other current techniques for creation of hemodialysis access.

Methods

Between January 1, 1999 and December 31, 2003, 44 wrist AVFs were converted to PTFE (4-7 mm Gore-Tex stretch) grafts. No patients were lost to follow up, varying from 3 months to 5 years. Causes of failure of the initial AVF were dialysis needle puncture complication (45%), lack of maturation (17%), fistula thrombosis (13%), poor arterial inflow (8%), and deep vein location due to obesity (17%). Vascular anatomy and surgical planning was assisted by preoperative duplex Doppler examination in all cases. The graft was anastomosed to the cephalic vein as distal as possible, dictated by the size of the vein of 5 mm or larger and the absence of proximal stenotic segments. The anastomosis configuration varied from end graft to end vein, when large (7 mm), to end graft to spatulated vein, or angled graft to vein bifurcation patch. The cephalic vein at the wrist anastomosis, when patent, was suture-ligated though a separate small incision.

The remaining portion of the cephalic vein, when long enough, was used for dialysis needle punctures until the graft portion had been incorporated, thereby avoiding temporary central vein dialysis catheter placement.

Actuarial patient, graft and clot free survival data were analyzed using the Kaplan-Meier technique. The analysis included the computation of 95% confidence intervals (CI) for the survival estimates.

Results

Twelve-month patient, graft and clot free survival for the 44 patients were 90% (CI: 0.79-1.00), 89% (0.79-1.00) and 79% (0.65-0.95), respectively. (Fig. 1). Corresponding two-year survival statistics were 75% (0.57-1.00), 83% (0.69-1.00) and 54% (0.36-0.83). The tick marks on the curves indicate patient censoring times for each survival category.

However, the long-term patient survival was predicted below 20% by 36 months (Fig. 1), reflecting the high mortality in the dialysis population in general and the high co-morbid conditions in this study specific subgroup of patients.

In contrast to patient survival, the analysis predicted graft and clot free survival statistics between three and five year of 80% and 55%, respectively. Therefore, the majority of patients are expected to die with functioning grafts.

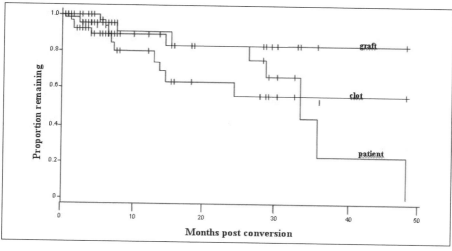

Figure 1:   Patient, graft and clot free survival for 44 patients with primary AVF converted to PTFE grafts. The tick marks on the curves indicate individual events for each survival category.

Discussion

The two stage hemodialysis access procedure, first by native vein AVF at the wrist, followed by a loop forearm PTFE graft to the enlarged vein, results in graft and clot free survival exceeding that of any other vascular access procedure used. Currently the AVF conversion is most commonly performed in the setting of failing or malfunctioning AVF. In the authors' experience about 15% of the authors AVFs are converted to PTFE grafts. This concept could apply to a large portion of the ESRD predialysis population. To become effective, much education and understanding from referring physicians and the patients and their families are needed. Early referral (6-12 months) is preferred to allow vein enlargement, a prerequisite for two-stage access procedure success. Also, a second planned delayed surgery with graft placement does not represent a failure but rather a means to improve overall dialysis access outcome.

Access for dialysis has evolved into a subspecialty bridging over many medico-socio-economic issues. Outcome improvements result from maximizing all aspects of dialysis care including early referral, surgical evaluation and technique, optimal utilization of each access site, excellence in dialysis puncture technique, and surveillance of established access.

DISCUSSION

Vascular Access for Hemodialysis IX
May 6-7, 2004
Lake Buena Vista, Florida

May 6, 2004
Abstract Session II

Dr. Ingemar Davidson
"Conversion of Failed Native Vein Fistulas to PTFE Grafts Yields 90% Access Function at One Year"

Comment: I think that with the basilic veins there is a higher patency rate with a two stage procedure. An AVF first, followed six or eight weeks later by the basilic vein transposition.

Question: What percentage of the patients require a catheter?

Davidson: I was afraid you would ask that. I don't know. I would think about half of them but I just don't know. The hardest part is to convince the patient to operate twice and the nephrologist to understand that this is not a failure.

Question: It is a nice technique but why wouldn't you just resite your fistula more proximally? In that setting where you have a very dilated vein, you usually have a concommitantly dilated artery?

Davidson: I do that every time I can. Most of the time if you run into a short segment of the vein that is not long enough for dialysis puncture, then you would do this. I agree completely with you. That is my first choice.

21

OUTCOMES OF VASCULAR ACCESS PROCEDURES IN PATIENTS COMMENCING HAEMODIALYSIS

Charles Marshall Fisher FRACS
Head, Department of Vascular Surgery
Royal North Shore Hospital
St Leonards 2065
Sydney, Australia
Telephone: 61 2 9926 8058
FAX: 61 2 9926 7007
E-mail: cfisher@doh.health.nsw.gov.au

Introduction

Establishment and maintenance of permanent haemodialysis access remains a major clinical problem with significant morbidity and mortality associated with the extended use of temporary central venous catheters as well as considerable resources consumed in undertaking interventions for problematic access.

Methods

A previous review[1] evaluated the outcomes of surgical intervention to establish vascular access for patients commencing haemodialysis. A further review has now been undertaken with an extended period of follow-up and with the review restricted to those patients registered with the ANZDATA Registry and those local patients known to have commenced haemodialysis.

The previous review analysed a cohort of 197 patients undergoing initial surgery for haemodialysis access between January 1994 and March 2001. The period of assessment of patency has been extended to the end of April 2004 although no additional patients were included. Patients and operations were originally identified from the Departmental database with additional review of medical records, surgeons' records as well as the ANZDATA Registry, the national database for dialysis and transplantation when required.

The current review is restricted to the 158 patients recorded in the ANZDATA database between March 1994 and September 2003 as well as a further 3 patients known to have commenced haemodialysis but not yet registered in the ANZDATA Registry. Thirty-six patients from the previous review have therefore been excluded. The reasons for exclusion were: 6 patients previously on permanent haemodialysis were misclassified as newly commencing haemodialysis, 5 transferred to CAPD without commencing haemodialysis although the original surgery was undertaken when the management plan was for the patient to undergo haemodialysis and of the remainder, 9 were lost to follow-up, 7 died and 9 remained alive but not on yet haemodialysis. None of these 25 patients were recorded in the ANZDATA Registry as having received haemodialysis. To be formally registered, so as to exclude patients receiving temporary haemodialysis and recovering renal function or transferring to CAPD, patients must remain on haemodialysis for 60 days. However, any registered patients dying within the 60 days remain registered.

Almost all operations were performed by or under the direct care of a single vascular surgeon with a small proportion of procedures undertaken by other vascular surgeons in the Unit with experience and interest in haemodialysis access surgery.

Data was analysed from the date of commencement of haemodialysis, although initial haemodialysis need not necessarily have been via the created access. When access surgery was undertaken after the commencement of haemodialysis, then the date of surgery was used rather than the date of initial haemodialysis. Patency is defined as patent access with flows, pressures and ease of cannulation such that successful haemodialysis was achieved and maintained. Primary patency is defined as patency maintained without surgical reintervention. Secondary patency is defined as patency maintained with repeat surgical intervention including thrombectomy and revision. Primary access failure is defined as the abandonment of access due to failure to mature (for arteriovenous fistulae) or other reasons including steal or the need to undergo any further surgical intervention. Secondary access failure is defined as loss of the access despite surgical intervention. Revisions of autogenous access using prosthetic patches are classified as revisions but when long interposition prosthetic grafts are placed, the access is deemed to have failed and a new prosthetic access placed. Similarly, when short interposition grafts are used to revise prosthetic access patency is defined as maintained, but when long segment grafts eg lengths greater than half the existing prosthetic length, then the access is deemed to have failed and new access created.

Radiological procedures were not included in this review, were typically infrequently undertaken in highly selected patients, and were generally not successful in providing definitive treatment with surgical intervention usually following. Thus the estimates of the duration of primary and secondary patency would not be expected to be significantly altered by the inclusion or exclusion of these procedures.

Access type was classified according to the material used for the access rather than the configuration. Hence autogenous access comprises radio-cephalic, brachio-basilic and brachio-cephalic fistulae as well as saphenous vein grafts transplanted to the arm. Prosthetic accesses are those using prosthetic interposition grafts between arteries and grafts. Expanded PTFE with standard wall thickness was uniformly frequently used other than a small number of hybrid polyurethane grafts. All grafts were 6mm internal diameter with no tapered or flared grafts used.

The policy of placement was for autogenous access using radio-cephalic arteriovenous fistulae to be created in the non-dominant arm whenever possible. When it was judged that such access was unable to be created then alternate access was considered, usually placement of an arteriovenous graft in the non-dominant forearm. Creation of an arteriovenous fistula in the dominant arm as primary arm was occasionally undertaken but the limitation of dominant arm function whilst cannulated or the possibility of patient self-cannulation with up 20% of Australian haemodialysis patients dialysing in their own homes generally precluded this as a first choice access. The local experience of apparently reasonable secondary patencies for prosthetic access in the forearm as well as a perception of more difficult cannulation, more frequent steal phenomena and more frequent aneurysm formation with brachio-cephalic or transposed brachio-basilic fistulae meant that prosthetic access in the forearm was typically used as primary access when it was judged that a radio-cephalic fistula, if established, would be unlikely to mature as well as following failed radio-cephalic fistulae. Transplanted long saphenous veins were occasionally used early in the review period but were discontinued because of occasional leg wound problems, the requirement for general anaesthesia as well as the development of stenosis due to intimal hyperplasia. This latter complication was problematic because unlike that associated with prosthetic access that develops at the graft-vein anastomosis, intimal hyperplasia in vein grafts may develop at any point in the graft and hence repair, particularly in the presence of thrombosis, was more difficult.

Baseline co-morbidities were those recorded by the ANZDATA Registry and for the three patients not yet registered, classification was made using the same criteria.

Results

The final disposition and censoring of patients is shown in Table I. Baseline demographics, co-morbidities and final disposition and other features are shown in Tables II, III, IV for all patients and classified according to the initial and final accesses placed. The differences in proportions of patients receiving transplants and differences in age were less when patients were classified according to final rather than initial access type. The differences in numbers of operations performed and accesses placed were increased when patients were classified according to final access with patients with failed autogenous access expected to more likely receive prosthetic access subsequently than patients with failed prosthetic access to then receive autogenous access.

Table I.

Disposition of patients (n=161) at closure of review period	
Alive and well on haemodialysis	58 (36%)
Died	53 (33%)
Transplanted	40 (25%)
Transfer to CAPD	10 (6%)
Lost to follow-up	0 (0%)

Table II.

Baseline Demographics and Co-morbidities	
Male	92 (57%)
Transplanted	40 (25%)
Mean (median) age (years)	60 (63)
T/F to CAPD	10 (6%)
Died	53 (33%)
CAL	14 (9%)
IHD	55 (34%)
PAD	28 (18%)
Cerebrovascular	21 (13%)
Diabetes	31 (20%)
Hypertension	141 (91%)
Median (mean) pt follow-up (months)	39 (42)
First access median (mean) prim follow-up (months)	12 (23)
First access median (mean) secondary follow-up (months)	24 (29)
Mean (median) number accesses	1.4 (1)
Mean (median) number total operations	2.7 (2)

Patient survival is shown in Figure 1. As noted above, only 36% of patients remained alive and well and on haemodialysis at closure of the review period 37 months after the period when initial surgery was undertaken. Patients considered for transplantation were more likely to be younger and with less major co-morbidities and would have been expected to be censored by receiving a transplant whereas older, less fit patient with higher expected morbidity would be expected to remain on haemodialysis whilst they remained alive.

The secondary patencies of initial and primary and secondary accesses of all accesses placed are shown in Figures 2, 3 and 4 and the types and distribution of accesses placed shown in Tables V. There was no significant difference in median secondary patencies between autogenous and prosthetic access on Kaplan-Meier analysis, although it should be noted that the shapes of the curves differ.

The outcomes of revisions of accesses are summarised in Table VI and shows that similar proportions of prosthetic and autogenous accesses remained patent as

Table III.

Baseline Demographics, Co-morbidities and Final Disposition			
	Initial Access		
	Autogenous (n=115)	Prosthetic (n=46)	P
Male	64%	39%	0.003
Transplanted	30%	13%	0.03
Mean (median) age (years)	58 (62)	63 (68)	0.07 (0.08)
T/F to CAPD	6%	7%	0.92
Died	30%	39%	0.29
CAL	7%	13%	0.22
IHD	32%	39%	0.40
PAD	15%	26%	0.09
Cerebrovascular	11%	17%	0.30
Diabetes	18%	28%	0.16
Hypertension	91%	91%	0.99
Median (mean) pt follow-up (months)	39 (42)	38 (41)	(0.77)
First access median (mean) prim follow-up (months)	11 (24)	13 (20)	(0.40)
First access median (mean) secondary follow-up (months)	19 (30)	27 (29)	(0.92)
Mean (median) number accesses	1.5 (1)	1.3 (1)	0.20
Mean (median) number operations	2.4 (2)	3.3 (2)	0.06

can be seen in the survival charts, but that far more revisions were required for prosthetic accesses to maintain that patency. Although a much greater proportion of autogenous accesses remained revision free, a smaller proportion remained revision free and patent suggesting that many autogenous accesses considered unsatisfactory were abandoned without further attempts to improve patency.

Cox regression was applied to factors possibly associated with secondary patency of first accesses placed and patient survival and is shown in Tables VII and VIII. Only female sex was associated with increased access failure and access type in particular was not. Only increased age was associated with increased patient mortality on multivariate analysis and initial use of prosthetic access was not.

Conclusions

The previous review undertaken analysed the results of a cohort of patients identified from a surgical database. The overall patencies for autogenous access were similar to many reported series with prosthetic access patencies much higher than in other series. In that review, access patencies were calculated from the date of surgery rather

Table IV.

Demographics, Co-morbidities and Final Disposition

| | Final Access | | |
	Autogenous (n=85)	Prosthetic (n=76)	P
Male	69%	43%	0.001
Transplanted	31%	18%	0.07
Median (mean) age (years)*	66 (62)	70 (65)	(0.15)
T/F to CAPD	6%	7%	0.85
Died	29%	37%	0.32
CAL	6%	12%	0.18
IHD	28%	41%	0.09
PAD	11%	26%	0.01
Cerebrovascular	11%	16%	0.33
Diabetes	18%	25%	0.25
Hypertension	95%	87%	0.06
Median (mean) pt follow-up (months)	37 (40)	40 (43)	(0.52)
First access median (mean) primary follow-up (months)	20 (30)	7 (15)	(<0.001)
First access median (mean) secondary follow-up (months)	34 (37)	10 (20)	(<0.001)
Median (mean) number accesses	1 (1.12)	3 (1.76)	(<0.001)
Median (mean) number operations	1 (1.67)	3 (3.82)	(<0.001)

*Age at last follow-up

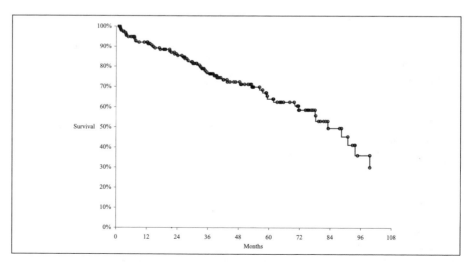

Figure 1:   Patient survival from commencement of haemodialysis. Data shown for points with SEM<10% and for n>5. Censored patients shown.

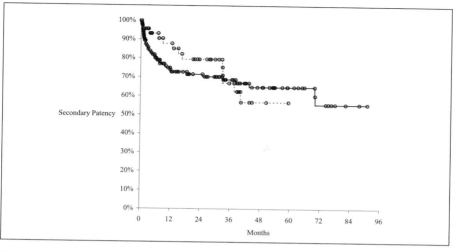

Figure 2:   Secondary patencies for first created prosthetic (——) and autogenous accesses. (____) Censored accesses shown. Points shown
for data with seem<10% and >5 accesses.

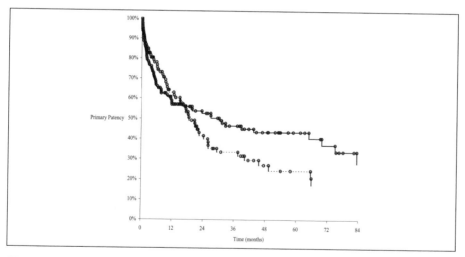

Figure 3:   Primary patencies for all created prosthetic (——) and autogenous
accesses. (____) Censored accesses shown. Points shown for
data with seem<10% and >5 accesses.

the date of cannulation or commencement of haemodialysis. However, these
patients may possibly have had better apparent access patencies due to potentially short follow-up as well as inclusion of patency times prior to commencement
of haemodialysis. On the other hand, all procedures were necessarily assessed
including those accesses failing prior to the commencement to haemodialysis.
Furthermore, not all patients who underwent surgery commenced haemodialysis,
with some patients either dying before commencing haemodialysis, choosing not

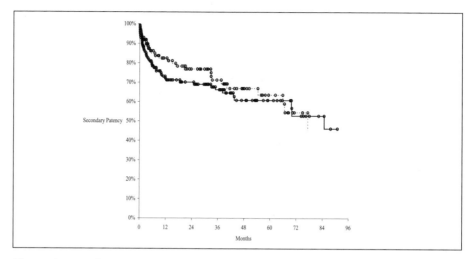

Figure 4:   Secondary patencies for all created prosthetic (———) and autoge-
             nous accesses. (___) Censored accesses shown. Points shown for
             data with seem<10% and >5 accesses.

Table V.

Distribution of accesses placed

	Initial (n=161)	Subsequent (n=68)	Final (n=161)
Autogenous	115 (71%)	15 (22%)	85 (53%)
Prosthetic	46 (29%)	53 (78%)	76 (47%)

Table VI.

	Autogenous	Prosthetic
Number created	130	99
Remaining Patent	85 (65%)	70 (71%)
Accesses Revised	35 (27%)	52 (53%)
Accesses Revised and Remaining Patent	16 (46%)	19 (37%)
Total Revisions	53	150
Accesses Revision Free	95 (73%)	47 (47%)
Accesses Revision Free and Patent	65 (68%)	38 (81%)

to undergo haemodialysis, receiving a transplant or converting to CAPD. These
patients and accesses may possibly have a worse outcome than those commencing haemodialysis.

The current review used patients registered with the national ANZDATA Registry
in September 2003 as well as 3 local patients not yet registered. Patency was assessed
from the date of haemodialysis when haemodialysis was commenced after access
surgery. It is arguable what is the most appropriate method of assessment of patency
but the methods used in this study to assess patency as well as classification of access
are consistent with many other reports, although comparison can be problematic.

Table VII.

Univariate Analysis of Factors Associated with Secondary Patency of First Access Placed

	Coefficient	SE	p	Hazard Ratio	95% CI	
COAD	0.38	0.41	0.35	1.46	0.66	3.26
IHD	0.32	0.29	0.26	1.38	0.79	2.41
PVD	0.45	0.32	0.16	1.57	0.83	2.95
Cerebral	0.06	0.41	0.88	1.06	0.48	2.36
Diabetes	-0.21	0.35	0.55	0.81	0.41	1.62
Hypertension	-0.41	0.48	0.38	0.66	0.26	1.68
Age (yrs)	0.00	0.01	0.98	1.00	0.98	1.02
Sex	-0.62	0.28	0.03	0.54	0.31	0.94
Fistula	-0.09	0.31	0.77	0.91	0.49	1.69
Radial access	-0.26	0.34	0.45	0.77	0.40	1.51

*only factor significant on multi-variate analysis

Table VIII.

Univariate Analysis of Factors Associated with Patient Survival

	Coefficient	SE	P	Hazard Ratio	95% CI	
COAD	0.81	0.39	0.04	2.26	1.05	4.83
IHD	0.72	0.28	0.01	2.06	1.19	3.55
PVD	0.39	0.31	0.21	1.48	0.80	2.74
Cerebral	0.74	0.31	0.02	2.10	1.14	3.88
Diabetes	0.32	0.31	0.31	1.37	0.74	2.53
Hypertension	-0.22	0.61	0.71	0.80	0.24	2.62
Age*	0.06	0.01	<0.001	1.06	1.03	1.09
Sex	-0.52	0.28	0.06	0.60	0.35	1.03
Fistula	0.35	0.29	0.23	1.42	0.80	2.51
Radial access	0.21	0.31	0.50	1.23	0.67	2.28

*only factor significant on multi-variate analysis

Definition of primary, assisted primary and secondary patency is well defined for peripheral arterial reconstructive surgery and recently guidelines for the reporting of results for renal dialysis access surgery has been proposed in the United States[2]. Nonetheless, many authors continue to report data that do not appear to follow these guidelines, are internally inconsistent and difficult to compare with other results. Examples include exclusions of fistulae failing to mature, failure to distinguish sites and types of autogenous access, failure to exclude patent but non-functional accesses, failure to include accesses removed for steal, aneurysm or infection, failure to define elective two-stage fistulae procedures such as transloca-tion of basilic veins as failure of primary patency, use of interval rather than over-all patency, and failure to distinguish prior haemodialysis status of patients as either initial or long-term.

The current recommendations[3] for creation of permanent haemodialysis of a high rate of autogenous usage are at least in part based on the perception of poor long-term results using prosthetic access. The current review shows a secondary patency similar to or higher than that for autogenous access is achievable using prosthetic access although significantly more interventions were required to maintain that patency. Data was not kept on the need for temporary central venous cannulation, although the author would contend that the morbidity and occasional mortality associated with the use of central catheters is at least in part a function the duration that the catheter is in situ for as well as the need for line changes. The morbidity of short-term perioperative cannulation such as may be required when patients present with thrombosed but salvageable access is low and much less than that associated with longer-term cannulation such as may be required whilst accesses mature.

It is contended that part of the benefit of autogenous access is a lower rate of complications. This is certainly true for radio-cephalic fistulae but there is possibly a higher rate of steal, aneurysm formation and revision required for autogenous access not using radio-cephalic fistulae ie. brachio-basilic, brachio-cephalic fistulae or saphenous vein based access. Most authors appear to have increased the rate of autogenous access usage by increased rates of utilisation of the latter accesses rather than improving the numbers or patencies of radio-cephalic fistulae. However, this is difficult to determine from the literature as the types of autogenous access are not always defined and complications or revision rates are usually not linked to the type of autogenous access. The current review has a very high proportion of functioning radio-cephalic fistulae with a low rate of revision and complications.

Furthermore, the type of access placed could be classified according to the haemodynamics as fistulae ie direct arterio-venous anastomosis or as interposition grafts rather than the vessel wall. The haemodynamics of the two forms of access are quite different, although clearly prosthetic grafts have different compliance to native vein and are lined by pseudo-intima rather than intima.

It also been suggested that the initial use of prosthetic access is associated with significantly increased mortality. Furthermore, use of autogenous access in these patients would only be expected to be associated with improved survival if the mortality was directly due to the prosthetic access or its complications rather than pre-existing patient related factors. An association between initial or final access type and mortality was not observed in this review on univariate analysis, with only age significantly associated with mortality in a multivariate model. Thus the proposition that prosthetic access should be avoided for this reason is not supported by the current data. Furthermore, there were significant baseline differences between patients receiving prosthetic and autogenous access with those receiving autogenous access more likely to be male and subsequently receive a transplant. There was also a strong trend (p=0.07) for these patients to be younger. It may therefore be argued that the baseline differences between patients receiving different accesses and not merely surgeon choice is partly responsible for the choice of initial access used. When patients were classified according to final access, the difference in gender (possible related to anatomical size of the vessels) is clearly present but other differences are less apparent.

More surgical interventions are required to maintain secondary patency for prosthetic access. Although the reasons for failure of patency of access were not formally classified and the decision to abandon access clinically rather than protocol based, the most common cause of early primary failure of autogenous access was failure to mature whereas thrombosis or intimal hyperplasia accounted for most primary failures for prosthetic access. The primary patency of prosthetic access exceeded that for autogenous access for the first fifteen months after access placement or commencement of haemodialysis. Because of the mechanism of failure of the access ie. the cephalic vein being judged unlikely to ultimately mature, less subsequent salvage procedures were undertaken on autogenous accesses, the access adjudged to have failed and reconstruction of alternate access undertaken.

No routine vein mapping was undertaken during this period. Fistulography and duplex were selectively used for autogenous accesses failing to mature to identify adequate sized but non-accessible veins that could be mobilised. Problems with established accesses were identified by low flow or increasing venous pressure. The patients generally underwent angiographic assessment and occasionally ultrasound. Routine ultrasound assessment of accesses was not undertaken. Stenoses at venous anastomoses of stenosed access grafts were repaired surgically rather than dilated. Some authors have suggested that routine pre-operative vessel assessment with ultrasound and routine access assessment such as with flow studies improve outcomes. In the current review, the long-term patency of accesses both prosthetic and autogenous is high. Pre-operative scanning may have increased the success of autogenous access by correctly identifying veins unlikely to mature but utilisation of autogenous access may have fallen. Assisted primary patency may have been increased by routine access surveillance but it is less clear that secondary patency would be increased by routine surveillance. Furthermore, some studies have suggested that routine surveillance results in a much greater rate of intervention with associated increased costs.

The decision to abandon autogenous access was not usually made until haemodialysis commenced with only three fistulae abandoned after surgery but before haemodialysis. In the current review, there is a high rate of early failure of autogenous access, with 18 of 37 failures of initially placed autogenous access occurring within 90 days of commencement of haemodialysis. These accesses were placed a median of only 18 days prior to commencing haemodialysis. Should these accesses been deemed to have failed prior to haemodialysis commencing, then the apparent patency rates for autogenous access may have been much higher.

References

1. Fisher CM, Neale NL. Outcome of surgery for vascular access in patients commencing haemodialysis. *Eur J Vasc Endovasc Surg.* 2003;73: 615-20.
2. Sidawy AN, Gray R, Besarab A, et al. Recommended standards for reports dealing with arteriovenous hemodialysis access. *J Vasc Surg.* 2002;35:603-10.
3. NKF-DOQI clinical practice guidelines for vascular access: Guideline 29: Goals of access placement: Maximising primary A-V fistulae. *Am J Kidney Dis.* 2001;37(Suppl 1):75-85.

22

TO THIGH OR NOT TO THIGH, SHOULD A PROSTHETIC GRAFT BE PLACED?

Marc H. Glickman, MD[1], Howard E. Katzman, MD[2],
Jeffrey H. Lawson, MD, PhD[3]

Vascular & Transplant Specialists, Eastern Virginia Medical School,
Norfolk, Virginia.
Cedars Medical Center, Miami, Florida
Duke University Medical School, Durham, North Carolina

CONTACT INFORMATION FOR ALL AUTHORS
Marc H. Glickman, MD
Vascular & Transplant Specialists
880 Kempsville Road, Suite 1000
Norfolk, VA 23502
Phone: 757-466-6513
Fax: 757-466-8698
Email: mglickman@vascularandtransplant.com

Howard E. Katzman, MD
Surgical Group of Miami
1321 N.W. 14th St., Suite #306
Miami, FL 33125
Phone: 305-324-4840
Fax: 305-545-9562
Email: hkatzman4@adelphia.net

Jeffrey H. Lawson, MD, PhD
Duke Univ. Medical Center
RM 479 MSRB Research Dr., Box 2622
Durham, NC 27710
Phone: 919-681-6432
Fax: 919-681-1094
Email: lawso006@mc.duke.edu

SUPPORT:

All authors received reimbursement from Hancock Jaffe Laboratories, Inc., for costs of conducting the clinical investigation for the MVB graft. None of the authors have a direct financial relationship with Hancock Jaffe Laboratories or a financial interest in the Mesenteric Vein Bioprosthetic graft.

Introduction

The increasing longevity of end stage renal disease (ESRD) patients has influenced the likelihood that multiple hemoaccess sites and a variety of access options will be utilized during the course of a patient's treatment. The necessity of providing a means of continued hemoaccess after preferred upper extremity sites become unavailable has prompted some to advise that when upper extremity sites have been exhausted, the lower extremity should be considered as an access site.[1]

Clinical experience using prosthetic hemoaccess grafts in the lower extremity has been variable; however, much of the reported experience has resulted in the thigh being avoided as an access site in most cases. Several studies have described the significant effort required to maintain lower extremity polytetraflouroethylene (PTFE) grafts due to higher rates of graft complications and infection in particular, with 16% to 41% of grafts infected.[2-7] Some have recommended that the thigh be avoided and that these patients be treated with tunneled dialysis catheters. Unacceptable complication rates observed with cryopreserved femoral vein are responsible for the conclusion that the routine use of cryopreserved femoral vein in the thigh position should be avoided.[8] In contrast, several publications report patency and complication rates for PTFE grafts in the thigh comparable to upper extremity grafts, prompting one author to conclude "the femoral artery – vein graft should be regarded as an alternative means for both primary or secondary haemodialysis access."[9,10]

The ProCol® bovine mesenteric vein bioprosthesis (MVB) is an alternative graft material designed to demonstrate compliance and handling properties similar to native vein. Acceptable patency and complication rates have been achieved in challenging vascular access patients with the Mesenteric Vein Bioprosthesis[11-15]. In this prospective study, the MVB graft is evaluated in the thigh position after one or more prior synthetic access grafts have already failed.

Methods

Between October 1999 and February 2002, 52 patients were enrolled in a study to evaluate the MVB as an access conduit. This study was conducted at three participating sites under an Investigational Device Exemption approved by the Food and Drug Administration. The protocol was approved by each center's Institutional Review Board prior to initiating the study at each site and all subjects gave informed consent. Criteria for patient inclusion in the study were; a history of a prior failed synthetic graft(s), in addition to any native fistula or catheter-based access, and the absence of systemic septic disease or preexisting localized infection at the time of implant. Enrollment at the participating investigational sites was: Vascular & Transplant Specialist, Eastern Virginia Medical School, Norfolk, Virginia, (n=22), Cedars Medical Center, Miami, Florida (n=15); Duke University Medical Center, Durham, North Carolina (n=13) All subjects received a 6-mm MVB (ProCol® graft, Hancock Jaffe Laboratories, Inc., Irvine, CA).

Follow-up examinations were performed 6 weeks, 6 months, and 12 months postoperatively and at six-month intervals thereafter by a combination of the implanting surgeon, nephrologists or dialysis clinic nurse in charge. Graft patency rates were generated using the Kaplan-Meier survival curve analysis. All patients were included in the intent to treat group for analysis with censoring at the time of death, lost to follow-up, or withdrawal. Definitions for primary and secondary patency were taken from the recommended standards for reports dealing with arteriovenous hemodialysis accesses.[16] Complications, graft interventions, total number of events, the linearized rate (events/graft year), and the number of grafts with events were computed. Statistical analyses were performed using SAS® (version 8.2, Cary, NC).

Results

Fifty-two grafts were implanted in 52 patients. Patient demographics were largely female (67%) and African American (65%). The mean patient age was 49.5 ±14.2 yrs. Forty-four percent of all patients entering the study were diabetic and 89% were hypertensive. All patients had a history of failed prostheses prior to entering this study; mean 2.7 ±1.4 prior synthetic grafts (range 1–6 grafts). In 13 cases (26%), a synthetic graft had previously been placed in the same lower extremity limb. Implant position was femoral artery-femoral vein (35), femoral artery- saphenous vein (15), femoral artery-iliac vein (1), and iliac artery-iliac vein (1).

Follow-up totaled 77.4 graft years (928.7 grafts months). Mean follow-up was18.6 months. Thirteen (25%) patients died prior to study completion of causes unrelated to the graft. Two of these patients died within the first 30 days and were excluded from the analysis leaving 50 patients in this study. Three patients withdrew from the study when a kidney transplant was received (n=1), a request was made to discontinue dialysis treatment (n=1), or the patient requested access at a different location (1). One patient could not be located and was considered lost to follow-up 18 months into the study.

Primary patency for the entire intent to treat group was 44.2% (12 mo), 22.8% (24 mo) and 19% (36 mo). Primary assisted patency rates were 52.5% (12mo), 43.9% (24 mo), and 39% (36 mo) (Fig. 1). Secondary patency 12, 24 and 36 months post implant was 70.9%, 69.0% and 64.9%, respectively (Fig. 2). Eighty-two percent of grafts implanted were successfully accessed. Nine grafts were abandoned without the graft ever being accessed for the following reasons; death (n=2), graft abandoned for infection (n=3), technical related to patient's anatomy (n=3) and early thrombosis due to hypotensive state followed by graft infection post intervention (n=1).

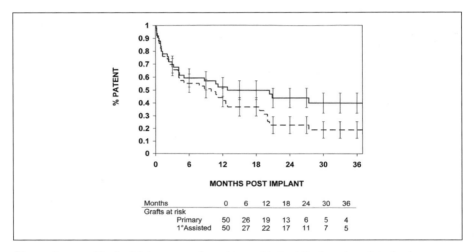

Figure 1:   Kaplin-Meier curve for primary (dotted line) and assisted primary (solid line) patency. Error Bars ± 1 Standard Error (Greenwood).

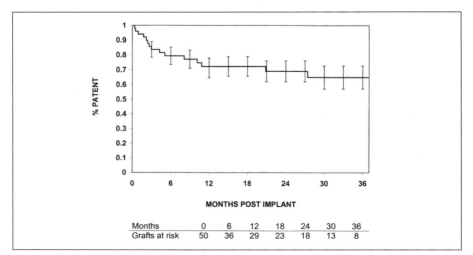

Figure 2:   Secondary patency by Kaplin-Meier analysis. Error Bars ± 1 Standard Error (Greenwood).

Twenty-four thrombotic events (0.31/graft yr) occurred in 17 grafts (34%). Seven (29%) of all thromboses occurred within 30 days of implant, four of which were salvaged. These early thrombosis were related to outflow stenosis (n=1), kinking at the anastomosis (n=1), hypotensive condition (n=2), and post cannulation compression (n=1). During the entire study, four grafts were abandoned for thrombosis directly related to a stenotic outflow vein, a fifth graft thrombosed and could not be salvaged due to the patient's hypercoagulable state and one graft thrombosed with no information available.

Complications other than thrombosis included infection in seven grafts (14%), five of which were secondary to wound infection. Two events occurred within the first 30 days and five were late events. Treatment was graft explant (n=5), ligation (n=1) and one access was revised and salvaged. Post cannulation bleeding (n=3) required the surgical repair of two grafts and a third access was ligated. One bleeding incident from an eroded area required revision of the affected area of the graft and replacement with an interposition graft. Another graft was repaired to control bleeding related to the patient's hypertensive condition. Two of the three grafts (6%) with pseudoaneurysmal dilatation were salvaged with an interposition graft and one was ligated. Post cannulation hematomas were evacuated (n=2) and slow healing wounds involving three grafts required evacuation or revision of the affected area. Overall complications occurred at a rate of 0.90/yr (Table I). Twenty-nine grafts (58%) were complication free.

Fifty-three interventions in 29 grafts were required to maintain graft patency (0.68/yr). Twenty assist angioplasties were performed in 13 grafts. Thrombectomies (n=12) were both percutaneous and surgical procedures. Graft revision with or without concurrent thrombectomy (n=21) was the most prevalent procedure accounting for 40% of all interventions.

Conclusions

Comparisons to patency rates in the published literature are often misleading as inclusion and censoring criteria impact calculations and results. Two recent publications utilized criteria comparable to the SVS reporting standards adopted for this

Table 1.   Graft complications – number of events requiring intervention and rate of occurrence. Total graft years for calculation of linearized rate is 77.4.

Complication	# Events	# Grafts	Event rate/yr
Thrombosis	24	17	0.31
Infection	7	7	0.09
Bleeding	5	5	0.07
Pseudoaneurysm / dilatation	4	3	0.05
Wound healing	3	3	0.04
Hematoma w/ evacuation	2	2	0.02
Steal symptoms	0	0	N/A
Seroma	0	0	N/A

study and offer data suitable for comparison. These studies reported cumulative patency rates at 24 months (54% and 40%) for studies of 116 and 63 PTFE grafts.[3,10] We achieved a superior patency rate (69.0%) at the same 24 month postoperative interval with the MVB graft. Furthermore, the intervention rate required to maintain the MVB grafts was lower (0.68 / yr) compared to 1.68 and 1.15 interventions/yr for PTFE.

Several authors have commented upon the greater number of technical failures in upper extremity grafts. In one study there were nearly twice as many technical failures, instances where a graft either could not be placed or failure was immediate, in the thigh position (6.8% of all procedures were technical failures) compared to upper extremity procedures.[10] In a group of 134 PTFE grafts, 28% experienced early thrombosis.[7] In this study of 50 MVB grafts, 14% thrombosed within 30 days of implant.

Graft infection is the complication most associated with lower extremity access and is often the reason why surgeons shy away from the groin area. In our study infection was reported in 14% of all grafts implanted yet this result is acceptable for this indication and is lower that most reports in the published literature (Figure 2.) Lower limb ischemia is also a serious issue in the ESRD population. In one study of 116 patients, 11% presented with ipsilateral limb ischemia after receiving a PTFE graft for access in the thigh requiring nine major limb amputations, and two graft ligations.[3] In our study there were no symptoms of steal, and no sequela of limb ischemia.

Alternative placements and the use of autologous material utilized in an effort to improve the outcome have offered mixed results and leave unresolved issues. In a recent report of 14 PTFE grafts placed in the suprapatellar location, avoiding the groin area, the rate of infection was reduced to 1 graft. However, a higher rate of abandonment due to thromboses resulted in only 18% of grafts still patent after 24 months.[17] Autologous femoral vein transposition has been explored as an alternative to synthetic graft placement. One recent study directly compared results for 17 patients with synthetic femoral loop grafts to 15 patients with autologous femoral vein transpositions. Although the occurrence of infection was similar for both

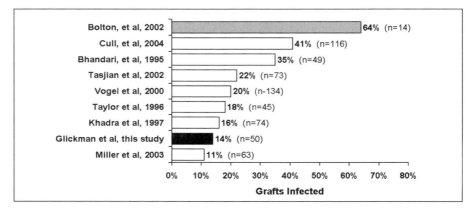

Figure 3:   Incidence of infection for thigh grafts per published literature. Cryopreserved femoral vein (gray), PTFE (white) and MVB – this study (black)

groups (35.3% vs 26.7%), infection was more likely to be resolved with medication in the autologous group. Symptoms of steal developed in 33% of femoral vein transposition patients, resulting in two banding procedures and the abandonment of one site.[18] Another analysis of 25 patients with transposed superficial femoral vein fistulas reported no infections but observed that a major impediment to the procedure was a high incidence of postoperative ischemia requiring that 8 of 25 patients undergo reoperation to correct the effects of a steal syndrome.[19]

In conclusion, by using the MVB graft, acceptable lower risk factors, improved patency rates and lower intervention rates, allow the thigh position to be utilized in these challenging, often high risk patients. Satisfactory cumulative patency was maintained with reasonable effort and an acceptable rate of complications.

References

1. Weiswasser JM, Kellicut D, Arora S, Sidawy A. Strategies of arteriovenous dialysis access. *Semin Vasc Surg.* 2004; 17(1):10-18.
2. Bhandari S, Wilkinson A, Sellars L. Saphenous vein forearm grafts and Gortex thigh grafts as alternative forms of vascular access. *Clinical Nephrol.* 1995; 44(5).325-328.
3. Cull JD, Cull DL, Taylor SM, et al. Prosthetic thigh arteriovenous access: Outcome with SVS/AAVS reporting standards. *J Vasc Surg.* 2004; 39(2).381-386.
4. Khadra MH, Dwyer AJ, Thompson JF. Advantages of polytetrafluoroethylene arteriovenous loops in the thigh for hemodialysis access. *Am J Surg.* 1997; 173(4).280-283.
5. Tashjian DB, Lipkowitz GS, Madden RL, et al. Safety and efficacy of femoral-based hemodialysis access grafts. *J Vasc Surg.* 2002; 35(4).691-693.
6. Taylor SM, Eaves GL, Weatherford DA, et al. Results and complications of arteriovenous access dialysis grafts in the lower extremity: A five year review. *Am Surg.* 1996; 62(3).188-191.
7. Vogel KM, Martino MA, O'Brien S, et al. Complications of lower extremity arteriovenous grafts in patients with end-stage renal disease. *South Med J* 2000; 93(3).593-595.
8. Bolton WD, Cull DL, Taylor SM, et al. The use of cryopreserved femoral vein grafts for hemodialysis access in patients at high risk for infection: A word of caution. *J Vasc Surg.* 2002; 36(3).464-468.
9. Korzets A, Ori Y, Baytner S, et al. The femoral artery-femoral vein polytetrafluoroethylene graft: a 14-year retrospective study. *Nephrol Dial Transplant.* 1998; 13(4).1215-1220.
10. Miller CD, Robbin ML, Barker J, Allon M. Comparison of arteriovenous grafts in the thigh and upper extremities in hemodialysis patients. *J Am Soc Nephrol.* 2003; 14(11).2942-2947.
11. Bacchini G, Del Vecchio L, Andrulli S. Survival of prosthetic grafts of different materials after impairment of a native arteriovenous fistula in hemodialysis patients. *ASAIO J.* 2001; 47(1).30-33.
12. Glickman MH, Lawson JH, Katzman HE, Schild AF, Fujitani RM. Challenges of hemodialysis access for high risk patients: Impact of mesenteric vein bioprosthetic graft. *J Vasc Access.* 2003; 4.73-80.

13. Hatzibaloglou A, Vesissaris I, Kaitzis D, et al. ProCol vascular bioprosthesis for vascular access: midterm results. *Journal of Vascular Access.* 2004; 5.

14. Senkaya I, Aytac II, Eercan AK, et al. The graft selection for haemodialysis. *Vasa.* 2003; 32(4).209-213.

15. Scher LA, Katzman HE. Alternative graft materials for hemodialysis access. *Semin Vasc Surg.* 2004; 17(1).19-24.

16. Sidawy AN, Gray R, Besarab A, at al. Recommended standards for reports dealing with arteriovenous hemodialysis accesses. *J Vasc Surg.* 2002; 35(3).603-610.

17. Flarup S, Hadimieri H. Arteriovenous PTFE dialysis access in the lower extremity: a new approach. *Ann Vasc Surg.* 2003; 17(5).581-584.

18. Hazinedaroglu SM, Tuzuner A, Demirer S, et al. Femoral vein transposition versus femoral loop grafts for hemodialysis: a prospective evaluation. *Transplant Proc.* 2004; 36:65-67.

19. Gradman WS, Cohen W, Haji-Aghaii M. Arteriovenous fistula construction in the thigh with transposed superficial femoral vein: Our initial experience. *J Vasc Surg.* 2001; 33(5).968-975.

DISCUSSION

Vascular Access for Hemodialysis IX
May 6-7, 2004
Lake Buena Vista, Florida

May 7, 2004
Abstract Session III

Dr. Marc Glickman
"To Thigh or Not to Thigh, Should a Prosthetic Graft be Placed?"

Question: You said there was no seromas but that certainly is an area that there is a lot of lymphatics. Did you have any persistent lymphatic leaks?

Glickman: None.

Question: You had no incidences of steal or significant ischemia. What criteria do you use to screen patients and rule out those that are not candidates?

Glickman: Palpable pulses and a full arterial examination. We do not place the graft in an area where they may undergo a segmental angioplasty. The majority of our patients, if they have SFA stenosis, they have had a pretty aggressive vascular workup to make sure their vascular status is adequate.

Question: Where do you find these patients? Diabetics with previous amputations?

Glickman: We service an area of, for example we have 1,800 covered lives. We have a very large dialysis population. We service 44 dialysis units.

Question: When you have to do a revision around a pseudoaneurysm, what material do you use for the revision? Do you use Procol or Goretex?

Glickman: I use Procol for all of these. This was within the study and we continue to use Procol for that to maintain that compliance within the graft.

Question: What is the difference between primary and primary assisted versus secondary?

Glickman: Primary patency rate is patency of a graft without any type of interventions. It ends when a graft does occlude or when its first occlusion occurs without any type of intervention. Primary assisted patency is after interventions that we do to maintain graft patency without any events of thrombosed. So all of those grafts, none of those grafts have thrombosis. Some of those thrombosis grafts require interventions, angioplastys, etc. Secondary patency is graft functionality. In other words, how long is the survival of that graft? You saw in our study 67% of those grafts survived for 36 months.

Question: Which is more expensive, Procol or PTFE?

Glickman: Procol is more expensive but I think that our patency rates are better. In the data that we have seen over and over again for the complicated patient, probably it is well worth the cost. I think it is not only the cost today, it is cost in the future. That is what we are most concerned about. It may cost $400 more today but you are preventing thousands of dollars worth of complications and lives.

23

EXPANDED POLYTETRAFLUOROETHYLENE AND NITINOL STENT-GRAFT FOR SALVAGE TREATMENT OF VASCULAR ACCESS SITES: INITIAL EXPERIENCE

John Ross, MD

Address correspondence to
John R. Ross, MD,
PO Box 908, Bamberg, SC 29003;
telephone: 803-245-4327; fax: 803-245-6276; e-mail:
JRRsurgery@aol.com

Introduction

Obtaining vascular access for long-term hemodialysis without insertion of a central venous catheter is a challenge in many patients with end-stage renal disease (ESRD), especially those who are morbidly obese and those in whom several arteriovenous (AV) grafts have failed. In such patients, because of the presence of venous stenosis, the only appropriate outflow vein for an AV graft may be centrally located, a condition that presents a considerable surgical dilemma.

In the past 15 years, several new endovascular techniques, including placement of stents and stent-grafts (covered stents), have been used in attempts to restore the patency of AV access grafts. Results have been variable, partly because of differences in the materials and techniques used and the locations of stenoses within the vascular grafts.[1] Uncovered stents were first employed to treat venous stenosis in dialysis shunts in 1989.[2] Since then, use of these devices has been found to be safe, but patency rates have generally been no higher than those obtained with percutaneous transluminal angioplasty (PTA).[3-5] However, several authors have noted that insertion of a stent was successful in salvaging AV access grafts in patients in whom angioplasty and multiple surgical revisions had failed.[6-8]

Clinical experience with covered stents in the treatment of access problems has so far been limited to case reports and small series. Again, results have been equivocal. In a series of 20 patients,[9] stent-grafts covered with polyester were found to be safe and effective in salvaging vascular access grafts in the upper arm. In a series of 14 patients, Sapoval et al[10] found that polyester-covered stents were useful in treating angioplasty-induced ruptures in dialysis accesses; however, the devices did not prevent stenosis and there was an inflammatory reaction of unknown origin.

Treatment of pseudoaneurysms in dialysis grafts by insertion of stents covered with polyethylene terephthalate was reported to prolong the functional life of the grafts in three cases described by Silas and Bettmann[11] and in a series of 10 patients reported by Najibi et al.[12]

Rabindranauth and Shindelman,[11] Quinn et al,[12] and Masuda et al[13] all constructed stent-grafts by suturing an expanded polytetrafluoroethylene (ePTFE) vascular graft to the outside of a metallic stent. These covered grafts were then used to treat pseudoaneurysms, vascular ruptures, and stenoses in patients with ESRD receiving dialysis. Rabindranauth and Shindelman[12] described two patients in whom pseudoaneurysms were successfully excluded by use of these devices and patency was retained during a follow-up period of up to 6 months. In a series of 17 patients, Quinn et al[12] had a technical success rate of 100% for insertion of ePTFE-covered stents used to treat ruptures, stenoses associated with an aneurysm, and occlusive disease and central stenoses not responsive to angioplasty. Although patency rates were similar to those achieved with PTA and uncovered stents, the authors noted that they had used early generation stent-graft technology and suggested that future stent-grafts could yield better results. Masuda et al[13] inserted a customized stent covered with ePTFE at the venous end of an AV fistula to create an access pathway in eight patients who had a mean of 3.8 failed vascular accesses. There were two early failures, but three of the remaining six grafts were patent for more than a year and two grafts were still functioning 22 and 13 months, respectively, after insertion.

A self-expanding, longitudinally flexible stent-graft consisting of a nitinol support system and an ePTFE lining (VIABAHN Endoprosthesis, W.L. Gore & Associates, Inc., Flagstaff, AZ) is now available. This endoprosthesis has been found to be effective in treating occlusion due to diffuse iliofemoral disease,[14] as well as true aneurysms of the subclavian artery in patients with connective tissue disorders.[15] A novel procedure uses the Viabahn device in combination with a special surgical approach in an attempt to meet outflow vein challenges and salvage the AV access in patients undergoing long-term dialysis. The procedure includes a no-suture venous anastomosis and an outflow vein technique employing both the endoprosthesis and a newly implanted ePTFE vascular graft. We here describe our initial experience with this procedure in a series of 11 patients.

Methods

Beginning in April 2003, patients were considered for insertion of a Viabahn endoprosthesis if they had a failing or failed AV access graft, potential for sufficient venous outflow and a willingness and ability to comply with required preoperative and postoperative clinical evaluations. Patients in whom standard procedures for treating the access (for example, implantation of a jump graft or use of PTA) could be used and those allergic to contrast media were excluded from the series. In addition, patients were not included unless they were found to have a central outflow vein of at least 7 mm in diameter that could be reached with a Viabahn device, adequate inflow (systolic blood pressure greater than 140 mmHg), and a brachial artery of at least 3.5 mm in diameter for the arterial anastomosis. All patients who underwent insertion of a Viabahn endoprosthesis provided written informed consent to the procedure.

The insertion procedure (Figure 1) is performed under fluoroscopic control and with the patient under local anesthesia. It begins with a cut-down identification of a small vein in the axilla. An 18-gauge cannulation needle is used to access the small vein, and a 0.035-inch guidewire is placed centrally. The cannulation needle is removed, followed by a 7Fr sheath to introduce contrast. Angiovenography is performed to locate any stenoses; ensure that the vein is at least 7 mm in diameter if necessary, PTA is applied.

Next, a segment of the brachial artery above the elbow is identified. A new 6-mm ePTFE graft is tunneled from the antecubital area to the axilla. A Viabahn endoprosthesis (7 mm by 15 cm) is threaded over the backloaded wire through the graft and into the outflow vein. When the device is positioned so that it overlaps the ePTFE graft by 2.5 to approximately 3 cm, it is deployed. The anastomosis between the

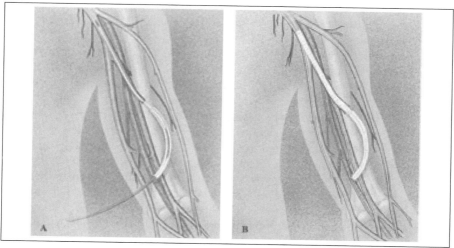

Figure 1:   Procedure for insertion of a Viabahn endoprosthesis. (A) The Viabahn device is inserted over a guidewire, through the tunneled vascular graft, and into a small vein. The distal end of the device is positioned in a central vein, and the overlap between the device and the vascular graft is about 3 cm. (B) The Viabahn is deployed and inflated with a balloon, creating a sealed, sutureless anastomosis between the device and the vein and between the device and the vascular graft. A standard suture anastomosis is made between the vascular graft and the brachial artery.

endoprosthesis and vascular graft is sutureless. The medial portion of the stent-graft extends into the outflow vein having a diameter of at least 7 mm.

A 7-mm PTA balloon is used to complete expansion of the Viabahn device. Two seals are immediately created: one at the interface between the endoprosthesis and the vascular graft (as a result of their 1-cm difference in diameter) and one at the interface between the endoprosthesis and the axillary vein. Venography through the vascular graft is performed to verify complete deployment of the stent-graft and identify any areas of stricture. Such areas are treated by balloon catheter application. A standard suture technique is used for the anastomosis between the proximal portion of the vascular graft and the brachial artery. Routine clinical examinations and duplex ultrasound assessments were performed approximately 3, 6, and 12 months postoperatively. Data from the patients' records were compiled and entered into a dedicated computer database.

Follow-up in this series consisted of postprocedure ultrasonographic assessments. Data from the patients' records were compiled and entered into a database for analysis. Patency rates were calculated by using survival analysis.

Results

Eleven patients (age range, 42 to 81 years) underwent the Viabahn insertion procedure. All patients had diabetes and hypertension, most were obese, and one was positive for human immunodeficiency virus. Overall, the patients had a mean of 2.5 previously failed access grafts (range, 0 to 5).

No complications occurred during insertion of the Viabahn device. The initial success rate (patency) after insertion was 100%. Hemodialysis was resumed after the usual maturation time for vascular access grafts. Cannulation of the Viabahn device is not recommended, but in most cases, it is positioned too deeply to be reached by a cannulation needle.

The postoperative follow-up time in the series thus far ranges from 4 to 11 months (mean, 6.8). Five patients have had no complications or graft-patency problems (4 to 8 months after the procedure). One patient died of causes unrelated to vascular access 7 months postoperatively, without experiencing access problems. Central stenosis developed in two patients and was treated successfully by PTA. Another patient also required PTA. Thrombosis developed in a patient with a known coagulopathy; PTA thrombectomy was successful in reestablishing patency and no stenosis was observed. A mild ischemic hand syndrome developed in another patient 2 months after the procedure, and the graft was ligated. This problem was assumed to be the result of lost inflow because the artery chosen was too small to handle both the flow to the hand and that to the graft. There was one graft infection, which was treated by segmental resection.

As shown in Figure 2, the primary patency rate for access salvage in this series was 100% at 3 months (11 patients) and 82% at 6 months (7 patients; 95% confidence interval [CI], 58% to 100%). The graft in the one patient who has had the Viabahn device in place for 11 months is patent.

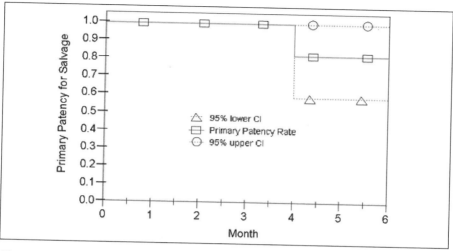

Figure 2:   Results of survival analysis showing primary patency (to 6 months) for salvage of vascular graft dialysis access in 11 patients who underwent insertion of a Viabahn endoprosthesis. CI denotes confidence interval.

Conclusions

Use of the Viabahn Endoprosthesis made it possible for the patients in this series to continue to undergo hemodialysis through the same limb and obviated the need for catheters. The patency of the vascular access grafts during the post-procedure observation period was satisfactory. Additional research is required to assess the long-term effectiveness and safety of the Viabahn endoprosthesis in AV access salvage.

References

1. Bush RL, Lin PL, Lumsden AB. Management of thrombosed dialysis access: thrombectomy versus thrombolysis. *Semin Vasc Surg.* 2004; 17.32-39.
2. Gunther RW, Vorwerk D, Bohndorf K. Venous stenoses in dialysis shunts: treatment with self-expanding metallic stents. *Radiology.* 1989; 170.401-405.
3. Patel RI, Peck SH, Cooper SG, et al. Patency of Wallstents placed across the venous anatomosis of hemodialysis grafts after percutaneous recanalization. *Radiology.* 1998; 209.365-370.
4. Hoffer EK, Sultan S, Herskowitz MM, Daniels ID, Sclafani SJ. Prospective randomized trial of a metallic intravascular stent in hemodialysis graft maintenance. *J Vasc Interv Radiol.* 1997; 8.965-973.
5. Vorwerk D, Guenther RW, Mann H, et al. Venous stenosis and occlusion in hemodialysis shunts: follow-up results of stent placement in 65 patients. *Radiology.* 1995; 195.140-146.

6. Zaleski GX, Funaki B, Rosenblum J, Theoharis J, Leef J. Metallic stents deployed in synthetic arteriovenous hemodialysis grafts. *AJR Am J Roentgenol.* 2001; 176.1515-1519.

7. Gray RJ, Horton KM, Dolmatch BL, et al. Use of Wallstents for hemodialysis access-related venous stenoses and occlusions untreatable with balloon angioplasty. *Radiology.* 1995; 195.479-484.

8. Hood DB, Yellin AE, Richman MF, Weaver FA, Katz MD. Hemodialysis graft salvage with endoluminal stents. *Am Surg.* 1994; 60.733-737.

9. Farber A, Barbey MM, Grunert JH, Gmelin E. Access-related venous stenoses and occlusions: treatment with percutaneous transluminal angioplasty and Dacron-covered stents. *Cardiovasc Intervent Radiol.* 1999; 33.214-218.

10. Sapoval MR, Turmel-Rodrigues LA, Raynaud AC, Bourquelot P, Rodrigue H, Gaux JC. Cragg covered stents in hemodialysis access: initial and midterm results. *J Vasc Interv Radiol.* 1996; 7.335-342.

11. Rabindranauth P, Shindelman L. Transluminal stent-graft repair for pseudoaneurysm of PTFE hemodialysis grafts. *J Endovasc Surg.* 1988; 5.138-141.

12. Quinn SF, Kim J, Sheley RC. Transluminally placed endovascular grafts for venous lesions in patients on hemodialysis. *Cardiovasc Intervent Radiol.* 2003; 26.365-369.

13. Masuda EM, Kistner RL, Eklof B, Lipman RA, Balkin PW, Kamida CB. Stent-graft arteriovenous fistula: an endovascular technique in hemodialysis access. *J Endovasc Surg.* 1998; 5.18-23.

14. Lammer J, Dake MD, Bleyn J, et al. Peripheral arterial obstruction: Prospective study of treatment with a transluminally placed self-expanding stent graft. *Radiology* 2000;217:95-104.

15. Kasirajan K, Matteson B, Marek JM, Langsfeld M. Covered stents for true subclavian aneurysms in patients with degenerative connective tissue disorders. *J Endovasc Ther.* 2003; 10.647-652.

DISCUSSION

Vascular Access for Hemodialysis IX
May 6-7, 2004
Lake Buena Vista, Florida

May 7, 2004
Abstract Session III

Dr. John Ross
"Nitinol/ePTFE Stent-Graft Treatment of Venous Stenosis in Patients Undergoing Hemodialysis"

Question: I have not done this and it would be hard for us to do this in our center not the surgeons typically doing this part of it. So either we have to figure out a way to have our angiographers do it and transfer them to the O.R. quickly or learn how to do it ourselves.

Ross: Or you can send the patients to us! We are set up in our operating room to do this.

24

THE ADVANTAGE OF INTERRUPTED NITINOL CLIPS IN THE CREATION OF AUTOLOGOUS ARTERIOVENOUS FISTULAE—ONE CENTER'S EXPERIENCE FROM A CONTROLLED, PROSPECTIVE, RANDOMIZED, MULTI-CENTER STUDY

A. Frederick Schild, MD, FACS
Neyton M. Baltodano, MD
Moises Salama, MD

University of Miami School of Medicine
Jackson Memorial Hospital
DeWitt Daughtry Family Department of Surgery
P.O. Box 012440 (R-440)
Miami, FL 33101
East Tower #3016-A
(305) 585-5286 TEL
(305) 585-3794 FAX
Fschild@med.miami.edu

Introduction

The rising population of end-stage renal disease (ESRD) patients is cause for significant concern. In 1995, public and private sources made payments for ESRD of more than 13 billion dollars, with 17% of that amount associated with dialysis access morbidity[1]. There are nearly 400,000 people in the Medicare End Stage Renal Disease Program[2] and, with the ESRD patient population growing by at 7.8% each year[3], it is estimated that the number of patients with ESRD will nearly double by the year 2010.

There are several options for surgically created accesses including autologous arteriovenous fistulae (AVF) and arteriovenous grafts. While both are considered acceptable forms of access, arteriovenous fistulae have been reported to have both superior patency and revision rates compared to those of arteriovenous grafts. This data, coupled with the 1997 recommendations from the National Kidney Foundation's Kidney Disease Outcomes Initiative (K-DOQI)[4], has sparked increased pressure to perform a higher percentage of arteriovenous fistulae (K-DOQI recommends that a) 50% of all new accesses should be AVF, b) 40% of prevalent ESRD patients undergoing dialysis access should have AVF, and c) all patients with previously failed accesses should be re-evaluated for primary AVF).

Many published papers have discussed strategies for increasing both fistula adoption and survival, including earlier referral, pre-operative vein mapping, and aggressive maintenance. Based on our own experience with AVFs, we believe that suturing technique is also an important factor affecting both short and long term AVF survival. However, there has long been debate regarding the ideal suturing technique for vascular anastomoses. Nobel Prize recipient Alexis Carrel first described the vascular anastomosis using a modified interrupted/continuous technique (triangulation of three continuously sutured segments of a vascular anastomosis). Since that time, there has been polarization resulting in the acceptance of both the interrupted and continuous suturing techniques for various types of vascular anastomoses including peripheral vascular, general vascular, and cardiovascular.

More recently, several studies[5,6] have demonstrated a significant difference in both the scientific and clinical outcomes based on the differences between the interrupted and continuous suturing techniques. Unfortunately, most surgeons have abandoned the interrupted technique because, historically, it has been both more time consuming and technically challenging due mainly to additional knot-tying and suture management issues. However, recent advances in shape-memory alloy technology have resulted in the development, introduction, and adoption of a new anastomotic clip that both preserves routine suturing practices and eliminates the historic time and technical issues long associated with the interrupted suturing technique[7].

This report represents one center's contribution to the Comparison Of Maturity, Patency, And Related Economics (COMPARE) Study, which is a controlled, prospective, randomized, multi-center trial comparing the outcomes of AVF created using either interrupted U-CLIP™ Anastomotic Devices or continuous suture.

Methods

Between January 2003 and April 2004, prospective patients requiring dialysis access procedures were screened at the University of Miami Jackson Memorial

Hospital Vascular Access Clinic. Patients meeting the inclusion criteria required a forearm arteriovenous access procedure, were referred by a nephrologist, had adequate blood vessel flow for primary dialysis access, required dialysis access within six months, had target vein diameter > 2.5 mm, and had signed an informed consent form. Exclusion criteria included a failed previous access attempt in the target arm, active gastrointestinal bleeding, active infection or fever > 100° F, short life expectancy (< 1 year) due to other illnesses such as cancer or pulmonary, hepatic or renal disease, skin conditions that could interfere with fistula maturity and/or access, severe uncontrolled systemic hypertension (systolic pressure > 240 mm Hg within one month), history of intravenous drug use, edema, lesions, or skin breakdown of the target arm, participation in another investigational protocol related to AV access, or unwillingness or inability to comply with any protocol requirements. Immediately prior to surgery, the anastomotic technique of patients was randomized to either continuous polypropylene suture (PROLENE™, Ethicon, Inc., Somerville, NJ) or interrupted nitinol clips (U-CLIP™ Anastomotic Device, Coalescent Surgical, Inc, Sunnyvale, CA).

The U-CLIP™ Anastomotic Device (Figure 1) consists of three main components: a vascular needle, a flexible member, and a nitinol clip. The vascular needle is available in several sizes to accommodate surgeon preference and tissue requirements. The flexible member is constructed of several braided strands of nitinol wire that lend some rigidity that helps during placement and deployment. The nitinol clip, when deployed, serves as a knot by approximating vessel edges under consistent tension. The U-CLIP™ is applied using a standard vascular needle driver, much the same way as standard continuous suture. When the nitinol clip is pulled into position and contains tissue from both anastomotic edges, the proximal end is compressed by the needle driver, activating the clip's release from the needle and flexible member. The clip then returns to its knotted, or closed position based on its previously determined shape memory geometry. A typical anastomosis requires between 10 and 12 clips to complete. The learning curve appears to be very short (~ 5 anastomoses) and requires an understanding of clip sizing, spacing, geometry, and tissue thickness.

Intraoperative exclusions included the presence of inadequate vein and/or artery, requirement to perform a side-to-side anastomosis, heavily calcified arteries potentially affecting flow and/or dialysis efficiency, or unexpected intraoperative findings creating an unreasonable intra-operative risk, or an increased probability of postoperative complications in terms of recovery.

Transit Time Flow Measurements were taken by a Butterfly flow meter (Medi-Stim, Oslo, Norway) intraoperatively to confirm initial flow adequacy. Flow measurements were obtained of both the vein and artery prior to and immediately after creation of the anastomosis. Patient follow-up consisted of return office visits at one, two, six, and twelve months where duplex ultrasound was used to measure

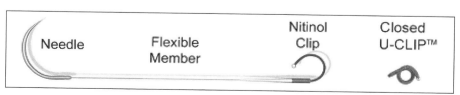

Figure 1:   U-CLIP™ Anastomotic Device.

Brachial Artery Flow Rate in ml/min and confirmation of maturity and patency was recorded on the Case Report Forms (CRFs).

Fistula maturity was defined as confirmed ability to dialyze by the dialysis clinic and the duration of primary patency was measured from the time of access placement to the time of first intervention, subsequent procedure, or failure. Comprehensive data was recorded regarding all post-operative events including but not limited to complications (hematoma, infection, etc.), interventions (branch ligation, percutaneous transluminal angioplasty, etc.), revisions (elevations, transpositions, etc.), replacements (arteriovenous fistula, arteriovenous graft, vascular catheter, etc.), and deaths.

Statistical Methods

Maturity of AVF and events were compared using a one-sided t test. Patency of AVF was compared using both a one-sided t test and Kaplan-Meier survival analysis. Demographic and intraoperative data were compared using a pooled two-sample t test. Differences where $P < 0.05$ were considered significant.

Results

A total of 31 patents have undergone surgery for the creation of arteriovenous fistulae (Table 1). Mean follow-up was 95 days (range 2-388). In terms of demographics, there were no significant differences in race, gender, or BMI, although there was a trend toward more diabetics in the U-CLIP™ group (42% vs. 18%, $P=0.12$). Procedurally, there were no significant differences in vein diameter or anastomotic

Table 1.   Demographic and Procedural Data.

Gender	U-CLIP™	Continuous Suture	Significance
Male	14	17	NS
Female	0	0	NS
Race			
White	1	1	NS
African American	7	8	NS
Hispanic	6	6	NS
Other	0	2	NS
Diabetic	6 (43%)	3 (18%)	NS
Average Body Mass Index (BMI)	26.48	25.61	NS
Average Vein Diameter (mm)	3.0	2.8	NS
Average Anastomotic Time (min)	16.1	16.4	NS
Average Intraoperative Venous			
Flow Rate (ml/min)	214	174	NS

time. Intraoperative, post-anastomosis venous flow measurements were higher in the U-CLIP™ group, although the difference failed to achieve significance.

Brachial artery flow rates at early (4-8 week) and late (6-12 months) follow-up were also higher for the U-CLIP™ group, but also failed to achieve significance with only our small subset of patients. There was a trend toward improved maturation (83.3% vs. 69.2%, $P=0.20$) (Figure 2) and improved primary patency (42.9% vs. 28.6%, $P=0.29$) (Figures 3 and 4) in the U-CLIP™ group. Secondary and cumulative patency values are similar as there were no successful interventions to reestablish patency of mature AVFs. Total events were lower for the U-CLIP™ group and also trended toward significance (4 vs. 8, $P=0.17$). Although the differ-

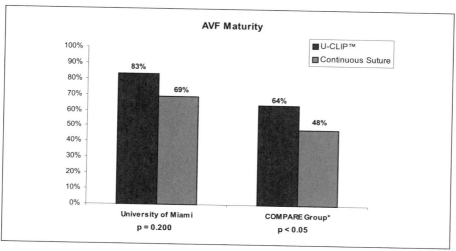

Figure 2:   AVF Maturity (*Published results from abstract accepted for presentation at 2004 Annual Meeting of the Society for Vascular Surgery and subsequent publication in the Journal of Vascular Surgery).

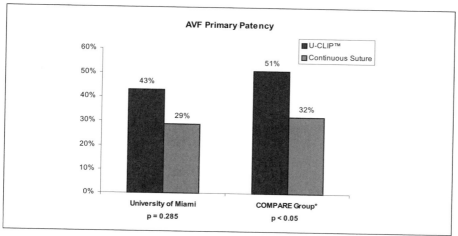

Figure 3:   AVF Primary Patency (*Published results from abstract accepted for presentation at 2004 Annual Meeting of the Society for Vascular Surgery and subsequent publication in the Journal of Vascular Surgery).

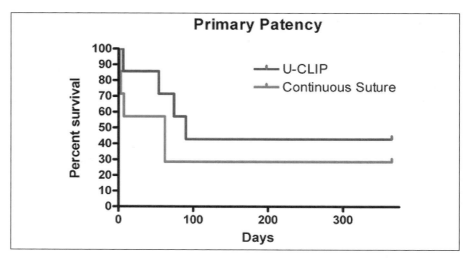

Figure 4:   Kaplan-Meier Analysis.

ence was not significant, dialysis availability, in terms of patient days, was also higher in the U-CLIP™ group (184 vs. 156, $P=0.58$).

Discussion

The data from our center demonstrated only a trend toward an improvement in maturity, patency, and events within the U-CLIP™ group. However, when we compared our results with the entire sample of patients from the multiple centers (Glickman M, Berman S, Dickerman R, et al. COMPARE Study in Arteriovenous Fistula Anastomoses: Preliminary Results from a Controlled, Prospective, Randomized, Multi-Center Study; abstract accepted for presentation at the 2004 Annual Meeting of the Society for Vascular Surgery), we found that our results were consistent and that the U-CLIP™ group demonstrated a statistically significant improvement in the areas of maturity, patency, and events (Figures 2 and 3) in the overall study.

Our multicenter data is also consistent with other studies that demonstrate both the scientific and clinical superiority of the interrupted technique for vascular anastomosis. Several scientific studies have closely examined the effects of compliance on both the regional hemodynamics and wall mechanics surrounding the anastomotic site[8,9]. These studies have demonstrated a statistically significant difference in compliance profiles that affects pressure pulse wave propagation in the vessel, leads to areas of flow separation and turbulence, and ultimately alters wall shear which has been shown to modify the biological response of the endothelial layer. In addition, interrupted anastomoses were also shown to generate better para-anastomotic compliance profiles that may reduce development of intimal hyperplasia.

One recently published retrospective, non-randomized multi-center study[6] evaluating the effect of suture technique (interrupted vs. continuous) on AVF patency demonstrated a statistically significant improvement in primary, secondary, and overall access patency in the interrupted group. A second recently published study[10] demonstrated a statistically significant improvement in the maturity as well as 12, 24, and 36 month primary patency of forearm AVFs created with the U-CLIP™ when compared to conventional continuous polypropylene sutures.

Because of its compliant nature, we believe that the interrupted anastomosis has the ability to expand, allowing the vein of an AVF to enlarge at its point of origin, completely free of anastomotic restriction. On the other hand, a continuously sutured anastomosis serves as a focal point of constriction, thus restricting the expansion of the anastomosis and initially limiting the enlargement of the AVF's vein at its origin. Our intraoperative and postoperative flow data support this hypothesis as flow rates were higher in the U-CLIP™ group at each measurement. This increased flow rate may be responsible for potentially earlier maturation and subsequent cannulation of AVFs created with the U-CLIP™. This earlier maturation facilitates faster removal of the temporary dialysis catheter, thus alleviating possible morbidities, including a high incidence of both infection and venous stenosis.

Because there were fewer overall events in the U-CLIP™ group, it is reasonable to conclude that the maintenance costs of AVFs in that group were lower as well. The U-CLIP™ group demonstrated a 39% relative decrease in event related morbidity (28.6% vs. 47.1%). Using $8,000 for the annualized cost of vascular access morbidity[11], the U-CLIP™ group demonstrated a potential savings of $3,137 per patient year, clearly indicating its cost-effectiveness.

Conclusion

In our study, interrupted anastomoses created with the U-CLIP™ demonstrated trends toward increased maturity, increased flow rates, increased patency, and event-free post-operative course when compared to continuously sutured controls. Inferred adverse event related costs were also lower in the U-CLIP™ group. In our opinion, the U-CLIP™ provides a superior clinical and economic means of anastomosis in vascular access surgery.

References

1. U.S. Renal Data System: *U.S. Renal Data System 1997 Annual Report* (chapt X). Washington, D.C., 1997, pp 143-161.
2. U.S. Renal Data System: *USRDS 2003 Annual Data Report: Atlas of End-Stage Renal Disease in the United States, National Institutes of Health, National Institute of Diabetes and Digestive and Kidney Diseases* (chapt 2). Bethesda, MD, 2003, pp 47-60.
3. Sidawy A, Gray R, Besarab A, et al. Recommended standards for reports dealing with arteriovenous hemodialysis accesses. *J Vasc Surg.* 2002; 35.603-610.
4. NKF-DOQI clinical practice guidelines for vascular access. National Kidney Foundation-Dialysis Outcomes Quality Initiative. *Am J Kidney Dis.* 1997; 30.S150-191.

5. Gerdisch M, Hinkamp T, Ainsworth S. Blood flow pattern and anastomotic compliance for interrupted versus continuous coronary bypass grafts. *Heart Surg Forum.* 2002; 6(2). 65-71

6. Shenoy S, Miller A, Petersen F, et al. A multicenter study of permanent hemodialysis access patency: Beneficial effect of clipped vascular anastomotic technique. *J Vasc Surg.* 2003; 38.229-235.

7. Hill A, Maroney T, Virmani R. Facilitated coronary anastomosis using a nitinol U-Clip device. *J Thorac Cardiovasc Surg.* 2001; 121.859-870.

8. Baguneid M, Goldner S, Pulford P, et al. A comparison of anastomotic compliance profiles after vascular anastomosis: nonpenetrating clips versus standard sutures. *J Vasc Surg.* 2001; 19.812-820.

9. Ballyk P, Walsh C, Butany J, Ojha M. Compliance mismatch may promote graft-artery intimal hyperplasia by altering suture-line stresses. *Journal of Biomechanics.* 1998; 31.229-237.

10. Lin PH, Bush RL, Nelson JC, et al. A prospective evaluation of interrupted nitinol surgical clips in arteriovenous fistula for hemodialysis. *Am J Surg.* 2003 Dec; 186(6).625-630.

11. McKarley P, Wingard RL, Shyr Y, Pettus W, Hakim RM, Ikizler TA. Vascular access blood flow monitoring reduces access morbidity and costs. *Kidney Int.* 2001; 60.1164-1172.

DISCUSSION

Vascular Access for Hemodialysis IX
May 6-7, 2004
Lake Buena Vista, Florida

May 6, 2004
Abstract Session 1

Dr. Frederick Schild
"The advantage of Interrupted Nitinol Clips in the Creation of Autologous Arteriovenous Fistulae – One Center's Experience from a Controlled, Prospective, Randomized, Multi Center Study"

Question: What is the length of your anastomosis? Why did you exclude HIV patients?

Schild: We excluded HIV positive patients because in our experience in Miami many of them have been drug users or many of them have been sick for a long time and their veins were all probably used up and it made it very difficult. As far as the size of the anastomosis, it depends on the size of the artery but it is usually about close to a centimeter.

Question: What do you think is the difference between the U-clip and the interrupted prolene?

Schild: The difference between the u-clip and the interrupted prolene is that you don't have to tie it if you space it correctly. I think it is easier to use. It is very quick. I think it gives probably a little better anastomosis. However, if you want to sit and tie an interrupted prolene, okay. Well you put the u-clip spacing about the same amount as you would put your spacing in a running suture. As I say there is a short learning curve, you learn exactly how far apart you can do this without causing it to leak or anything. Very few of these have oozing after the anastomosis.

Question: Do you think there is a physiologic advantage to the U-clips and what happens if the anastomosis requires angioplasty?

Schild: With this interrupted anastomosis there is compliance that you don't have with the running suture. It also helps the velocity because you have this compliance since it's interrupted. There has been a tremendous amount of literature that shows an interrupted anastomosis is superior to a running anastomosis. As far as angioplasty, I don't have any personal experience with that but I do not anticipate a problem with that.

25

THE USE OF CUTTING
BALLOON ANGIOPLASTY IN NATIVE
DIALYSIS FISTULAS

D. Beckett M.B.B.S, P.M. Crowe FFRRCSI FRCR,
M.J. Henderson MRCP FRCR, T. Wilmink MD MPhil FRCS

Correspondence:
P.M Crowe
Department of Radiology, Birmingham Heartlands Hospital,
Bordesley Green East, Birmingham B9 5SS, United Kingdom
dr_p_crowe@yahoo.co.uk
Telephone: +(44) 121 424 0287
Fax: +(44) 121 766 6919

Introduction:

Vascular access use is integral in the management of patients with end stage renal failure. Permanent access is achieved by arteriovenous fistula formation or by the placement of a synthetic graft. Vascular access has been shown to differ between the United States and Europe[1] (Table 1).

Venous stenoses in haemodialysis fistulas are a common cause of shunt dysfunction. The presence of fibrous strands incorporated into the vessel neointimal layer and repeated needle trauma have been implicated. Percutaneous interventional procedures provide a successful alternative to surgical reintervention. The technical success of conventional angioplasty is approximately 80%[2]. Failure of percutaneous transluminal angioplasty in the majority of patients is due to residual venous

Table 1.   Arteriovenous fistula, graft and catheter use among prevalent haemodialysis patients within the US and Europe. Results from the DOPPS[1].

	AVF	Grafts	Catheters
US	24%	58%	18%
Europe	80%	10%	10%

stenoses (Fig. 1). The use of high pressure balloon angioplasty has been used in this clinical setting. Stent placement, atherectomy and laser treatment have been used as alternative methods. Conventional angioplasty and high pressure balloon dilatation are painful.

Cutting Balloon angioplasty was initially approved for use in coronary angioplasty. Initial work by Vorwerk[3, 4] has lead to its increasing use within radiology. Vessel dilatation at low pressure and increased luminal diameters secondary to greater plaque compression rather than vessel wall expansion, in conjunction with a low complication rate have made it an attractive alternative or conjunct to conventional angioplasty[5]. Atherotomy relieves hoop stress by the placement of precisely controlled incisions within the vessel intima (Fig. 2, 3). We describe our early experience of the Peripheral Cutting Balloon[TM] (Boston Scientific) in native dialysis fistulas.

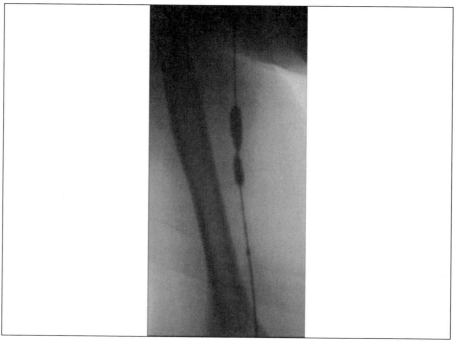

Figure 1:   Figure 1. Conventional balloon angioplasty of venous run off stenosis. Waisting of angioplasty balloon is demonstrated.

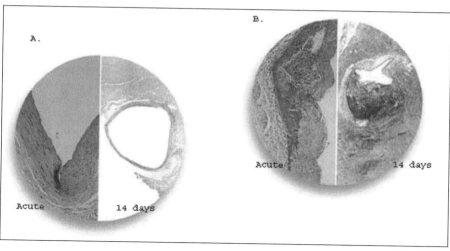

Figure 2:   Histological slides from porcine artery. A: Results from porcine
artery overstretched by 30% with PCB. B: Results of porcine artery
overstretched by 30% with traditional angioplasty. Sharp intimal incisions are seen with the PCB without irregular dissection. Courtesy
of Boston Scientific Corp.

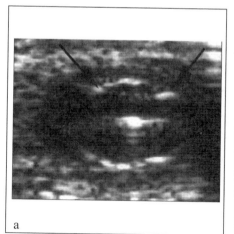
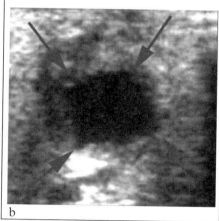

Figure 3:   a) Axial ultrasound through stenotic lesion shows inflated cutting
balloon with atherotomes seen (arrows). Courtesy Dr. Kieran
McBride, Queen Margaret Hospital, Dunfermline, Fife.

b) Axial ultrasound following peripheral cutting balloon angioplasty
shows intimal incisions (arrows). Courtesy Dr. Kieran McBride,
Queen Margaret Hospital, Dunfermline, Fife.

Methods:

Nine patients (10 interventions) underwent cutting angioplasty of native renal dialysis fistulas stenoses. Patient age ranged from 26-78 years (3 female and 6 male). There was 1 re-intervention. All interventions were above elbow venous stenoses.

Indications:

This is a non-randomised study to test the technical success and safety of the cutting balloon. Our early experience is described. All patients had reduced haemodialysis flow rates and venous stenosis >30% on venography.

In 4 cases, cutting balloon angioplasty was used after conventional angioplasty when residual waisting/ stenosis was >30% (residual waisting limited by pain during conventional angioplasty n=1). Cutting Balloon angioplasty was followed by conventional angioplasty in 3 cases when the cutting balloons used were under sized. In 3 cases peripheral cutting balloon angioplasty was the only treatment technique used.

Technique:

A 6-F (n=10) introducer sheath was inserted into the vein. The cutting balloon was inserted across the stenotic segment over a 0.018" guide wire (Figure 4). Atherotome length was 1cm. The balloon was inflated to a maximum pressure of 10 atm. Single or multiple inflations were performed to cover the entire length of stenosis. Cutting balloons with diameters of 5mm (n=5), 5.5mm (n=2), 6mm (n=2), and 7mm (n=1) were used. Diameter was approximated to the normal venous diameter adjacent to the stenotic segment on venography and oversized by 1mm.

Cutting balloon angioplasty was followed in 3 patients by conventional angioplasty (5.5mm cutting balloon followed by 6mm diameter conventional balloon angioplasty, 5mm diameter cutting balloon followed by 7mm diameter conventional balloon angioplasty, and 7mm diameter cutting balloon followed by 8mm diameter conventional angioplasty). Conventional balloon pressures of 10-15 atm were used.

Results:

The cutting balloon could be advanced across the stenosis in all cases. Initial technical success defined as a residual stenosis less than 30% was achieved in 90%. Failure defined as residual stenosis >30% was seen in one patient, associated with balloon rupture and minor contrast extravasation.

In 3 of the 4 cases in which cutting balloon angioplasty followed insufficient conventional balloon angioplasty, cutting angioplasty resulted in a reduction in the residual stenosis <30%. All cutting balloon angioplasty of venous lesions were well tolerated and relatively painless.

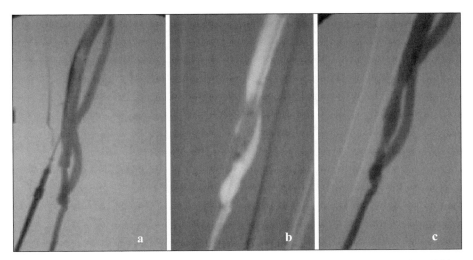

Figure 4:   a) Venogram demonstrates >50% venous stenosis in a native AVF.
b) 5mm diameter cutting balloon is inflated across the stenosis over a 0.018" guide.
c) Post peripheral cutting balloon angioplasty. Immediate venography shows good technical success.

In one case, minor local contrast extravasation was seen. Rupture of the cutting balloon was seen in 1 case. No difficulty in balloon retrieval was encountered. No thrombosis was seen within the 1st week following intervention. As a late sequlae, at 6 weeks, 1 case of aneurysmal dilatation of the venous limb was demonstrated (Figure 5).

Patient follow up was for 1-21months. One death from coronary vascular disease was seen at 3 months. Primary patency was 90% at the end of the procedure and 60% at 2 months (aneurysm n=1, re-stenosis n=3). Five remain patent at the end of the study (21 months, 4 months, 3 months, 3 months, and 2 months).

Conclusion:

The Peripheral Cutting Balloon^{TM} (Boston Scientific) is effective in management of native arteriovenous fistula stenosis. Indications for the use of peripheral cutting balloon angioplasty included: recurrent venous stenosis, resistant stenosis and patients in whom angioplasty pain and discomfort featured heavily. Complications included one balloon rupture and minor self-limiting contrast extravasation, without clinical consequence. One case of post-angioplasty aneurysmal dilation of the venous limb was described. We conclude that cutting balloon angioplasty is a relatively safe and effective intervention for resistant stenoses in native fistulas and causes significantly less pain than standard or high pressure PTA. Further work is needed to assess long term patency.

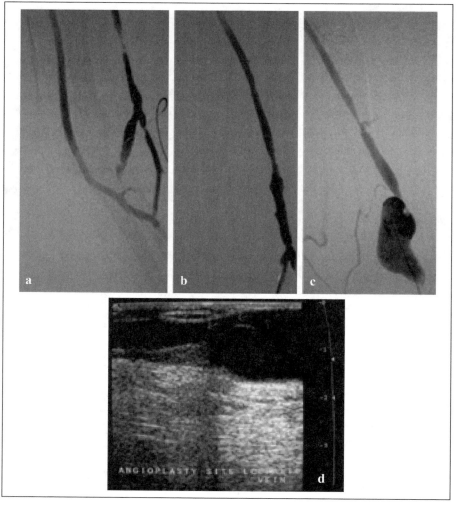

Figure 5:   a) Initial venogram demonstrates a venous stenosis of within the cephalic vein.

b) Venogram following peripheral cutting balloon angioplasty reveals good initial technical success. A degree of residual waisting is noted.

c) Venogram at 6 weeks reveals aneurysmal dilatation at the site of initial angioplasty.

d) Ultrasound image demonstrating venous aneurysm at the angioplasty site (left cephalic vein).

References:

1. Pisoni R.L, Young E.W, Dykstra D.M, Greenwood R.N, Hecking E, Gillespie B, et al. Vascular access use in Europe and the United States: Results from the DOPPS. *Kidney Int.* 2002; 61. 305-316.

2. Beathard G. Percutaneous Transvenous angioplasty in the treatment of vascular access stenosis. *Kidney Int.* 1992; 42. 1390-1397.

3. Vorwerk D, Adam G, Müller-Leisse C, Günther R.W. Haemodialysis fistulas and grafts: use of cutting balloons to dilate venous stenoses. *Radiology.* 1996; 201. 864-867.

4. Vorwerk D, Günther R.W, Schürmann K, Sieberth H. Use of a cutting balloon for dilatation of a resistant venous stenosis of a haemodialysis fistula. *Cardiovasc Intervent Radiol.* 1995; 18. 62-64.

5. Hara H, Nakamura M, Asahara T, Nishida T, Yamaguchi T. Intravascular ultrasonic comparisons of mechanisms of vasodilatation of cutting balloon angioplasty versus conventional balloon angioplasty. *Am J Cardiol.* 2002; 89(11). 1253-6.

DISCUSSION

Vascular Access for Hemodialysis IX
May 6-7, 2004
Lake Buena Vista, Florida

May 7, 2004
Abstract Session III

Dr. David Beckett
"The Use of Cutting Balloon Angioplasty in Native Dialysis fistulas"

Question: Have you had the opportunity to go back and reangioplasty with the standard balloon after these have restenosed?

Beckett: We have found with the conventional balloon angioplasties that we have had to go back but only at the same setting having ballooned with a cutting balloon.

Question: I was just wondering if it was easier at a remote time to have a standard angioplasty following the breaking of the intima with the cutting balloon.

Beckett: We have not done that yet, no.

26

THE TRANSPOSED BRACHIOBASILIC FISTULA – GOOD RESULTS IN DIFFICULT SITUATIONS

Ewan Macaulay MD*, Elena Saw MB*, Wendy Craig MB*, Lorraine Close RN*, Ann Humphrey MRCP**.

Department of Vascular Surgery* and Nephrology**, Aberdeen Royal Infirmary, Aberdeen, United Kingdom.

Corresponding Author:
Mr Ewan Macaulay
Consultant Vascular Surgeon
Ward 36
Aberdeen Royal Infirmary
Aberdeen
Scotland
AB25 2ZN
Phone 01224 559446
Fax 01224 552553
Ewan.Macaulay@arh.grampian.scot.nhs.uk

Introduction

The number of patients receiving haemodialysis is increasing rapidly worldwide[1,2]. The method of vascular access appears to vary remarkably both between and within countries particularly with regard to the number of synthetic grafts used[3]. A consensus has now been reached that the best form of vascular access for haemodialysis is an autogenous arteriovenous fistula[3,4] and targets have now been issued on both sides of the Atlantic[5,6]. Some centers are able to claim autogenous fistula rates of greater than 90%[7] whilst in others it may be as low 30%[8]. These differences may reflect patient groups[9,10,11,12] as well as practice. In an elderly population, a large percentage of whom have significant co-morbidities, with poor quality forearm veins and arteries, it is difficult to fashion a native fistula.

The transposed brachiobasilic fistula has the advantages that it uses a vein that has seldom been previously punctured and has good arterial inflow. Reluctance to adopt this technique may reflect concerns over the wide variation in patency rates reported in the literature. Dagher[13], with the longest documented study of transposed brachiobasilic fistulae, reports functional patency rates of 70% at 8 years. Hossny[14] also reports secondary patency rates of 82.8% at 2 years. In contrast, Rivers et al.[15] and Elcheroth et al.[16] report, respectively, 49% 30 month cumulative patency, and 49.2% 4 year cumulative patency rates. Differences in technique may also cause concern, with a variety of one and two stage procedures described utilizing both superificialisation and tunneling of the vein[7,8].

In 2001, the transposed brachiobasilic fistula was introduced to our institution. This report describes our results and compares them to those obtained for brachiocephalic fistulae formed over the same period. We aim here to illustrate the valuable contribution of this access technique to the vascular surgeon's patency rates, particularly for patients for whom access has been difficult.

Methods

Setting   The study took place in Aberdeen Royal Infirmary, the referral centere for renal access surgery, covering the population of 507,000 living in the Grampian region and Orkney and Shetland Islands of Scotland. The fistula service is staffed by five surgeons, one of whom does over 50% of the caseload and who performs the majority of the complex access procedures. Repeated "snapshot" audits have shown that at any one time there are about 160 patients on long term haemodialysis with an autogenous fistula in 80%, a synthetic fistula in 10%, a temporary central venous catheter in 10% and a permanent catheter in only one patient.

Audit method   The routine use of the transposed brachiobasilic fistula was introduced to our institution in 2001. The period from 1st April 2001 to 31st July 2003 was examined. All surgical data was prospectively audited. Fistula usage and problems were recorded on the patients dialysis record and retrospectively retrieved. As well as primary, primary assisted and secondary haemodynamic patency, factors recorded included age, sex, diabetic status and number of previous fistulae. Using standard criteria[17,18] primary patency was defined as haemodynamic patency with no interventions to assist patency. Primary assisted patency was defined as haemodynamic patency maintained by a surgical or radiological intervention without fistula thrombosis and secondary patency was defined as restoration of patency in a thrombosed fistula without major modification or replacement of the fistula. Data was analysed using the Statistical Package for Social Sciences (SPSS, version 11.5).

Surgical technique   The transposed brachiobasilic fistulae were fashioned using a single step technique. This involved harvesting the basilic vein from antecubital fossa to axilla and then tunneling the vein laterally before anastomosing to the brachial artery.

The brachiocephalic fistulae were formed in a standard fashion utilizing a transverse antecubital fossa incision and anastomosing the median cephalic vein to the brachial artery. If the median cephalic vein was unsuitable the cephalic vein was mobilized via a separate incision and swung medially.

Results

During the audited period, 171 patients received 258 new site fistulas of which 45 (17.4%) were synthetic and 213 (82.6%) autogenous. Of the autogenous fistulae, 92 (35.7% of all fistulae) brachiocephalic and 32 (12.4% of all fistulae) transposed brachiobasilic fistulae were formed in 109 patients (62 male, 27 diabetics) with a median age of 69 (range 15 to 87) years. Fourteen patients had more than one fistula formed during the audited period: 3 patients had two brachiocephalic fistulae, 9 patients had a brachiocephalic and transposed brachiobasilic fistula, one patient had two brachiobasilic fistulae formed and one patient had two brachiocephalic and one transposed fistula. For analysis between groups the site of the first fistula formed during the audited period was used. There were no differences in sex distribution (Chi-square = 0.10, p = 0.919), age (Mann-Whitney U = 830, p = 0.11) or diabetic status (Chi-Square = 3.48, p = 0.06) between the two groups (Table 1). Brachiocephalic fistulae were more likely (Chi-Square 2 d.f. = 11.69; p = 0.003) to be primary fistulas (Table 2).

Overall primary patency was 94% at 30 days and 65% at 1 year. Overall primary assisted patency (94% at 30 days, 79 % at one year) was similar to secondary patency (96% at 30 days and 77% at one year) with no differences (Log rank test p >0.05) between the 2 groups of fistulae (Figures 1 – 3).

Table 1.   Demographics of patients undergoing autogenous fistula formation.
*Chi-square test. **Mann-Whitney U test.

	Brachiocephalic (n = 84)	Transposed brachiobasilic (n = 25)	P
Male	48 (57%)	14 (56%)	0.9*
Diabetic	18 (21%)	10 (40%)	0.06*
Age (median (SD))	69 (13)	66 (18)	0.11**

Table 2.   Number of fistula by procedure.

Number of fistula	Brachiocephalic (n = 92)	Transposed Brachiobasilic (n=32)
Primary	60 (65.2%)	10 (31.3%)
Secondary	16 (17.4%)	9 (28.1%)
Tertiary or greater	16 (17.4%)	13 (40.6%)

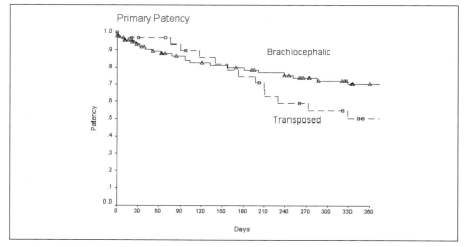

Number at risk												
Brachiocephalic	92	75	69	63	60	58	56	52	50	45	41	37	34
Transposed	32	29	28	26	23	22	20	18	15	14	13	11	9

Figure 1:   Primary patency for brachiocephalic and transposed brachiobasilic fistulae to 360 days. At 360 days the standard error is 5% for brachiocephalic and 9.9% for the transposed fistulae. No significant difference (Log rank test 3.09, p = 0.08)

Fifty eight of the 92 (63%) brachiocephalic fistulae and 25 of 32 (78%) transposed fistulae were successfully needled (Table 3).

Conclusions

This paper has examined our initial experience with a single stage transposed brachiobasilic fistula and has shown similar results to those for brachiocephalic fistulae performed in our institution, with patency rates between the two extremes described in the literature. First mentioned by Cascardo et al[19], and fully described by Dagher et al[20] in 1976, the transposed procedure involves mobilization, distal division and superficial tunneling and transposition of the basilic vein with distal end-to-side anastomosis with the brachial artery. The procedure is technically feasible in over 95%

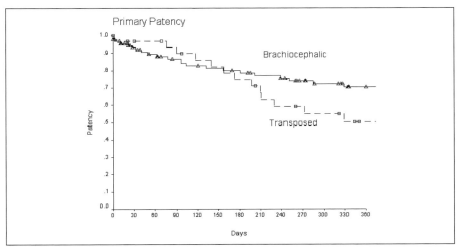

Number at risk

Brachiocephalic	92	75	69	63	61	59	57	54	53	48	45	42	38
Transposed	32	29	28	27	26	25	23	21	20	19	18	15	13

Figure 2:   Primary assisted patency for brachiocephalic and transposed brachiobasilic fistulae to 360 days. At 360 days the standard error is
4.6% for brachiocephalic and 9.1% for the transposed fistulae. No
significant difference (Log rank test 2.83, p = 0.09).

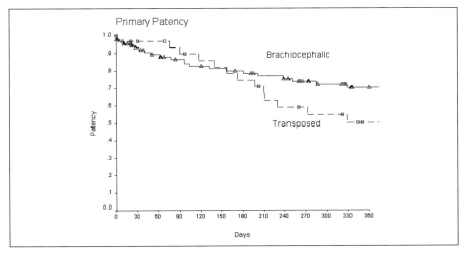

Number at risk

Brachiocephalic	92	77	70	64	62	60	58	55	54	49	45	42	38
Transposed	32	29	28	27	26	26	23	21	20	19	18	15	13

Figure 3:   Secondary patency for brachiocephalic and transposed brachiobasilic fistulae to 360 days. At 360 days the standard error is 4.8% for
brachiocephalic and 9.0% for the transposed fistulae. No significant
difference (Log rank test 2.03, p = 0.15).

Table 3.   Causes of failure to initiate haemodialysis.

	Brachiocephalic (n=92)	Transposed Brachiobasilic (n=32)
Successfully needled	58 (63%)	25 (78%)
Causes of failure to access		
Early occlusion	5 (5%)	1 (3%)
Less than 6 weeks mature at censoring	4 (4%)	
Failure to develop	8 (9%)	1 (3%)
Pre-dialysis patient	10 (11%)	3 (9%)
Patient death prior to maturity	7 (8%)	2 (6%)

cases[15]. The advantages include a long, straight, easily accessible conduit with high flows, one anastomosis, and maintenance of anatomic continuity at its venous end with the axillary vein. As already mentioned, variations on the technique exist, the most simple and common being simple elevation of the basilic vein[21]. Staged procedures can be used for superficialising the vein[22]. Endoscopic techiniques have also been utilized to reduce incision length[23]. In this series, we used a single stage technique, with tunneling of the vein, which has the advantage of requiring only one procedure and places the vein in the best position for easy needling.

Because of the extensive nature of the surgery, we try to avoid performing the transposed procedure. We will often attempt a more distal autogenous fistula or a brachiocephalic using sub-optimal vein initially and the transposed fistula is reserved as a second, or third line measure. In addition, we routinely use duplex scanning prior to placement of a transposed fistula but only selectively prior to brachiocephalic fistula formation. These factors probably explain the better initial patency rates seen in our transposed fistula group.

A patent brachiocephalic fistula appears, however, to be more durable, with 87% primary patency at 3 months and 70% at one year compared to 93% and 50% respectively for the transposed fistula. This suggests that, despite being successfully used, problems occur with the transposed fistula within a short period. This may be due to an initial learning curve in using these fistulas but may also reflect problems with transposing the vein, possibly reflected in the different techniques and results reported from different institutions[21,22,23].

Other than standard clinical monitoring on dialysis, we do not currently perform routine fistula surveillance. Primary (70% at one year) and secondary (79%) patency rates in the brachiocephalic group suggest that it would be difficult to demonstrate an improvement in outcome by surveying this group. In the transposed group, primary (50%) and secondary (72%) patency rates suggest that surveillance may be advantageous, - although the 69% primary assisted rate indicates that clinical surveillance is effective at identifying at risk fistulae prior to thrombosis. The literature is currently inconclusive[24] with regard to routine surveillance, particularly in autogenous fistulae. However, our data suggest that in precious fistulae, such as the transposed basilic, there may be benefit. Furthermore, we have not examined temporary line insertion rates and it is possible that a surveillance program, by allowing early endovascular intervention, might reduce these events.

We have used brachiocephalic fistulae as our standard in this elderly group of patients and because of the lesser surgery will opt for this if at all possible. The two techniques are therefore complimentary with transposition being reserved for patients who have exhausted other arm autogenous sites. It could be argued that a synthetic fistula placed in the forearm will preserve the upper arm sites for future access and that good patency rates have been obtained. However, a forearm synthetic fistula usually utilizes the vein near the elbow which is important in the formation of both brachiocephalic and transposed brachiobasilic fistulae. In contrast to this, an upper arm synthetic graft can be successfully fashioned even after failure of both a brachiocephalic and transposed fistula in that limb[25]. In fact, in our experience, when forming an upper arm graft after failure the vein, which is mobilized proximal to the previous dissection, is dilated and arterialized making the anastomosis relatively straightforward. We have not compared our results to those of arm synthetic grafts in our institution. This is principally because we have reserved synthetic grafts for patients who have failed all attempts to place an autogenous fistula or for those in whom an indwelling line is not possible to place or contraindicated because it would utilize our last remaining central venous site. These situations are not comparable. However, Matsura et al[26] demonstrated the superiority of the transposed fistula over the synthetic graft.

Many of the publications quoting high patency rates for both autogenous and synthetic fistulae were looking at a younger, fitter population and the results cannot be extrapolated to the modern dialysis era. For example, the initial studies of Dagher's fistulae, carried out in the late seventies[13,20] had a population of mean age 44 with no diabetics. Similarly, the results of Hossny[14], whose population had a mean age of 49, with 86.7% and 82.8% 1 and 2 year patency rates, and Humphries et al.'s cohort[27], which included pediatric patients, are incomparable. It is widely acknowledged that comorbid medical conditions impact on the failure rates of access[28], not least that of diabetes[11]. In this series despite an aggressive policy for formation of forearm autogenous fistulas if possible, almost two thirds of the brachiocephalic fistulae were first fistulae and 9 of 109 patients died within 8 weeks of fistula formation. This reflects our patient population who are elderly with a high incidence of diabetes, obesity and vascular disease. A more detailed, longitudinal study would be required to examine the patency rates of different fistulae accounting for these factors in the relevant population, in order to determine the optimal management.

By using the brachiocephalic group as our standard we have been able to demonstrate that a single step transposed brachiobasilic fistula gives acceptable results. We believe this remains a useful technique in the armamentarium of the access surgeon which does not compromise further access placement.

References

1. Moeller S, Gioberge S, Brown G. ESRD patients in 2001: global overview of patients, treatment modalities and development trends. *Nephrol Dial Transplant.* 2002; 17. 2071-2076

2. US Renal Data System USRDS 2003 Annual Data Report: atlas of end-stage renal disease in the United States. Bethesda, MD, National Institutes of Health, National Institute of Diabetes and Digestive and Kidney Diseases, 2003.

3. Rodriguez JA, Armadans L, Ferrer E, et al. The function of permanent vascular access. *Nephrol Dial Transplant.* 2000; 15. 402-408.

4. Schuman ES, Gross GF, Hayes JF, Standage BA. Long term patency of polytetra fluoroethylene graft fistulas. *Am J Surg.* 1988; 155. 644-646.

5. The Renal Association. *Treatment of adults and children with renal failure: standards and audit measures.* 3rd Edition, London. Renal Association and Royal College of Physicians, August 2002.

6. NKF-K/DOQI clinical practice guidelines for vascular access: Update 2000. *Am J Kidney Dis.* 2001; 37(S1). S137-S181.

7. Buckhart CM, Cikrit DF. Arteriovenous fistulae for haemodialysis. *Semin Vasc Surg.* 1997; 10(3). 162-165.

8. Gibson KD, Gillen DL, Caps MT, et al. Vascular access survival and incidence of revisions: a comparison of prosthetic grafts, simple autogenous fistulas and venous transposition fistulas from the United States Renal Data System Dialysis Morbidity and Mortality Study. *J Vasc Surg.* 2001; 34. 694-700.

9. Lindner A, Charra B, Sherrard DJ, Scribner BH. Accelerated atherosclerosis is prolonged maintenance haemodialysis. *N Engl J Med.* 1974; 290. 697.

10. Wetzig G, Gough I, Furnival C. One hundred cases of arteriovenous fistula for haemodialysis access: the effect of cigarette smoking on patency. *Aust N Z J Surg* 1985; 55. 551-554.

11. Hodges T, Fillinger M, Zwolak R, et al. Longitudinal comparison of dialysis access methods: risk factors for failure. *J Vasc Surg,* 1997; 26. 1009-1019.

12. Leaf D, Macrae H, Grant E, et al. Isometric exercise increases the size of forearm veins in patients with chronic renal failure. *Am J Med Sci.* 2003; 325. 115-119.

13. Dagher FJ. The upper arm av haemoaccess: longterm follow-up. *J Cardiovas Surg.* 1986; 24(4). 447-449.

14. Hossny A. Brachiobasilic arteriovenous fistula: different surgical technques-dtheir effects on fistula patency and dialysis-related complications. *J Vasc Surg.* 2003; 37. 821-826.

15. Rivers SP, Scher LA, Sheehan E, Lynn R, Veith FJ. Basilic vein transposition: and underused autologous alternative to prosthtic dialysis angioaccess. *J Vasc Surg.* 1993; 18. 391-396.

16. Elcheroth J, de Pauw L, Kinneart P. Elbow arteriovenous fistulas for chronic haemodialysis. *Br J Surg.* 1994; 81(7). 982-984.

17. Rutherford RB Baker JD, Ernst C, et al. Recommended standards for reports dealing with lower extremity ischemia: revised version. *J Vasc Surg.* 1997; 26. 517-538.

18. Sidaway AN, Gray R, Besarab A, et al. Recommended standards for reports dealing with arteriovenous haemodialysis accesses. *J Vasc Surg.* 2002; 35. 603-610.

19. Cascardo S, Acchiardo S, Bevan E, Popowniak K, Nakamoto S. Proximal arteriovenous fistulae for haemodialysis when radial arteries are not available. *Proc Eur Dial Transplant Assoc.* 1970; 7. 42.

20. Dagher FJ, Gelber RL, Ramos EJ, Salder J. The use of the basilic vein and brachial artery as an avf for long term dialysis. *J Surg Res.* 1976; 20. 373-376.

21. Davis JN, Howell CG, Humphries AL. Haemodialysis access: elevated basilic vein arteriovenous fistula. *J Pediatr Surg.* 1986; 21. 1182-1183.

22. Zielinski CM, Mittal SK, Anderson P, et al. Delayed superficialisation of the barchiobasilic fistula: technique and initial experience. *Arch Surg.* 2001; 136. 929-932.

23. Hayakawa K, Tsuha M, Aoyagi T, et al. New method to create arteriovenous fistula in the arm with an endoscopic technique. *J Vasc Surg.* 2002; 36. 635-638.

24. Mills JL, Berman SS. Postoperative surveillance of dialysis access. In:Berman SS (Ed) *Vascular Access in Clinical Practice;* Marcel Dekker Press, New York, 2002; 107-123.

25. Berman SS. Construction of prosthetic arteriovenous grafts for hemodialysis. In: Berman SS (Ed) *Vascular Access in Clinical Practice;* Marcel Dekker Press, New York, 2002; 65-105.

26. Matsura JH, Rosenthal D, Clark M, et al. Transposed basilic vein versus polytetrafluoroethylene for brachial axillary arteriovenous fistulas. *Am J Surg.* 1998; 176. 219-221.

27. Humphries AL, Colborn GL, Wynn JJ. Elevated basilic vein arteriovenous fistula. *Am J Surg.* 1999; 177. 489-491.

28. Abularradge CJ, Sidaway AN, Weiswasser JM, White PW, Arora S. Medical factors affecting patency of arteriovenous access. *Semin Vasc Surg.* 2004; 17(1). 19-24.

DISCUSSION

Vascular Access for Hemodialysis IX
May 6-7, 2004
Lake Buena Vista, Florida

May 7, 2004
Abstract Session III

Dr. Ewan Macaulay
"The Transposed Bracio-Basilic Fistula – Good Results in Difficult Situations"

Question: I just would like to reemphasize, and I guess it is relatively obvious, but when you are doing a brachialcephalic or a radialcephalic to use the median antecubial vein as a conduit below the elbow. It is quite frequently a very nice vein and adds to the fistula.

Macaulay: I think if you are going to use the median antecubital it is quite nice to take it down to the trifurcation. It goes down in the deep vein there and you can often, if you do not have enough length, get an extra little length. The other thing is the trifurcation, if you are worried that the vein is quite small you can take it and use the trifurcation to fashion the hood to place it onto the artery.

Question: Did I understand you to say that if your brachialbasilic fistula thromboses that you do not try to declot it or did I misunderstand?

Macaulay: They are usually precious fistulas and we do try to declot them. We do not have an awful lot of luck doing it, no.

Comment: I must say when I thrombectomize a fistulae, I use pituitary curette or gynecologic curette. I am very aggressive with mechanical manipulation and I like to salvage them that way. I have had real good success. It is very brutal if you watch it but in fact one of the most difficult part of a thrombosed fistula is that the thrombus is very adherent to the wall and mechanical manipulation with a curette can give those back to you on occasion.

Question: I noticed that you took your incision across the elbow down to the forearm. Have you had any functional abnormalities, any problems?

Macaulay: No, we have had no problems with it at all. We actually had very little incidence of superficial nerve damage. We have not had any problems with hematomas. None of these patients have been returned to us for anything like that. I think the reason for that is because I use an interrupted nylon closure and if there is a little bit of soakage it just comes through the stitches.

Comment: Since I am in a contrarian mood, I will express an opposite point of view. I only take it down to where the vein divides into the median antecubital and the basilic. The vein is quite large there and if I extend the incision up to the axilla I get plenty of room to do the access. It works very nicely.

Comment: Any fistula, which has been working for over three/four months without any problem, you can successfully declot it. We do it all the time. I agree with you completely Mitch, that the clot is very adherent. The second reason is most often the fistula clots and a revision is necessary because there is an underlying problem that upstream there is some stenosis somewhere. If you try to find the stenosis, we can easily patch that stenosis also using a vein patch.

Comment: Absolutely. Sometimes you need to make multiple incisions over the access if it is a well developed access to get to the stenosis.

27

RADIATION THERAPY FOR IMPROVED DIALYSIS PATENCY—SAFETY AND FEASIBILITY

C. Keith Ozaki, M.D., Scott A. Berceli, M.D., Ph.D.,
Anne S. Irwin, R.N., Thomas S. Huber, M.D., Ph.D.,
James M. Seeger, M.D., Timothy S. Flynn, M.D.,
W. Anthony Lee, M.D., Jatinder R. Palta, Ph.D.,
Nancy P. Mendenhall, M.D., Robert A. Zlotecki, M.D., Ph.D.

Departments of Surgery and Radiation Oncology, University of Florida College of Medicine and the Malcom Randall VAMC, Gainesville, FL

Address correspondence to:
C. Keith Ozaki, M.D.
PO Box 100286
Gainesville, Florida 32610-0286
(352)376-1611, extension 6470
fax: (352)271-4510
email: ozaki@surgery.ufl.edu

Supported in part by a grant from W. L. Gore & Associates, Inc.

Introduction

Low dose radiation can lethally target rapidly dividing cells, such as those in the venous anastomotic hyperplastic lesions that lead to prosthetic arteriovenous dialysis graft failure. Vascular brachytherapy attenuates restenosis after specific coronary interventions[1], though such technically sophisticated approaches may not transfer well to the clinical scenario of the newly placed prosthetic dialysis access grafts. External beam radiation therapy offers a less clinically cumbersome approach to potentially abrogate prosthetic dialysis access graft venous anastomotic intimal hyperplasia.

Thus, after demonstrating proof-of-principle in a canine model[2], we secured a United States Food and Drug Administration investigation device exemption (FDA IDE) to test the hypothesis that single fraction early post-operative external beam radiation therapy is safe and feasible in the human setting of prosthetic dialysis access grafts. Based on discussions with the FDA, this was accomplished via a prospective, five patient clinical trial, and was a pre-requisite to a planned prospective, multi-center randomized clinical trial to evaluate the efficacy of this approach to extend the durability of dialysis access grafts.

Methods

This study was initiated after securing appropriate institutional certifications, including approval from the University of Florida Human Use of Radioisotopes and Radiation Committee, the University of Florida Health Science Center Institutional Review Board, and the FDA (IDE #G000225).

From November 2000 until January 2002 five patients were prospectively enrolled from the Malcom Randall VAMC Vascular Surgery Clinic. Eligibility criteria included renal failure requiring hemodialysis, age > 18 years, need for new forearm expanded polytetrafluoroethylene (ePTFE) graft, hemodialysis access expected to be used for at least 1 year, and evaluation and approval by both a vascular surgeon and radiation oncologist. Patients with known collagen vascular disease, prior radiation treatment to the limb, pregnancy, life expectancy less than one year, comorbid illnesses that would preclude one year follow-up, ongoing treatment with steroids, or prisoners were excluded from enrollment.

The clinical practice of the involved vascular surgeons has been previously reported[3]. In summary, prosthetic permanent access conduits are placed only after options for autogenous fistulas have been exhausted. All patients underwent placement of a forearm 6 mm standard wall ePTFE (W.L. Gore & Associates, Inc.) arteriovenous graft. Four radiopaque standard surgical clips were placed immediately adjacent around the perimeter of the venous anastomosis to guide post-operative radiation therapy.

Within 24 hours post graft placement, a single fraction 8 Gy external beam radiation therapy dose was delivered using GMV photon to the venous anastomosis site through a single entrance portal. Dose was prescribed to the deepest point of the graft in a 4x6 cm field, utilizing bolus materials when indicated to optimize dmax dose point. The device used was a linear accelerator, manufactured by Varian

Associates (model number CLINAC 2100 C/D, serial number 522, software version 5.2). This unit has been approved by the FDA for use in the external beam radiation treatment of patients. Fluoroscopy was employed to verify the anastomotic area, and the field approved by the radiation oncologist prior to treatment.

Thereafter patients were examined in Vascular Surgery Clinic for clinical evidence of graft patency and wound complications at one week, and one, three and every six months postoperatively until study termination in July 2002. In addition patients were examined three times per week at their dialysis access centers. Wounds were scored by standardized radiation morbidity scoring (Radiation Therapy Oncology Group (RTOG) guidelines)[4]. This system rates radiation changes in the skin and subcutaneous tissues on a six level scale. Per protocol, angiograms were performed 1 and 6 months post-operatively. The region of minimum venous outflow luminal diameter immediately adjacent to the anastomosis was measured via two orthogonal projections. Percent stenosis was calculated as (1-(stenotic diameter/normal diameter)) X 100, with "normal diameter" being the diameter of the vein near the stenosis, excluding areas with post-stenotic dilatation. Complications and graft failures were managed according to standard clinical practice.

The primary endpoint was the combined complication rate of graft thrombosis, aneurysm formation, and significantly impaired wound healing within the first four months, a time frame dictated by the FDA. If these complications occurred in at least four patients within the first four months then the study was to be terminated. Secondary endpoints were primary and secondary patency, and maximal percent diameter reduction via angiography.

Results

All patients enrolled were male and between the ages of 59 and 71 (mean 64±3 SD). The brachial vein was the venous outflow in four patients due to the diminutive size of more superficial veins at the antecubital fossa, with the basilic serving as the outflow for the fifth. All five patients underwent graft placement and treatment as planned.

Mean and median follow up was 12 months (range 6-20 months). No patient suffered wound complications, and all RTOG scores were 0, indicating no clinically detectable skin or soft tissue changes over the period of the study (Figure 1). All patent grafts were suitable for cannulation within one-month post-operatively.

Table 1 summarizes the medium-term clinical patency and magnitude of outflow stenosis for these grafts. Patency corresponded directly with ability to dialyze via the graft. Primary patency did not extend past 8 months for any of the grafts. Of the four grafts that underwent secondary procedures, two had secondary patency greater than one year. Four of five grafts demonstrated evidence of venous outflow obstruction or failed as early as one month, and all three patent grafts studied at six months exhibited moderate to severe distal anastomotic narrowing.

Tissue retrieved from the venous outflow of patient #3 (five months after initial graft placement and radiation treatment) revealed intense venous intimal hyperplasia without discernable radiation induced changes (Figure 2).

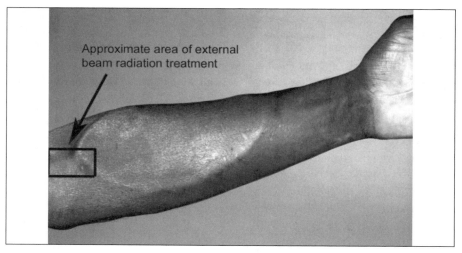

Approximate area of external beam radiation treatment

Figure 1:   Depiction of representative patient one month postoperatively, with illustration of treated (4x6 cm) area of venous anastomosis.

Table 1.   Summary of patency and angiographic results.

Patient	Primary Patency (months)	Assisted Primary Patency (months)	Secondary Patency (months)	% venous outflow stenosis @ 1 month	% venous outflow stenosis @ 6 months
#1	5	5	8 [5]*	0%	75%
#2	5	17	17 [1]	40%	40%
#3	0.5	0.5	0.5	NA	NA
#4	8	8	8.5 [1]	60%	50%
#5	1.5	1.5	>12 [1]	15%	(off HD)

*[ ] indicates number of interventions

Conclusions

Radiotherapy not only is useful in treating malignant conditions, but also has proven beneficial in preventing benign neoproliferative conditions such as skin keloids. Postoperative irradiation in single doses of 9 Gy within 24 to 72 hours have been shown to prevent keloid formation in 97% of cases[5] Additionally, radiation oncologists successfully utilize low dose electron beam radiotherapy to treat heterotopic bone formation, which is another benign neoproliferative condition similar to neointimal hyperplasia[6,7]. These studies have demonstrated that a single dose of radiation (7-8 Gy), or a high fractionated dose (10-20 Gy in 5-10 fractions), given peri-operatively significantly reduces the risk of heterotopic bone formation.

In the vascular system several human studies have used radiotherapy to prevent restenosis following balloon dilatation of atherosclerotic vascular lesions[1,8-14] and in prosthetic peripheral arterial bypasses[15].

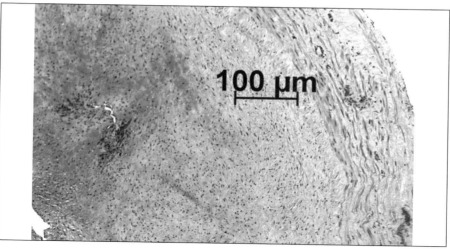

Figure 2:   Portion of ePTFE bridge graft venous outflow after graft failure. This venous cross section demonstrates a portion of the irradiated vein wall along the right hand side of the photo, with nearly occlusive neointimal hyperplasia. A small central residual vein lumen with some adjacent organizing thrombus is in the lower left corner.

After multiple large animal experiments[2,16,17], small series in humans have been reported that explore the role of radiation therapy for improved dialysis access patency[18-21]. One report involves primary ePTFE grafts[21]. In this randomized study from the Netherlands, 17 patients received 18 Gy in two 9 Gy fractions (8 failed to complete their planned treatment), and 25 patients randomized to the control group. No statistically significant clinical differences were found with radiation treatment, though patient accrual failed to meet expectations in the study.

Our approach stands in distinction to other groups by our use of a single, low dose fraction of electron beam irradiation. In addition to considerations related to the keloid and heterotopic bone dosage reports outlined above, in cell culture systems radiation causes a dose dependent inhibition of smooth muscle cell growth, with a low ED50 of 2-3 Gy[22]. *In vivo* small mammal studies also support use of single low dose ranges[23].

There are reports of endovascular brachytherapy as adjuncts to address dialysis access graft stenoses as opposed to external beam delivery[17,19,20]. Advantages of endovascular brachytherapy include dosage to a highly selective area with relatively less radiation to the surrounding tissues. In our series the arterial anastomosis was usually within the radiation treatment field. However, we selected external beam therapy since it is less operator dependent, can be performed in community settings where many dialysis access grafts are placed, and does not require invasive procedures that may otherwise jeopardize the newly placed ePTFE to a variety of complications. In addition, current external beam techniques permit precise dose delivery to specific target sites.

Although irradiation arrests cell proliferation in the short-term, chronic soft tissue injury including injury to the target vessel may occur. Fortunately, the dose responses and sensitivities to dose-fractionation are significantly disparate for these two effects[24,25]. Our lack of wound complications despite the recent vascular anastomoses and the presence of prosthetic materials in this high risk patient population supports this concept, and the reports of others[18,21].

The FDA required large animal safety and feasibility data prior to initiating the current study. In those experiments eight dogs underwent placement of 6-mm standard wall ePTFE grafts from the right common carotid artery to the left jugular vein tunneled around the posterior neck. This model functionally and anatomically mimicked human dialysis access grafts. In five treatment dogs the venous anastomosis received an 8 Gy irradiation dose immediately after surgery. Control dogs were not irradiated. All dogs underwent daily examinations to assess wound healing and graft patency. In that study shunt angiograms were completed 3 and 6 months postoperatively. Grafts were harvested after perfusion fixation per protocol at 3 and 6 months.

All incisions healed normally, though all dogs developed wound seromas that resolved spontaneously. At necropsy, both radiation treated and control grafts were well incorporated, and there were no aneurysms. One control graft thrombosed 4 months postoperatively, and angiogram and histology confirmed severe neointimal hyperplasia at the venous anastomosis. The remaining dogs with patent grafts developed similar amounts of intimal hyperplasia. Smooth muscle a-actin positive cells and proliferating cellular nuclear antigen studies showed no accelerated fibroproliferative response at radiation treated anastomoses. Skin incisions and soft tissues over irradiated anastomoses revealed no radiation induced changes on light microscopy, and no increase in apoptosis compared to controls. These results confirmed in a large animal model the feasibility and safety of a single early postoperative 8 Gy single fraction of external beam irradiation of the venous anastomosis.

The current human study confirms that early postoperative low dose external beam radiation therapy is safe (no significant wound complications) and feasible, though it must be acknowledged that the overall number of patients tested was small. Under the dosing conditions of this trial, there is no evidence to support the efficacy of radiation therapy for improved prosthetic dialysis access graft patency. The low durability of the grafts in this trial may be related to selection of patients with poor venous anatomy for permanent access. In view of the low patency results and other recent reports[21], we are currently re-evaluating the next phase, a randomized clinical trial.

References

1. Sheppard R, Eisenberg MJ, Donath D, Meerkin D. Intracoronary brachytherapy for the prevention of restenosis after percutaneous coronary revascularization. *Am Heart J.* 2003; 146:775-786.

2. Rectenwald JE, Pretus HA, Seeger JM, Huber TS, Mendenhall NP, Zlotecki RA, Palta JR, Li ZF, Hook SY, Sarac TP, Welborn MB, Klingman NV, Abouhamze ZS, Ozaki CK. External-beam radiation therapy for improved dialysis access patency: feasibility and early safety. *Radiat Res.* 2001; 156:53-60.

3. Huber TS, Ozaki CK, Flynn TC, Lee WA, Berceli SA, Hirneise CM, Carlton LM, Carter JW, Ross EA, Seeger JM. Prospective validation of an algorithm to maximize native arteriovenous fistulae for chronic hemodialysis access. *J Vasc Surg.* 2002; 36:452-459.

4. Cox JD, Stetz J, Pajak TF. Toxicity criteria of the Radiation Therapy Oncology Group (RTOG) and the European Organization for Research and Treatment of Cancer (EORTC). *Int J Radiat Oncol Biol Phys.* 1995; 31:1341-1346.

5. Lo TC, Seckel BR, Salzman FA, Wright KA. Single-dose electron beam irradiation in treatment and prevention of keloids and hypertrophic scars. *Radiother Oncol.* 1990; 19:267-272.

6. Pellegrini C, Konski AK, Gastel JA, Rubin P, Evarts CM. Prevention of heterotopic bone ossification with irradiation after total hip arthroplasty. *Journal of Bone and Joint Surgery.* 1992; 74A:186-200.

7. Pellegrini-VD J, Gregoritch SJ. Preoperative irradiation for prevention of heterotopic ossification following total hip arthroplasty. *J Bone Joint Surg Am.* 1996; 78:870-881.

8. Verin V, Urban P, Popowski Y, Schwager M, Nouet P, Dorsaz PA, Chatelain P, Kurtz JM, Rutishauser W. Feasibility of intracoronary beta-irradiation to reduce restenosis after balloon angioplasty. A clinical pilot study [see comments]. *Circulation.* 1997; 95:1138-1144.

9. Nori D, Parikh S, Moni J. Management of peripheral vascular disease: innovative approaches using radiation therapy. *Int J Radiat Oncol Biol Phys.* 1996; 36:847-856.

10. Waksman R. Local catheter-based intracoronary radiation therapy for restenosis. *Am J Cardiol.* 1996; 78:23-28.

11. Schopohl B, Leirmann D, Pohlit LJ, Heyd R, Strassmann G, Bauersachs R, Schulte HD, Rahl CG, Manegold KH, Kollath J, Bottcher HD. 192IR endovascular brachytherapy for avoidance of intimal hyperplasia after percutaneous transluminal angioplasty and stent implantation in peripheral vessels: 6 years of experience. *Int J Radiat Oncol Biol Phys.* 1996; 36:835-840.

12. Liermann D, Bottcher HD, Kollath J, Schopohl B, Strassmann G, Strecker EP, Breddin KH. Prophylactic endovascular radiotherapy to prevent intimal hyperplasia after stent implantation in femoropopliteal arteries. *Cardiovasc Intervent Radiol.* 1994; 17:12-16.

13. Bottcher HD, Schopohl B, Liermann D, Kollath J, Adamietz IA. Endovascular irradiation—a new method to avoid recurrent stenosis after stent implantation in peripheral arteries: technique and preliminary results. *Int J Radiat Oncol Biol Phys.* 1994; 29:183-186.

14. Popma JJ, Suntharalingam M, Lansky AJ, Heuser RR, Speiser B, Teirstein PS, Massullo V, Bass T, Henderson R, Silber S, von Rottkay P, Bonan R, Ho KK, Osattin A, Kuntz RE. Randomized trial of 90Sr/90Y beta-radiation versus placebo control for treatment of in-stent restenosis. *Circulation.* 2002; 106:1090-1096.

15. Hofmann WJ, Kopp M, Sedlmayer F, Trubel W, Kogelnik HD, Magometschnigg H. External beam radiation for prevention of intimal hyperplasia in peripheral arterial bypasses. *Int J Radiat Oncol Biol Phys.* 2003; 56:1180-1183.

16. Kelly BS, Narayana A, Heffelfinger SC, Denman D, Miller MA, Elson H, Armstrong J, Karle W, Nanayakkara N, Roy-Chaudhury P. External beam radiation attenuates venous neointimal hyperplasia in a pig model of arteriovenous polytetrafluoroethylene (PTFE) graft stenosis. *Int J Radiat Oncol Biol Phys.* 2002; 54:263-269.

17. Sun S, Beitler JJ, Ohki T, Calderon TM, Schechner R, Yaparpalvi R, Berman JW, Tellis VA, Greenstein SM. Inhibitory effect of brachytherapy on intimal hyperplasia in arteriovenous fistula. *J Surg Res.* 2003; 115:200-208.

18. Parikh S, Nori D, Rogers D, Charytan C, Osian A, Al Saloum M, Cavallo G. External beam radiation therapy to prevent postangioplasty dialysis access restenosis: a feasibility study. *Cardiovasc Radiat Med.* 1999; 1:36-41.

19. Cohen GS, Freeman H, Ringold MA, Putnam SG, Ball DS, Silverman C, Schulman G. External beam irradiation as an adjunctive treatment in failing dialysis shunts. *J Vasc Interv Radiol.* 2000; 11:321-326.

20. El Sharouni SY, Smits HF, Wust AF, Battermann JJ, Blankestijn PJ. Endovascular brachytherapy in arteriovenous grafts for haemodialysis does not prevent development of stenosis. *Radiother Oncol.* 1998; 49:199-200.

21. van Tongeren RB, Levendag PC, Coen VL, Schmitz PI, Gescher FM, Vernhout RM, Wittens CH, Bruijninckx CM. External beam radiation therapy to prevent anastomotic intimal hyperplasia in prosthetic arteriovenous fistulas: results of a randomized trial. *Radiother Oncol.* 2003; 69:73-77.

22. Gajdusek CM, Tian H, London S, Zhou D, Rasey J, Mayberg MR. Gamma radiation effect on vascular smooth muscle cells in culture. *Int J Radiat Oncol Biol Phys.* 1996; 36:821-828.

23. Mayberg MR, Luo Z, London S, Gajdusek C, Rasey JS. Radiation inhibition of intimal hyperplasia after arterial injury. *Radiat Res.* 1995; 142:212-220.

24. El Naggar AM, El Baz LM, Carsten AL, Chanana AD, Cronkite EP. Radiation-induced damage to blood vessels: a study of dose—effect relationship with time after X-irradiation. *Int J Radiat Biol Relat Stud Phys Chem Med.* 1978; 34:359-366.

25. Lindsay S, Kohn HI, Dakin RL, Jew J. Aortic arteriosclerosis in the dog after aortic x-irradiation. *Circ Res.* 1962; 10:51-59.

DISCUSSION

Vascular Access for Hemodialysis IX
May 6-7, 2004
Lake Buena Vista, Florida

May 7, 2004
Abstract Session III

Dr. C Keith Ozaki
"Radiation Therapy for Improved Dialysis Patency – Safety and Feasibility"

Question: One of the problems with the basic biology is that when you use radiation on a neo-intimal lesion after it has been treated with, say angioplasty, you are actually using the radiation on active tissue. You are actually radiating the tissue that has yet to become active, therefore, it is similar to treating a tumor with radiation. It is not going to have an effect.

Ozaki: Yes I agree and that has always been my view of intimal hyperplasia and radiation. Radiation would target actively dividing cells. The radiation oncologist on our team argued that there were other examples where pre-emptive radiation actually had an impact on that neointimal response and they site the heterotopic bone formation literature as well as keloid formation. In those clinical scenarios, they can actually give the radiation preoperatively and have an impact on that neo-proliferative response. Obviously, the results of this study is more consistent with the idea that radiation really only impacts actively dividing cells.

Question: Maybe I missed it. Did you in your large animal model look at varying times opposed to implantation of radiating the outflow vein?

Ozaki: We did all of our radiation in the large animal study within 24 hours and we did postoperative surveillance by angiograms at three and six months in that study.

Question: So if you could redesign your study prior to going to your prospective trial, would you make changes?

Ozaki: I have been skeptical that this would not work. But we had a lot of enthusiasm at our institution. We wanted to ensure that the study was done well. In view of this report as well as another report that came out last year from the Netherlands, right now I do not think it is promising enough to devote much effort toward this strategy for this problem. Other approaches may be more fruitful.

Comment/Question: I know you guys have a 92% autogenous vein use, but that brachial vein was so beautiful. Have you tried using the brachial vein for access?

Ozaki: Only as the outflow for a prosthetic graft. We have not used it as far as transposing or anything like that.

28

CASE PRESENTATION: IV TUNNELED CATHETER PLACEMENT VIA A DIRECT TRANSLUMBAR APPROACH

Daniel A. Siragusa, MD
(Assistant Professor, Department of Radiology, University of Florida Health Science Center – Jacksonville)

Ricardo Cruzado-Ceballos, MD
(Vascular/Interventional Radiology Fellow, University of Florida Health Science Center – Jacksonville)

H. Martin Northup, MD
(Professor, Department of Radiology, University of Florida Health Science Center – Jacksonville)

Corresponding Author:
Daniel A. Siragusa, MD
Shands Hospital – Jacksonville
Department of Radiology
655 West 8th Street
Jacksonville, FL 32209
(904) 244-4224 (phone)
(904) 244-5845 (fax)
Daniel.Siragusa@jax.ufl.edu

Introduction

United States Renal Data System (USRDS) data show an almost exponential growth in the hemodialysis population over the past decade.[1] As this population ages and we continue to improve medical care of chronic disease states such as diabetes, hypertension, and cardiovascular disease, there will be an ever increasing number of patients who have difficulty maintaining functional access for dialysis. USRDS 2003 data indicate that during the 1999-2001 period, approximately 855 patients died in the US due to lack of sufficient vascular access.[1] This statistic has improved from prior years, but is still unacceptably high. In the future, we need to not only be aggressive in maintaining existing access, but we must also be aggressive in pursuing new access sites and modalities. We present an index case of translumbar tunneled dialysis catheter placement to introduce a more in-depth discussion of this access modality.

Materials and Methods

Our patient is a 37 yo AA male who had exhausted all upper extremity surgically placed accesses. Additionally, his bilateral subclavian and internal jugular veins all had long segment occlusions (figure 1). A surgically placed groin AV graft had recently failed despite aggressive attempts at maintenance. Only one femoral vein remained open at the time of the procedure. After a multidisciplinary discussion of the options available, it was decided to place an IVC tunneled catheter via a direct, translumbar approach, leaving the remaining femoral site untouched to allow for another attempt at graft placement.

After appropriate informed consent was obtained, the patient was placed supine on the angiography table. A flush venogram of the IVC was done to ensure sufficient patency for catheter placement (figure 2). An infra-renal IVC access site was identified with a Sos Omniflush catheter, and the flush catheter was positioned with the loop in the mid-infrarenal IVC and secured in place. The patient was then administered general anesthesia.

After rolling the patient into the prone position, a right posterior oblique approach was identified approximately 8cm right of the mid-line and just above the iliac crest, and a 21-gauge needle from an Accustick II set was used to access the IVC using the previously placed catheter as a target (figure 3). After access was obtained with the needle, the 0.018 wire from the set was introduced, and the reinforced transition dilator was introduced in the IVC over the 0.018 wire. After exchange of the 0.018 wire for an 0.035 Amplatz wire, the tract was serially dilated, and a 16 french peel-away sheath was placed into the IVC. A subcutaneous tract was then made from the right flank, and a Maxid™ dialysis catheter was tunneled from the right flank to the IVC access site. The catheter was then placed into the IVC through the peel-away sheath using standard technique. We then advanced the catheter until its tip lay within the right atrium (figure 4). Standard post-procedure suturing and dressings were then applied, and we awakened the patient from anesthesia.

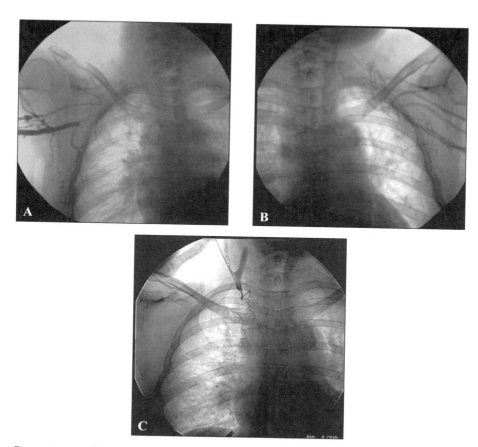

Figure 1:   Venograms of upper body central veins. (A) Right subclavian venous
             occlusion. (B) Left subclavian venous occlusion. (C) Right internal
             jugular occlusion. The left internal jugular vein was occluded on
             ultrasound examination.

Discussion

In every dialysis population, there exist a small subset of patients from whom maintaining reliable vascular access is a challenge. These patients exhaust their more
conventional access sites and require more advanced access techniques. The
translumbar placement of a long-term vascular access catheter directly into the IVC
was first described by Kenney, et al in 1985.[2] They reported a patient with short-gut
syndrome for whom the catheter was placed for long-term TPN. Since then, there
have been multiple reports and case series of patients for whom this technique has
been used for TPN, chemotherapy, bone marrow transplant, stem cell harvest via
apheresis and hemodialysis. Most patients are able to have this performed with
moderate sedation; however occasionally some patients, such as our example or
children, require the use of general anesthesia.

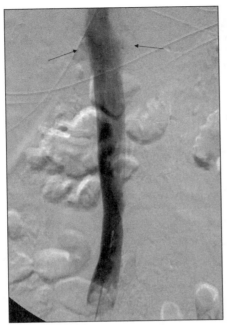

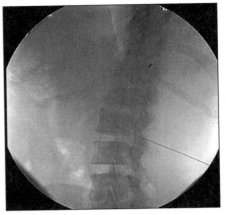

Figure 3:   21-gauge needle from an Accustick II set was used to access the IVC using the previously placed catheter as a target.

Figure 2:   Flush venogram of the IVC use to identify the renal veins (arrows).

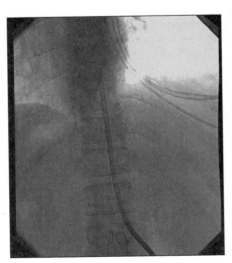

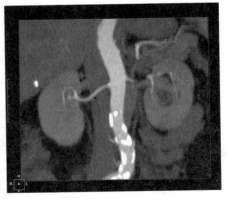

Figure 4:   Final dialysis catheter positioning with the tip in the right atrium.

Figure 5:   CT angiogram demonstrating the normal course of the right renal artery (arrow) as it passes behind the IVC at approximately the level of the right renal vein (arrowheads).

The first step in this procedure is identifying an appropriate site for accessing the IVC. While some physicians advocate forgoing venography, we prefer to perform an IVC venogram in order to identify the pertinent anatomy. The purpose of this venogram is to demonstrate that the IVC is patent and the positions of renal veins. Alternatively, ultrasound can be used for visualization of the IVC in some cases. It is important to remember that the right renal artery passes behind the IVC at approximately the level of the right renal vein (figure 5). Therefore, a mid-infrarenal IVC position is usually selected for the access point (usually at the L2-3 level). It is often helpful to position the loop of the flush catheter at the target position and secure it at the groin site. Other targets such as a guidewire or a pre-existing IVC filter have also been used.[3]

Next, we use an Accustick II set to obtain wire access to the IVC from the right back. The skin site we chose is approximately 8-10 cm to the right of midline and just above the iliac crest. This skin site allows for an angle of approach that accomplishes 3 things. First, the tract from the skin to the IVC is cephalad allowing for a non-acute entry angle into the IVC. Second, the more lateral starting position allows for avoidance of the paraspinal ligaments, which are very difficult to traverse with the dilators. Finally, this approach also allows for less acute angle from the eventual subcutaneous tunnel to the tract down to the IVC. The 21-gauge needle is advanced from the chosen skin site down to the IVC using the previously placed flush catheter and angled C-arm fluoroscopic guidance. The C-arm is angled in the RPO and cranial direction such that the view is directly down the needle (figure 6). Once the needle is started in the correct direction, the C-arm is rotated to the opposite oblique. The needle is then advanced until it is seen to reach the level of the flush catheter (figure 7). This technique allows for a minimal number of passes and prevents inadvertent double-wall puncture and passage of the needle into adjacent bowel.

When the needle position has been confirmed with aspiration and contrast injection, the 0.018 wire from the Accustick II set is advanced into the IVC and the reinforced transition dilator is advanced over the 0.018 wire into the IVC. All parts of the access set are then removed except for the outer sheath and an 0.035 Super Stiff Amplatz wire is introduced and advanced to the level of the right atrium (figure 8). Serial dilation is then performed over the Amplatz wire until an appropriate sized peel-away sheath can be inserted. It is often helpful to manually give the peel-away sheath a slight curve to allow for smoother entry in the IVC without kinking. Also, keep in mind that these catheters were not originally intended for this access route. Therefore, the peel-away sheath included in the kit may not be long enough to reach from the skin site down to the IVC. Therefore, make sure that you have longer peel-away sheaths available, especially for obese patients.

Once the peel-away sheath is in place, attention is then turned towards creating the subcutaneous tunnel. We prefer to tunnel our catheters to the right flank, preferably just anterior to the mid-axillary line. This allows for easy access by the patient for site-care and by the dialysis staff for treatments without excessive disrobing. In some patients, this requires a two-stage tunneling process. Accurate measurements are needed to make sure that the catheter chosen are long enough for the tunnel and to eventually extend up to the right atrium. Catheter lengths up to 45 cm (tip-to-cuff) may be needed. Once the catheter is tunneled from the flank to the site of the peel-away sheath, the catheter is introduced into the IVC using standard technique.

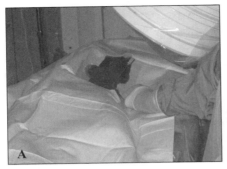

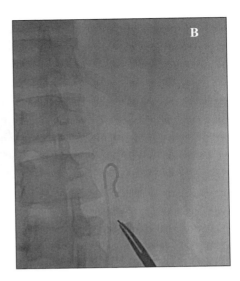

Figure 6:   The fluoroscopy C-arm (A) is angled in the RPO and cranial direction such that the fluoroscopic view (B) is directly down the needle.

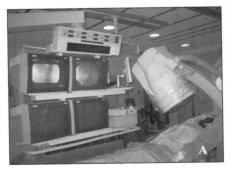

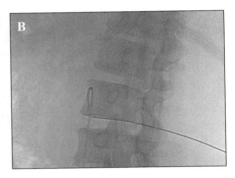

Figure 7:   The fluoroscopy C-arm is rotated to the opposite oblique (A). The needle is then advanced under fluoro until it is seen (B) to reach the level of the flush catheter.

Occasionally, guide wire assistance may be needed to attain accurate placement. Standard securement and heparin lock techniques are used. Finally, the flush catheter previously placed in the IVC is removed and groin pressure applied.

Results and Complications

Most series of patients demonstrate a 100% technical success rate with few periprocedural complications and initial flow rates in the 300-400ml/min range should be expected. The three main periprocedural complications are infection, bleeding, and perforation of a hollow viscus. Infection rates have been shown in several studies to be similar to those of tunneled catheters placed via traditional routes.[3,4,5] Periprocedural bleeding complications have been seen from both the IVC entry site and along the tract through the soft tissues down to the IVC and are estimated to be

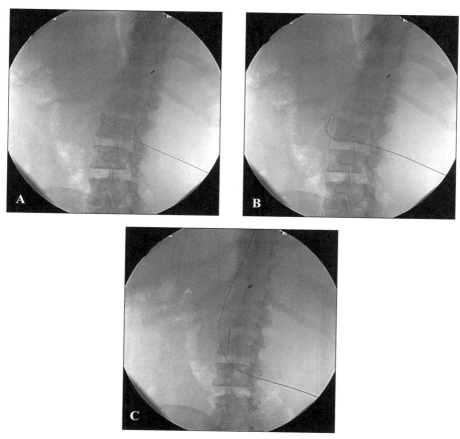

Figure 8:   Fluoroscopic images of (A) 0.018 wire from the Accustick II set has been advanced into the IVC and (B) the reinforced transition dilator is advanced over the 0.018 wire into the IVC. (C) Finally, an stiff Amplatz wire is introduced to use as a working wire.

less than 3.5%.[3,4,5,6,7] Most physicians performing this procedure also recommend that the first dialysis session post-catheter placement be performed without heparin, as there have been a few reported cases of delayed bleeding.[3] The perforation of a hollow viscus is a theoretical one and, to date, no report has been made of a patient having a clinically significant event related to this. Also, the use of a small gauge needle helps to minify the risk of a clinically significant event even if a bowel loop is entered.

Long-term patency rates are encouraging with primary patency of 55% at 6-months and 29% at one year. A life-table analysis performed by Bennett, et al demonstrated that the greatest decline in patency occurred in the first month after placement and was due to line sepsis or dislodgement. Sepsis in this group occurred more than 10 days after the placement of the catheter and was likely acquired after the procedure.[5] Overall, the most common long-term complication is infection and occurs with a rate of 2.8-3.4 episodes per 1000 catheter days, which is similar to the rates quoted for conventional access routes.[4,5,8] The next most common long-term

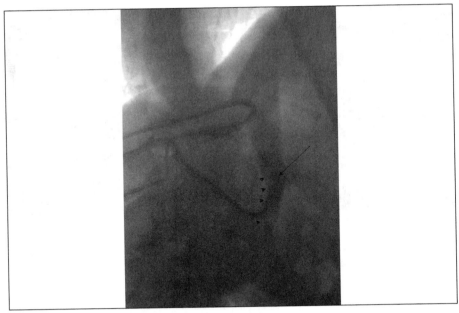

Figure 9:   This obese patient had almost complete migration of the catheter out of the IVC. This venogram demonstrates that the catheter tip (arrow) was just barely in the IVC (arrowheads). Luckily we were able to salvage this access and exchanged the catheter over a wire for a new one.

complication is catheter dysfunction due to clot or fibrin sheath formation and is estimated to occur at a rate of 3.3 per 1000 catheter days, again, similar to conventional routes.[3,4] This usually responds to outpatient fibrinolysis, but, if not, these catheters can be exchanged over a wire. Depending on the length of the subcutaneous tract, sometimes it is necessary to cut down on the supra-iliac skin site and create a new tunnel in order to perform the catheter exchange. IVC stenosis or thrombosis is a rare event. Catheter migrations are unusual events, but are clearly seen more often in patients with truncal obesity (figure 9).[3,6,9] While no definitive selection criteria on this risk factor have been identified, it should be considered and assessed before performing catheter placement via this route. Close monitoring of children with translumbar catheters also needs to be performed as they may migrate out of the IVC as the child grows.[8]

Conclusions

The translumbar insertion of dialysis catheters is a procedure that is recommended for those patients for whom more conventional access sites have been exhausted. It is a relatively safe and effective method of obtaining reliable vascular access that allows for the flow rates necessary for effective outpatient hemodialysis. Additionally, the long-term patency and complication rates are similar to those of jugular or subclavian lines.

References

1. U.S. Renal Data System, USRDS 2003 Annual Data Report: Atlas of End-Stage Renal Disease in the United States, National Institutes of Health, National Institute of Diabetes and Digestive and Kidney Diseases, Bethesda, MD. 2003.
2. Kenny PR, Dorfman GS, Denny DF. Percutaneous inferior vena cava cannulation for long-term parenteral nutrition. *Surgery.* 1985; 97:602-605.
3. Rajan DK, Croteau DL, Sturza SG, et al. Translumbar placement of inferior vena caval catheters: A solution for challenging hemodialysis access. *Radiographics.* 1998; 18:1155-1167.
4. Lund GB, Trerotola SO, Scheel PJ. Percutaneous translumbar inferior vena cava cannulation for hemodialysis. *Amer J Kid Dis.* 1995; 25(5):732-737.
5. Bennett JD, Papadouris D, Rankin RN, et al. Percutaneous inferior vena caval approach for long-term central venous access. *J Vasc Interv Radiol.* 1997; 8:851-855.
6. Biswal R, Nosher JL, Siegel RL, et al. Translumbar placement of paired hemodialysis catheters (Tesio Catheters) and follow-up in 10 patients. *Cardiovasc Intervent Rad.* 2000; 23(1):75-8.
7. Denny DF, Greenwood LH, Morse SS, et al. Inferior vena cava: Translumbar catheterization for central venous access. *Radiology.* 1989; 170:1013-1014.
8. Azizkhan RG, Taylor LA, Jaques PF, et al. Percutaneous translumbar and transhepatic inferior vena caval catheters for prolonged vascular access in children. *J Ped Surg.* 1992; 27(2):165-169.
9. Lund GB, Lieberman RP, Haire WD, et al. Translumbar inferior vena cava catheters for long-term venous access. *Radiology.* 1990; 174:31-35.

DISCUSSION

Vascular Access for Hemodialysis IX
May 6-7, 2004
Lake Buena Vista, Florida

May 7, 2004
Abstract Session III

Dr. Daniel Siragusa
"Case Presentation: IV Tunneled Catheter Placement via a Direct Translumbar Approach"

Question: How about caval thrombosis or stenosis?

Siragusa: It has been reported in one or two patients in the large series that have been done. The largest that I found was about 31 patients. But it is felt not to be a big deal because the amount of blood volume that is flowing through there, it is very difficult to have complete thrombosis.

Question: One other solution to this, especially for surgeons, or if you don't have high power interventional help, is to use the right gonadal vein in these patients. I have done this on three occasions successfully, to implant a tunneled catheter direct-ly by either a small flank incision into the right gonadal vein. This is another approach to deal with these patients with no other accesses.

Siragusa: Yeah, I've seen some of those as well in the literature.

29

NON-TUNNELED CATHETERS FOR HEMODIALYSIS: EIGHT-YEAR EXPERIENCE AT A SINGLE CENTER

Aslam Pervez, Mathews Joseph, Syed Asghar,
Fahim Zaman, Kenneth Abreo

Division of Nephrology
Department of Medicine
Louisiana State University Health Sciences Center
Shreveport, LA.

Address correspondence to:
ASLAM PERVEZ, M.D.
Assistant Professor
Division of Nephrology and Hypertension
Louisiana State University Health Sciences Center
1501 Kings Highway
Shreveport, LA 71130
Telephone: (318) 675-5914
Fax: (318) 675-5913
Email: aperve@lsuhsc.edu or apkhp@hotmail.com

Introduction

Non-tunneled hemodialysis (HD) catheter placement is a mandatory part of patient management in many clinical settings.[1] These catheters are commonly used for temporary vascular access in patients with acute renal failure who require hemodialysis (HD) and in ESRD patients who either have no vascular access, or have lost their vascular access due to infection, or are waiting for permanent access maturation.[2] The aim of the study was to evaluate the outcome and complications of non-tunneled catheter placement at our center. Herein, we describe our experience with the placement of non-tunneled dialysis catheters over the past eight years.

Methods

The computer database and paper records of all patients who received non-tunneled HD catheters placed by the Interventional Nephrology division at the Louisiana State University Health Sciences Center, Shreveport, LA between October 30, 1995 and January 22, 2004 (99 months) were reviewed. Demographic data, underlying diagnosis, indication for catheter placement, the date of catheter placement, site of venous access, procedural complications, and outcome were collected (Table 1). Exempt status was obtained from the Institutional Review Board for Human Investigation (IRB).

All procedures were performed by either one of six interventional nephrologists or by the nephrology fellow or resident with hands-on faculty supervision. Routine aseptic precautions were taken, including the use of maximal barrier precautions; e.g. sterile gloves, large sterile drape, sterile gown, cap, and mask. All patients received local anesthesia with 2% lidocaine. Internal jugular vein puncture was done with direct ultrasound (SiteRite, Dymax, Pittsburgh, Pennsylvania) guidance with a 7.5 MHz transducer covered with a sterile sheath. A mini stick kit (Boston Scientific, Medi-tech, Watertown, Massachusetts) was used (Figure 1). Ultrasound guidance was used in 10% of femoral cannulations. Fluoroscopy (OEC, Salt Lake City, Utah) was used in all internal jugular placements and in 8% of femoral placements.

Data analysis was performed using StatView software (SAS institute Inc., Cary, North Carolina). Analysis of variance (ANOVA) and descriptive analysis were used for demographic evaluations.

Table 1.   Patient Demographics.

Number of Patients	232
Male/Female	108 (47%)/124 (53%)
Whites/Blacks	33 (14%)/199 (86%)
Age (yrs. ± SD)	52 ± 15
BMI	26 ± 7

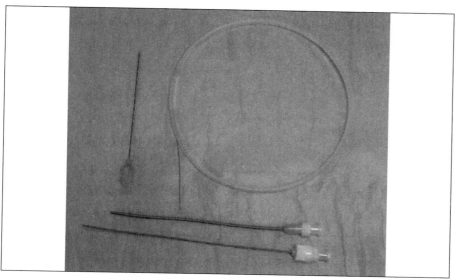

Figure 1:   Mini stick Kit. 21-gauge introducer needle, 0.018 in wire,
               3F and 5F catheters.

Results

Between 10/30/1995 and 01/22/2004, 650 non-tunneled HD catheters were placed
in 232 patients. Of these catheters, 79% were placed in the femoral and 21% in the
internal jugular veins. Two catheters were placed in the subclavian veins (Table 2).
There were 642 new catheters, and 8 were guide-wire changeovers. There were 108
males and 124 females; 199 African Americans and 33 Caucasians. The mean age
of the patients was 52 ± 15 years (range 17 - 92) and the mean BMI 26 ± 6.6 (range
11.8 – 62.4, median 25, mode 18). Nephrology fellows placed 75% of the catheters,
faculty 15%, and medicine residents 10%. Sixty-five percent of the catheters were
placed on the right side. The success rate was 97%. There were no major immediate complications. Inadvertent femoral arterial puncture occurred in 7 (1.1%) cases.
There was no instance of carotid artery puncture. There were 3 minor complications: one bleeding episode and two hematomas (Table 3).

Table 2.   Catheter Sites.

Catheter Site	Number (% of all catheters placed)
Total	650
Femoral	513 (79)
Internal Jugular	135 (21)
Subclavian	2 (0.3)

Table 3.   Complications.

Complications	Number (% of all catheters placed)
Total	11 (1.6)
Femoral Arterial Puncture	7 (1.1)
Hematoma	2 (0.3)
Excessive Bleeding	1 (0.2)
Deep venous thrombosis	1 (0.2)

Conclusion

Non-tunneled HD catheter placement is an essential part of patient management in many clinical settings. It is usually done using a landmark-guided technique. In some cases this technique does not work because external landmarks do not correlate with the exact location of the underlying vessels.[3–6] This is especially true for the internal jugular veins. Denys and Uretsky[7] assessed the position of internal jugular vein in 200 patients and found that in 5.5% of patients studied, the location of the internal jugular vein was not predicted by the external anatomical landmarks and in 8.5% of patients, the anatomy was sufficiently aberrant to complicate access placement by a blind method. At our institution, all internal jugular dialysis catheters are placed with ultrasound guidance, using a mini stick kit and fluoroscopy (Figure 2). This explains the extremely low incidence of complications such as carotid artery puncture or pneumothorax in our study. Landmark-guided technique is reasonably successful in femoral cannulations as the anatomy rarely varies.[8–10] However, in some patients who have had multiple prior catheters or grafts, the vascular anatomy and relationships are not reliable. Use of ultrasound guidance in these cases is necessary to complete the procedure with minimal trauma and complications. Sometimes, it may be difficult to advance the guide wire to a reasonable depth, necessitating the use of fluoroscopy. In such cases, a venogram should be done, and in many instances angioplasty of the stenosed vein may be needed in order to successfully place the catheter. On a few occasions, we have had

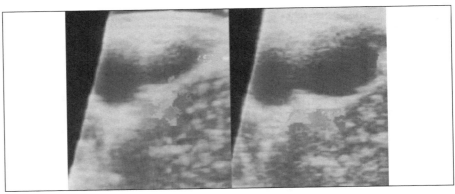

Figure 2:   Vein is compressible, artery is not (light pressure applied using ultrasound probe).

to dilate the vein with an 8 or 10 mm balloon prior for successful catheter placement (Figures 3 and 4).

Non-tunneled HD catheters are safe and easy to place with minimum risks. Use of ultrasound guidance with the mini stick kit is very helpful and minimizes complications in internal jugular and difficult femoral vein cannulation. In this cohort of patients the complications were infrequent. The overall initial success rate was 97%. There was only one documented DVT within the first three days of catheter placement. There was no incidence of pneumothorax or inadvertent arterial catheter placement.

In summary, the insertion of non-tunneled catheters for dialysis is a very safe procedure when done by dedicated interventional nephrologists. The simplicity, ease of placement, and relative safety of these catheters resulted in optimal accept-ance by both patients and physicians.

References

1. Oliver MJ. Acute dialysis catheters. *Seminars in Dialysis.* 2001; 14(6): 432-435.
2. Van Waeleghem JP. Vascular access in acute renal failure. *EDTNA ERCA J.* 2002; 29: Suppl 2:23-25.
3. Denys BG, Uretsky BF, Reddy PS. Ultrasound assisted cannulation of the internal jugular vein: a prospective comparison to the external landmark-guid-ed technique. *Circulation.* 1993; 87: 1557-1562.
4. Gadallah MF, White R, Vickers B, et al . Awareness of internal jugular, subcla-vian, superior vena cave and femoral vein anomalies may reduce morbidity of acute venous catheter procedures. *Clin Nephrol.* 1996; 44(5): 345-348.
5. Skolnick ML. The role of sonography in the placement and management of jugular and subclavian central venous catheters. *AJR.* 1994; 163: 291-295.
6. Kwon TH, Kim YL Cho DK. Ultrasound-guided cannulation of the femoral vein for acute hemodialysis access. *Nephrology Dial Transplant.* 1997; 12: 1009-1012.
7. Denys BG, Uretsky BF. Anatomical variation of internal jugular vein location: impact on central venous access. *Crit Care Med.* 1991; 19: 1516-1519.
8. Firek AF, Cutler RE, St. John Hammond PG. Reappraisal of femoral vein cannu-lation for temporary hemodialysis vascular access. *Nephron.* 1987; 47: 227-228.
9. Sznajder JI, Zveibil FR, Bitterman H, et al. Central vein catheterization, fail-ure and complication rates by three percutaneous approaches. *Arch Intern Med.* 1986; 146(2): 259-261.
10. Kairaitis LK, Gottlieb T. Outcome and complications of temporary hemodial-ysis catheters. *Nephrol Dial Transplant.* 1999: 14: 1710-1714.

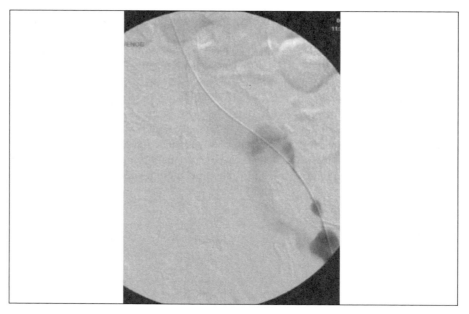

Figure 3:   Stenosed iliac vein from previous catheters.

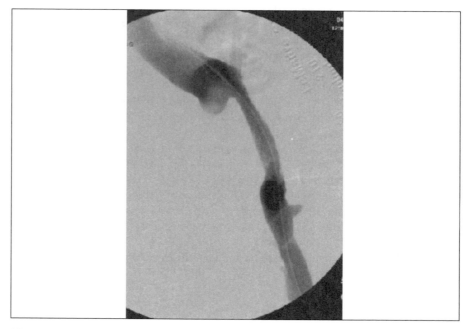

Figure 4:   The stenosed vein in figure 3 after angioplasty.

DISCUSSION

Vascular Access for Hemodialysis IX
May 6-7, 2004
Lake Buena Vista, Florida

May 7, 2004
Abstract Session III

Dr. Aslam Pervez
"Non-Tunneled Catheters for Hemodialysis (HD): Eight-Year Experience at a Single Center"

Question: How long do you leave your femoral temporary catheters in?

Pervez: Seven days maximum.

30

ACCESS REVISION BASED UPON FUNCTIONAL RATHER THAN ANATOMIC ABNORMALITIES: A CASE OF SUCCESSFUL EXPECTANT MANAGEMENT

David D. Oakes, MD, FACS
Steven S. Guest, MD

Stanford University School of Medicine
Stanford, California and
Santa Clara Valley Medical Center
San Jose, California

Address Correspondence To:
David D. Oakes, MD. FACS
Santa Clara Valley Medical Center
751 South Bascom Avenue
San Jose, California 95128
(408) 885-6060 FAX (408) 885-6054
e-mail: norma.desepte@hhs.co.santa-clara.ca.us

Introduction

The optimal timing of surgical revision of arteriovenous grafts remains controversial. Absolute indications for graft revision are inadequate dialysis (high recirculation) or graft thrombosis not correctable by interventional radiology. Some advocate revision as soon as an anatomic abnormality is detected by routine surveillance or by a fistulogram investigating early graft dysfunction.

Given that all grafts have a useful life measured in months or at most a few years, unnecessary surgical revision may lead to premature exhaustion of outflow veins, rendering future access difficult and, in some cases, eventually impossible. We therefore believe that grafts should not be surgically "corrected" solely because of anatomic abnormalities as long as dialytic function is adequate. The potential for long-term success of this expectant approach is illustrated in the following case.

Case Report

In July 1997 a 48-year-old diabetic male underwent placement of a straight bovine graft from the right radial artery to a large antecubital vein. Nine months later (May 1998) a fistulogram was performed because of elevated venous pressures. This showed a small cephalic vein in the upper arm (Figure 1 - straight open arrow); most of the outflow was retrograde via a large antecubital vein which drained into the basilic system (Figure 1- curved solid arrow). Also noted was a high-grade stenosis at the junction of the right subclavian and innominate veins, with a gradient of 22 mmHg (Figure 2a). This was reduced to 3 mmHg after balloon angioplasty. (Figure 2b)

In November 2000, another fistulogram was performed because of increased venous pressures. This showed complete occlusion of the cephalic vein about 2 cm proximal to the venous anastomosis (straight arrow), with all outflow going retrograde (curved arrow) (Figure 3). There was also re-stenosis of the central veins, with prominent venous collaterals (Figure 4).

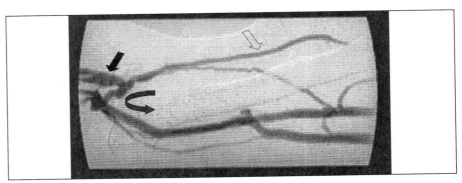

Figure 1:   Fistulogram from May 7, 1998, showing the graft (solid straight arrow) joining a small cephalic vein (straight open arrow). Most of the flow was retrograde via a large antecubital vein into the basilic system (curved arrow).

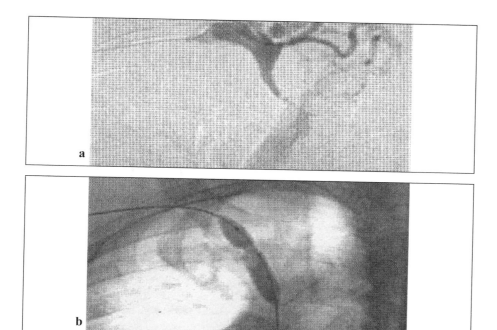

Figure 2:   (a) Fistulogram from May 7, 1998, showing high-grade stenosis at the junction of the right subclavian and innominate veins. The initial gradient was 22 mmHg. This was reduced to 3 mmHg after balloon angioplasty (b).

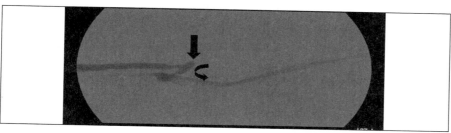

Figure 3:   Fistulogram on November 16, 2000, showing complete occlusion of the cephalic vein about 2 cm proximal to the venous anastomosis (straight arrow). Now all flow was retrograde via an antecubital vein into the basilic system (curved arrow). The patient was referred for surgical revision, but operation was deferred because dialytic function was satisfactory.

Because of occlusion of the cephalic vein and the presence of elevated venous pressures, the patient was referred for surgical revision. Operation would have required an interposition graft from the old graft to the basilic vein. Dialytic function was satisfactory, however, and we felt some of the increased venous pressure could be attributed to the central stenosis. We therefore recommended expectant

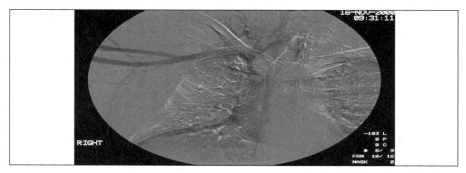

Figure 4:   Fistulogram on November 16, 2000, showing restenosis of central veins with prominent collaterals.

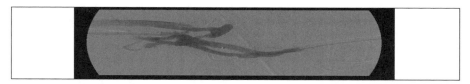

Figure 5:   Follow up study 16 months later (February 13, 2002) showing essentially no change in venous anatomy (compare Figure 3).

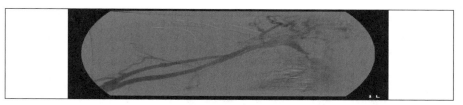

Figure 6:   Fistulogram on February 13, 2002, showing no change in central stenosis compared with November 23, 2002 (Figure 4).

management, arguing that delaying revision until graft thrombosis or loss of acceptable function would not appreciably complicate or compromise a future operation.

A followup fistulogram in February 2002 (16 months later) was essentially unchanged (Figures 5 and 6). Nevertheless the antecubital vein was dilated with an 8 mm balloon introduced via the femoral vein (Figure 7). This resulted in thrombosis of the graft, which resolved after overnight infusion of tissue plasminogen activator.

The graft provided adequate function until it thrombosed on May 21, 2003, 30 months after cephalic occlusion had first been documented. It was revised by placing an interposition graft from the original graft (Figure 8 – solid arrow) to the basilic vein (Figure 8 – open arrow). The operation was not complicated by having been delayed from November 2000.

The graft thrombosed in January 2004. It was successfully revised with a patch angioplasty and, in spite of complete occlusion of the central veins, was still functioning four months later at the time of this review.

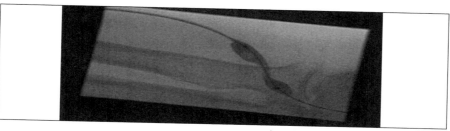

Figure 7:   In spite of stable anatomy, on February 13, 2002 the antecubital vein was dilated with an 8 mm balloon. This led to graft thrombosis, which resolved after overnight infusion of tissue plasminogen activator.

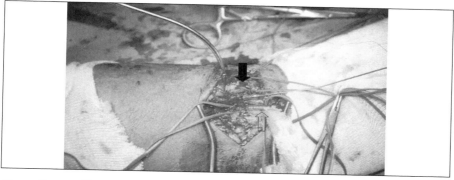

Figure 8:   The graft functioned well until May 21, 2003, 30 months after cephalic vein occlusion was first documented. This intra-operative photograph shows the graft (solid arrow) and a 5 mm basilic vein (open arrow). The two were joined by a 1.5 cm x 6 mm PTFE interposition graft.

Conclusions

Delaying surgical revision protected this patient's basilic vein from surgical trauma and from direct turbulent flow for 2 ½ years. The delay did not make the eventual operation in any way more difficult. We believe that expectant management significantly extended the life of this access.

Because balloon angioplasty can be performed without sacrificing venous length, we feel it is acceptable to use prophylactic intervention. On the other hand, surgical revision should be based upon functional rather than anatomic abnormalities in order to maximize the time vascular access can be maintained in any given patient.

We incidentally note that satisfactory vascular access has been maintained in this patient in spite of total occlusion at the junction of the right subclavian and innominate veins.

31

THE ROLE OF PATCH ANGIOPLASTY IN SALVAGING A FAILING BRESCIA FISTULAE WITH INFLOW STENOSIS

David D. Oakes, MD, FACS, Tej M. Singh, MD,
Steven S. Guest, MD

Stanford University School of Medicine
Stanford, California and
Santa Clara Valley Medical Center
San Jose, California

Address Correspondence To:
David D. Oakes, MD. FACS
Santa Clara Valley Medical Center
751 South Bascom Avenue
San Jose, California 95128
(408) 885-6060 FAX (408) 885-6054
e-mail: norma.desepte@hhs.co.santa-clara.ca.us

Introduction

A successful Brescia fistula creates a dilated, arterialized in situ vein, which is the optimal vascular conduit for hemodialysis. Once developed, these fistulae rarely fail, but, when they do, the failure is frequently secondary to inadequate inflow. This may be due to central arterial disease per se[1] but more commonly arises from stenosis of the juxta-anastomotic vein (the segment of vein adjacent to the anastomosis).[2–7]

Over the past 15 years we have developed a sequential approach for dealing with this problem. The following case illustrates one component of that strategy.

Case Report

A 40-year-old male presented in August 2001 with end stage renal disease. Hemodialysis was begun via a tunneled, cuffed catheter. On November 8, 2001 a left Brescia fistula was created. After three months the fistula was deemed usable. On April 9, 2002 it lost its thrill and bruit. By physical examination the vein was dilated and patent, but had no arterial inflow. The anastomosis was explored and a patch angioplasty performed using polytetrafluoroethylene (PTFE), crossing the original suture line. The fistula worked well for 5 months until decreased flows were again noted. A fistulogram on August 2, 2002 revealed a short, complete occlusion of the vein approximately 1-2 cm from the anastomosis (Figure 1- arrow). Balloon angioplasty was not possible. This area was explored on August 5, 2002 with the plan of performing a more proximal anastomosis, however, because the stenotic area is so localized, a second patch angioplasty was performed using PTFE.

The fistula functioned well for over a year until high recirculation values were noted. A fistulogram on September 23, 2003 showed "multiple tandem stenoses" (Figure 2). These were angioplastied, but without improvement in flow.

On December 8, 2003 the distal-most stenotic segment was explored surgically with the plan of performing a more proximal anastomosis. Once again a localized area of stenosis was found about one centimeter downstream from the previous patch. (Figure 2 - arrow). This new stenosis was slightly longer (3.5 cm), but with patent venous segments (>5.0 mm) both proximally and distally (Figures 3 and 4 – see 5.0 mm dilators). A third patch angioplasty was therefore performed (Figures 5a and 5b). The fistula was still functional 5 months later at the time of this review.

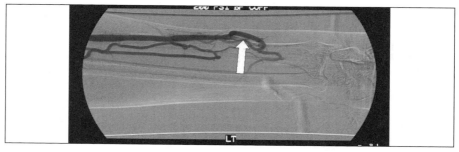

Figure 1:   Fistulogram from August 2, 2002 showing clot occluding the distal vein adjacent to the arterial venous anastomosis (arrow). The clot could not be crossed with a guide wire precluding balloon angioplasty. At operation a short stenotic segment was found which was repaired using a small patch of polytetrafluoroethylene (PTFE).

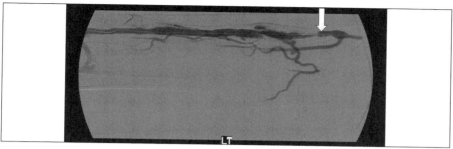

Figure 2:   Fistulogram from September 23, 2003. "Multiple tandem stenoses" were dilated angiographically without improvement in flow. The patient was therefore scheduled for surgical revision. The main stricture was just proximal to the patch placed on August 5, 2002. (arrow).

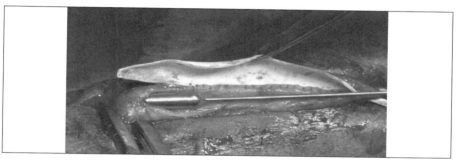

Figure 3:   Intraoperative photograph from December 8, 2003. The stricture has been opened longitudinally and is being patched with polytetrafluoroethylene. A metal dilator shows that the proximal vein is at least 5 mm in diameter.

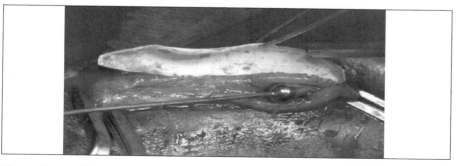

Figure 4:   Same as Figure 3, except that the dilator now shows that the distal vein is also greater than 5 mm.

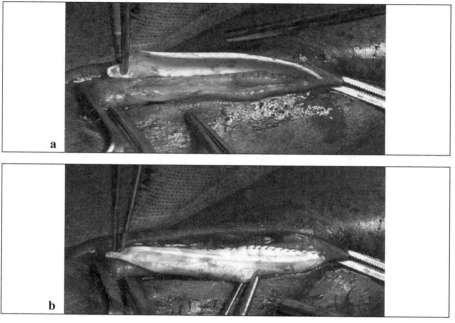

Figure 5:   This intraoperative photograph shows placement of a PTFE patch on December 8, 2003. a) Interior aspect of patch b) Outer aspect of patch.

Discussion

At one time dysfunctional Brescia fistulae were simply abandoned, but over the years we have learned that some can be successfully salvaged, especially if they develop an inflow problem after several months of use.[7] We originally recommended immediate surgical revision with the creation of a new, more proximal anastomosis for these patients, believing that the intimal trauma of surgery was less than that of balloon angioplasty. We now believe that balloon angioplasty should be attempted first. If unsuccessful, a more proximal anastomosis will still be possible.

In selected cases, such as described here, patch angioplasty of localized stenoses may allow fistula function in the long term and should be considered after balloon angioplasty and before a more proximal anastomosis is created. If the radial artery itself is too diseased, it may be possible to provide inflow to the distal vein by a graft from the brachial artery (Figures 6a and 6b).[8]

Conclusion

We feel that patch angioplasty has a role to play, after balloon angioplasty and before a more proximal anastomosis, in selected patients whose Brescia fistulae are failing secondary to a localized stenosis of the juxta-anastomotic vein. We currently recommend a sequential approach to this problem, considering at each step the appropriateness of each of the following techniques in the following order:

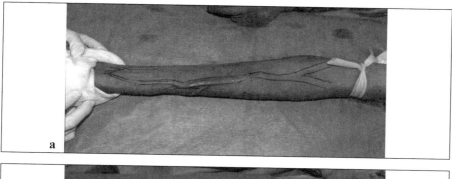

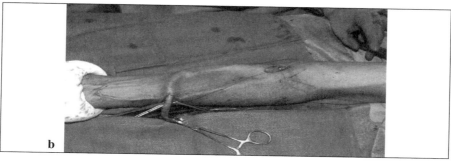

Figure 6:   These photographs show the technique of arterializing the distal vein by a graft from the brachial artery. a) Dilated superficial veins with inadequate inflow secondary to advanced disease of the radial artery. b) Bovine graft being tunneled from brachial artery to distal vein.

Balloon angioplasty

Patch angioplasty

More proximal anastomosis

Graft from the brachial artery to the distal-most part of the dilated vein

References

1. Oakes DD, Singh T, Guest SS. Late onset hand ischemia in a patient with a Brescia-Cimino fistula: an unusual cause for an unusual problem. In: Henry ML, Ed. *Vascular Access for Hemodialysis VIII.* Arlington Heights, Il: WL Gore and Associates and ACCESS Medical Press. 2002; 183-188.

2. Bone, GE, Pomajzi MJ. Management of dialysis fistula thrombosis. *Am J Surg.* 1979; 138:901-906.

3. Palder SB, Kirkman RL, Whittemore AD, Hakim RM, Lazarus JM, Tilney NL. Vascular access for hemodialysis: Patency rates and results of revision. *Ann Surg.* 1985; 202:235-239.

4. Haimov M. Circulatory access for hemodialysis. In: Rutherford RB, Ed. *Vascular Surgery.* Philadelphia-London-Toronto: WB Saunders Company; 1989; 1072-1085.

5. Marx AB, Landmann J, Harder FH. Surgery for vascular access. *Curr Probl Surg.* 1992; I:3-48.

6. Turmel-Rodrigues L, Pengloan J, Blanchier D, et al. Insufficient dialysis shunts: Improved long-term patency rates with close hemodynamic monitoring, repeat percutaneous balloon angioplasty, and stent placement. *Radiology.* 1993; 187:273-287.

7. Oakes DD, Sherck JP, Cobb LF. Surgical salvage of failed radiocephalic arteriovenous fistulae: techniques and results in 29 patients. *Kidney Int.* 1998;53:480-487.

8. Oakes DD, Adams GA, Sherck JP, Guest SS. A new operation utilizing inadequate Brescia fistulae to preserve more proximal veins. *J Vasc Surg.* 2002;36: 346-350.

32

OUTCOME AFTER AUTOGENOUS BRACHIAL-AXILLARY TRANSLOCATED SUPERFICIAL FEMORAL/POPLITEAL VEIN ACCESS

Thomas S. Huber, MD, PhD, Christa M. Hirneise, RN,
W. Anthony Lee, MD, Timothy C. Flynn, MD, James M. Seeger, MD

Division of Vascular and Endovascular Therapy
Department of Surgery
University of Florida College of Medicine
Gainesville, Florida

Correspondence:
Thomas S. Huber, MD, PhD
Division of Vascular and Endovascular Therapy
Department of Surgery
P.O. Box 100286
University of Florida College of Medicine
Gainesville, Florida 32610-0286
PH: 352-265-0605, FAX: 352-338-9818
E-mail: Huber@surgery.ufl.edu

Introduction

The optimal treatment for patients with "complex" or "tertiary" hemodialysis access problems remains unclear. This subset of patients poses a particularly difficult challenge in terms of maintaining sufficient access to assure adequate dialysis while minimizing the access related complications. The National Kidney Foundation Clinical Guidelines for Vascular Access (NKF/DOQI) have truly defined dialysis access care and have emphasized the benefits of autogenous configurations.[1] The NKF/DOQI recommended the autogenous radiocephalic and brachiocephalic accesses as the first two options and stated that the third option should be either an autogenous brachiobasilic or prosthetic access. However, they provide little guidance for patients with inadequate peripheral veins for autogenous access and those with multiple previous prosthetic failures. Unfortunately, it is anticipated that this subset of patients will increase given the expanding population of end stage renal disease (ESRD) patients and their improved life expectancies. Indeed, the United States Renal Data System reported that there were approximately 250,000 patients on hemodialysis in 2000 including 94,000 new patients while the mean life expectancy for ESRD patients between 50 – 54 years of age is > 5 years.[2] This report will review our published experience with the autogenous brachial-axillary translocated superficial femoral/popliteal vein access (SFV ACCESS) in a series of patients with complex hemodialysis access needs.[3]

Methods

Preoperative Evaluation   Patients referred for permanent hemodialysis were initially evaluated using our published algorithm designed to optimize the use of autogenous access.[4] Briefly, patients underwent upper extremity arterial and venous noninvasive imaging as their initial step. The arterial studies included standard pressure measurements and waveform analyses in addition to diameter measurements of the brachial and radial vessels at the elbow and wrist respectively. The venous noninasive imaging included assessment of both the diameter and quality of the cephalic and basilic veins and interrogation of the axillary and subclavian veins to rule out thromboses. Patients that were not candidates for one of the more traditional upper extremity autogenous accesses were considered candidates for a prosthetic access. Those without one of the traditional autogenous options and those with relative contraindications for a prosthetic access, usually from a history of multiple prosthetic access failures from early thrombosis or infection, were additionally considered for SFV ACCESS. These patients underwent further noninvasive imaging to confirm that the superficial femoral/popliteal vein was a suitable conduit, to confirm that their lower extremity arterial circulation was sufficient to heal the vein harvest incision (popliteal pressure > 50 mm Hg) and to determine that the saphenous vein was suitable to be used as a composite vein if the superficial femoral/popliteal vein was not sufficient or as a conduit for a distal revascularization/interval ligation (DRIL) procedure if postoperative hand ischemia developed.[5] The lower extremity arterial studies included pressure measurements with determination of ankle-brachial indices and waveform analyses. The diameter and quality of the saphenous and superficial/femoral popliteal veins were examined with duplex ultrasound. The superficial femoral/popliteal vein segments were considered suitable if their diameter was > 6 mm and there were no intraluminal defects. The arterial inflow and venous outflow on the upper extremity selected for the SFV ACCESS were further interrogated with a standard contrast arteriogram and venogram.

Operative Technique (Figure 1)   The brachial artery was exposed proximal to the antecubital fossa while the axillary vein was exposed in the axilla. It was usually necessary to remove all prior prosthetic accesses in the arm to facilitate exposure of the desired vessels and to create the tunnel for the vein graft. The superficial femoral/popliteal vein was exposed through an incision that extended from the inferior aspect of the femoral triangle to the above knee popliteal fossa on the lateral aspect of the sartorius muscle. The superficial femoral/popliteal vein was then dissected free caudally from its confluence with the profunda femoral vein to the mid popliteal fossa. The superficial femoral/popliteal vein was excised flush with the profunda femoral vein and immediately behind the patella in the mid popliteal fossa. A 30 cm segment of vein can be harvested using the outlined technique and this is usually sufficient to construct a brachial-axillary access that includes a generous lateral curve over the biceps muscle. The tunnel in the arm was created using a 6 mm semicircular tunneler, and the vein was passed through the tunnel non-distended and in a reversed orientation to maintain antegrade flow. The proximal and distal anastomoses were performed with 6-0 and 5-0 monofilament suture respectively while two #10 Jackson-Pratt drains were placed in the bed of the superficial femoral/popliteal vein harvest. The access and the ipsilateral upper extremity pulses were interrogated using both physical examination and continuous wave Doppler.

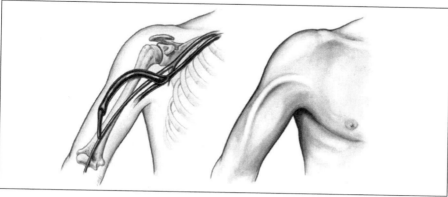

Figure 1:   The original artist's diagram of the autogenous brachial-axillary translocated superficial femoral/popliteal vein access (SFV ACCESS) is shown. The drawing depicts a composite configuration with saphenous and superficial femoral/popliteal vein although this has rarely been necessary in our more recent experience. As noted in the text, the SFV ACCESS has the appearance of a mature brachio-cephalic autogenous access (From Huber TS, et al. Use of superficial femoral vein for hemodialysis arteriovenous access. J Vasc Surg 31:1038-1041, 2000, with permission).

Notably, the traditional thrill used to confirm the adequacy of the access was not always present in the SFV ACCESS despite no technical defects and a patent ipsilateral central vein.

Postoperative Care   Patients were admitted to the hospital after the procedure and were closely monitored for the development of hand ischemia, wound infection/breakdown, and compartment syndrome. They were followed closely in the outpatient setting until the SFV ACCESS was suitable for cannulation although no set criteria were used to make this determination. Patients with mild to moderate (grade 1 – 2) hand ischemia were managed expectantly while those with severe (grade 3) ischemia underwent the DRIL procedure.[6] Patients that developed problems during dialysis from either reduced flows or elevated venous pressures underwent fistulogram and remedial treatment while those with thrombosed accesses underwent initial chemical lysis prior to revision.

Analyses and Statistics   The primary, primary assisted, and secondary functional patency rates for the SFV ACCESS were reported using the life table methods.[7] All continuous data were reported as the mean value + the standard deviation. Patient groups were compared using a Fisher's exact test and a p value < .05 was accepted as significant.

Results

A total of 30 patients underwent SFV ACCESS during the study period (11/98 – 12/03). The mean patient age was 54 + 15 years and the majority were female (67%) and Afro-American (63%) while a significant proportion were diabetic (50%) and obese (21%)(obese > 125% ideal body weight)). Diabetes (43%) and hypertension (23%) were the leading causes of ESRD. The patients had been on dialysis for 4 + 5 years (range 0 – 24 years) and had an average of 3 + 3 (range 0 – 17) previous permanent hemodialysis access procedures. The overwhelming majority of the patients were actively dialyzing through tunneled catheters (tunneled hemodialysis catheter – 90%, peritoneal dialysis catheter – 3%, prosthetic hemodialysis access – 7%).

The 30-day-in-hospital mortality rate was 3% while the 60-day mortality rate was 7%. One patient in the current study died prior to discharge due to a respiratory arrest while a second patient was readmitted in the early postoperative period with wound problems and had a fatal arrhythmia. Fifty seven percent of the patients experienced some type of perioperative complication and 38% required some type of remedial surgical procedure as a result of the complication. Significant hand ischemia developed in 43% of the patients (severity score 1 (mild) – 10%, 2 (moderate) – 7%, 3 (severe) – 27%) and required a DRIL procedure in 27% or all those with a severity score of 3. There were no significant differences in the incidence of hand ischemia between diabetics/non-diabetics (47% vs. 40%), males/females (20% vs. 55%, p = .12) and patients > 65 years /patients < 65 years (29% vs. 48%). Thigh wound complications and/or hematomas developed in 23% of the patients while arm wound complications and/or hematomas developed in 17%. There was a significant difference in the incidence of thigh complications and/or hematomas between obese/non obese patients (57% vs. 13%, p = .03), but not for the arm complications and/or hematomas (42% vs. 9%, p = .07). The mean hospital length of stay after the SFV ACCESS was 7 + 7 days while 7% of the patients were subsequently readmitted secondary to some type of perioperative complication for a total postoperative length of stay of 9 + 12 days. The SFV ACCESS was initially cannulated for dialysis at 7 + 1 weeks postoperatively.

The primary, primary assisted, and secondary patency rates for the SFV ACCESS were 96 + 4, 100 + 0, and 100 + 0 respectively at 6 months, 79 + 8%, 91 + 6%, and 100 + 0 % respectively at 12 months, and 67 + 13%, 86 + 9%, and 100 + 0 % respectively at 18 months **(Figure 2)**. The three accesses that thrombosed were all successfully treated with chemical lysis. No identifiable cause for the thrombosis was found in one case while critical stenoses were found in the superficial femoral/popliteal vein segment in the other two cases requiring open, surgical revision (interposition graft, vein patch angioplasty). The procedures to maintain patency among the "failing" accesses with critical stenoses included balloon angioplasty and interposition grafting in the superficial femoral/popliteal vein segment or central veins.

Discussion

The intermediate term functional patency rates for the SFV ACCESS are excellent although the procedure is associated with a significant cost in terms of perioperative morbidity and mortality. The patency rates are comparable to those reported for other autogenous accesses and significantly better than those usually reported for

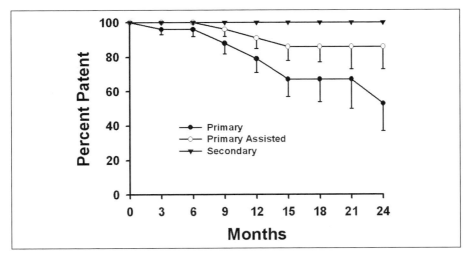

Figure 2: The primary, primary assisted, and secondary life table curves and their corresponding negative standard error bars are shown for the SFV ACCESS. The standard errors exceed 10% at 15 and 18 months respectively for the primary and primary assisted patency respectively. (From Huber TS, et al. Outcome after autogenous brachial-axillary translocated superficial-femoral/popliteal vein hemodialysis access. J Vasc Surg, in press, with permission).

prosthetic conduits. Furthermore, the results are even more impressive given the fact that the patient population had complex access problems with limited options and multiple prior procedures.

We have maintained a significant amount of enthusiasm for the SFV ACCESS despite the associated complications and contend that the characteristics of the vein and the excellent patency rates justify the procedure. The mean diameter of the superficial femoral/popliteal vein in adults is 7 mm at its midportion[8] and the wall is very thick relative to either the basilic or cephalic vein. Indeed, the SFV ACCESS has the appearance and handling characteristics of a mature, arterialized brachio-cephalic autogenous access. Additionally, the mortality rate in the current study, although significant, was comparable to that for our access practice as a whole and attests to the fact that ESRD patients are a modest operative risk despite what seems to be a fairly minimal procedure. Indeed, the annual, unadjusted death rate for all patients with ESRD across the United States is 177.6 per 1,000 patient years at risk.[2]

We would concede that the role of the SFV ACCESS in patients with complex access problems is debatable in light of the associated morbidity and mortality given the fact that there are other access alternatives. Essentially all of the patients in our series could have had a brachial-axillary prosthetic access, a tunneled catheter or a femoral-femoral inguinal access using either autogenous or prosthetic conduit. The study patients were considered for SFV ACCESS only if we felt that they would not derive significant additional benefit from a brachial artery based prosthetic access although this is obviously subjective. Furthermore, the use of temporary catheters increases the mortality for ESRD patients relative to autogenous or prosthetic accesses[9-11] while the infectious complications of thigh prosthetic accesses are significant and may be prohibitive.[12-15] Cull et al.[13] recently reported that incidence of infectious complications after 125 prosthetic thigh accesses was 41% while the 2 year primary patency rates were only 19% and concluded that tunneled catheters were a superior option. Notably, both Jackson[16] and Gradman et al.[17] have reported transposing the superficial femoral vein in the thigh to create an autogenous access. The patency rates reported by Gradman et al.[17] were excellent (12 months: primary - 73%; secondary - 86%) although the complication rates (major wound – 28%, remedial procedure for ischemia – 32%, major amputation – 4%) were significant and comparable to our series.

The algorithm defining our hierarchy of access configurations outlined in the Methods section reflects our current practice although the results of the study have forced us to reexamine the indications for the SFV ACCESS. The net effect is that we have become somewhat more conservative about recommending the procedure. Unfortunately, our univariate analyses did not allow us to identify the subsets of patients at risk for hand or wound complications with the exception of the increased incidence of thigh complications among obese patients. We presently reserve the procedure for compliant, good risk patients with a reasonable life expectancy and a suitable segment of saphenous vein that could be used for a DRIL procedure. Patients need to be compliant because those that require a DRIL procedure need long-term followup of the graft. There are no specific criteria to define a "good risk" patient other than plain surgical judgment. We have weighed the known preoperative risk factors for developing hand ischemia after a brachial artery based access into our decision process including female gender, peripheral vascular occlusive disease, age, and diabetes. The preoperative noninvasive and invasive arterial imaging studies have helped identify any significant arterial occlusive disease. However, none of the patients that developed hand ischemia had any evidence of discrete, hemodynamically significant arterial inflow lesions and very few had any evidence of forearm disease. We have also factored the patient's weight and body habitus into the decision algorithm due to the significant incidence of wound complications. Harvesting the superficial femoral/popliteal vein is significantly more challenging in obese patients and is associated with a greater incidence of thigh wound complications. Indeed, most of the prolonged hospital stays after the SFV ACCESS were due to thigh wound complications. Lastly, the criterion that the patients have a reasonable life expectancy simply represents an attempt to balance the cost of the procedure in terms of the perioperative morbidity and mortality and the benefit in terms of a successful access.

In conclusion, the intermediate term functional patency rates after SFV ACCESS are excellent although the magnitude of the procedure and the complication rates are significant. SFV ACCESS should only be considered for patients with limited access options.

References

1. National Kidney Foundation. K/DOQI Clinical Practice Guidelines for Vascular Access, 2000. *Am J Kidney Dis.* 2001; 37:S137-S181.
2. United States Renal Data System Annual Report 2002. Available from: URL: http://www.usrds.org/.
3. Huber TS, Hirneise CM, Lee WA, et al. Outcome after autogenous brachial-axillary translocated superficial femoral/popliteal vein hemodialysis access. *J Vasc Surg,* in press.
4. Huber TS, Ozaki CK, Flynn TC, et al. Prospective validation of an algorithm to maximize native arteriovenous fistulae for chronic hemodialysis access. *J Vasc Surg.* 2002;36:452-459.
5. Berman SS, Gentile AT, Glickman MH, et al. Distal revascularization-interval ligation for limb salvage and maintenance of dialysis access in ischemic steal syndrome. *J Vasc Surg.* 1997; 26:393-402.
6. Sidawy AN, Gray R, Besarab A, et al. Recommended standards for reports dealing with arteriovenous hemodialysis accesses. *J Vasc Surg.* 2002; 35:603-610.
7. Rutherford RB, Baker JD, Ernst C, et al. Recommended standards for reports dealing with lower extremity ischemia: revised version. *J Vasc Surg.* 1997; 26:517-538.
8. Hertzberg BS, Kliewer MA, DeLong DM, et al. Sonographic assessment of lower limb vein diameters: implications for the diagnosis and characterization of deep venous thrombosis. *AJR Am J Roentgenol.* 1997; 168:1253-1257.
9. Dhingra RK, Young EW, Hulbert-Shearon TE, et al. Type of vascular access and mortality in U.S. hemodialysis patients. *Kidney Int.* 2001; 60:1443-1451.
10. Xue JL, Dahl D, Ebben JP, Collins AJ. The association of initial hemodialysis access type with mortality outcomes in elderly Medicare ESRD patients. *Am J Kidney Dis.* 2003; 42:1013-1019.

11. Pastan S, Soucie JM, McClellan WM. Vascular access and increased risk of death among hemodialysis patients. *Kidney Int.* 2002; 62:620-626.

12. Bhandari S, Wilkinson A, Sellars L. Saphenous vein forearm grafts and gortex thigh grafts as alternative forms of vascular access. *Clin Nephrol.* 1995; 44:325-328.

13. Cull JD, Cull DL, Taylor SM, et al. Prosthetic thigh arteriovenous access: outcome with SVS/AAVS reporting standards. *J Vasc Surg.* 2004; 39:381-386.

14. Miller CD, Robbin ML, Barker J, et al. Comparison of arteriovenous grafts in the thigh and upper extremities in hemodialysis patients. *J Am Soc Nephrol.* 2003; 14:2942-2947.

15. Tashjian DB, Lipkowitz GS, Madden RL, et al. Safety and efficacy of femoral-based hemodialysis access grafts. *J Vasc Surg.* 2002; 35:691-693.

16. Jackson MR. The superficial femoral-popliteal vein transposition fistula: description of a new vascular access procedure. *J Am Coll Surg.* 2000; 191:581-584.

17. Gradman WS, Cohen W, Haji-Aghaii M. Arteriovenous fistula construction in the thigh with transposed superficial femoral vein: our initial experience. *J Vasc Surg.* 2001; 33:968-975.

33

USE OF TISSUE PLASMINOGEN ACTIVATOR (t-PA) IN PHARMACOMECHANICAL THROMBOLYSIS OF AUTOGENOUS ARTERIOVENOUS FISTULAS

Fahim Zaman MD, Aslam Pervez MD, Sara Murphy RN, Mashood Qadri MD and Kenneth Abreo MD

Departments of Medicine; Division of Nephrology
Louisiana State University Health Sciences Center; Shreveport LA

Address correspondence to:
Fahim Zaman MD
Department of Medicine
Division of Nephrology
Louisiana State University Health Sciences Center
1501 Kings Highway
Shreveport, LA 71130
Phone: (318) 675 7402
Fax: (318) 675 5913
E mail: fzaman @ lsuhsc.edu

Introduction

Vascular access creation and maintenance remain two of the most important and difficult issues in the management of patients on hemodialysis.[1, 2] Many centers across the United States have focused their efforts on trying to increase the proportion of autogenous arteriovenous fistula (AVF) for their hemodialysis patient population.[3] Thrombosis is the most common complication of AVF. Early thrombosis of AVF (within 4 weeks of creation) is usually not correctable and requires a new access. However, thrombosis of a functional AVF is seen due to an underlying critical stenosis that is potentially amenable to percutaneous transluminal angioplasty (PTA) or they fail secondary to technical problems related to cannulation or compression, which may be treated by thrombectomy alone. Herein, we describe our experience with the use of tissue plasminogen activator (t-PA) for thrombosed AVF.

Methods

The computer database and medical records of all patients who underwent thrombolysis of their AVF in the interventional nephrology vascular suite at the Louisiana State University Health Sciences Center (Shreveport, LA) between July 2002 and December 2003 were reviewed. Fifteen episodes of pharmacomechanical thrombolysis in 13 thrombosed AVF are reported (Table 1). The technique consists of instillation of t-PA along with manual maceration to dissolve the clot and then proceeds with percutaneous balloon angioplasty to correct the underlying stenosis. After confirming the location and extent of the clot by contrast injection and physical examination, a total of 2-4 mg of t-PA is injected with a 25 mm gauge needle at the proximal and distal part of the thrombus. The initial dose of the t-PA is based on the size of the thrombus as estimated on examination. Manual maceration of the thrombus is performed percutaneously. Upon restoration of blood flow, percutaneous transluminal angioplasty of stenosed areas is performed using standard techniques.

All the procedures were performed by one of three interventional nephrologists, or by the nephrology fellow under direct supervision of the faculty. Informed consent was obtained in all cases. A physical examination and review of all medications including allergies was done in every case. The patient's vital signs, including blood pressure, oxygen saturation, and electrocardiography were monitored continuously and recorded. All procedures were done under intravenous conscious sedation using Midazolam (Versed) and Fentanyl. Patients were kept in the recovery room postprocedure.

Results

Patient	Location of AVF	t-PA Dose (mg)	Number of Lesion	Result	Complication/ Comment
1	Left Upper Arm	3	2	Unsuccessful	Bleeding resolve without intervention
2	Left Forearm	2	1	Successful	None
3	Left Wrist	4	1	Unsuccessful	None
4	Left Upper Arm	2	1	Unsuccessful	Bleeding resolve without intervention
5*	Right Upper Arm	2	Not known	Successful	None
6	Left Upper Arm	2	Not known	Unsuccessful	None
7	Left Wrist	2	Not known	Unsuccessful	None
5*	Right Upper Arm	4	2	Successful	None
5*	Right Upper Arm	4	2	Successful	Stent placement for elastic lesion
8	Left Wrist	2	2	Successful	None
9	Left Upper Arm	2	1	Successful	None
10	Left Upper Arm	4	1	Successful	Bleeding resolve without intervention. Patient required one unit PRBC transfusion
11	Left Upper Arm	3	1	Successful	None
12	Right Upper Arm	2	1	Unsuccessful	None
13	Left Upper Arm	4	1	Successful	None

5*: (same patient on subsequent thrombolysis)

Discussion

Use of the thrombolytic agent (t-PA) followed by percutaneous balloon angioplasty was successful in 9 out of 15 attempts (60%). One patient required t-PA on 2 subsequent visits with a thrombosed AVF requiring intervention. One patient required blood transfusion for bleeding. No procedure related vascular access infections were noted. No patient underwent emergent surgery for intervention-related complication. The successful thrombolysis with t-PA along with balloon angioplasty prolongs vascular access patency without significant morbidity to patients.

The use of t-PA and recombinant t-PA have previously been described for thrombolysis of synthetic grafts and AVF.[4, 5] Results published in the literature by interventional radiologists and nephrologists for thrombosed AVF are encouraging. However most series reported in the literature consist of few patients. Statistically significant data with follow up such as published by Turmel-Rodrigues,[6] Haage[7] and Schon[8] has prompted renewed interest in this area of endovascular intervention for thrombosed AVF. The results published for thrombosed AVF in the surgical literature are varied, with some having comparable long term patency as compared to endovascular interventions. Ultrasonography for vein mapping is helpful prior to AVF creation to avoid access placement in unsuitable vessels. Extremity and central venography should be used in: 1) obese patients 2) prior central lines 3) failed first access 4) arm edema. Preoperative detection of critical stenotic lesions by active investigation of vascular access dysfunction and surveillance before thrombosis offers the best chance of salvage.

Randomized controlled trials with long term follow up between the two techniques is needed to establish the most effective means of maintaining access patency and provide us with statistically reliable patency rates.

References

1. Schwab SJ, Harrington JT, King AJ, Singh A, Levey AS, Roher R, Al Shohaib S, Meyer K, Rohrer, Perrone RD. Vascular access for hemodialysis. *Kidney Int.* 1999;Vol.55: p2078-2090.
2. Hakim R, Himmelfarb J. Hemodialysis access failure: A call to action. *Kidney Int.* 1999;vol.54: p1029-1040.
3. Culp K, Flanigan M, Taylor L, Rothstein M. Vascular access thrombosis in new hemodialysis patients. *Am J Kidney Dis.* 1995;vol.26: p341-346.
4. Boobes Y, al-Hassan H, Neglen P, Obeid K, Denour N. Recombinant tissue plasminogen activator to declot dialysis fistulas. *J Nephrol.* 1997 Mar-Aprl; 10(2): 107-110.
5. Ahmed A, Shapiro WB, Porush JG. The use of tissue plasminogen activator to declot arteriovenous accesses in hemodialysis patients. *Am J Kidney Dis.*1993 Jan; 21(1): 38-43
6. Turmel-Rodrigues L, Pengloan J, Rodrigue H, Brillet G, Lataste A, Pierre D, Jourdan JL, Blanchard D. Treatment of failed native arterio-venous fistulae for hemodialysis by interventional radiology. *Kidney Int.* 2000;57: 1124-1140.
7. Haage P, Vorwerk D, Wildberger JE, Piroth W, Schuermann K, Guenther RW. Percutaneous treatment of thrombosed primary arteriovenous hemodialysis access fistulae. *Kidney Int.* 2000; 57: 1169-1175.
8. Schon D, Mishler R. Salvage of occluded arteriovenous fistulae. *Am J Kidney Dis.* 2000;36: 804-810.

34

IN-VIVO COMPARISON OF AKÓNYA ELIMINATOR™, A NEW NON-ROTATIONAL MECHANICAL THROMBECTOMY DEVICE WITH THE ARROW-TREROTOLA PTD: PRELIMINARY OBSERVATIONS IN A SWINE MODEL

András Kónya, MD, PhD and Kenneth C. Wright, PhD

Section of Vascular and Interventional Radiology,
Division of Diagnostic Imaging,
The University of Texas M. D. Anderson Cancer Center,
Houston, Texas

Supported in part by grants from the John S. Dunn Research
Foundation and by grant NIH-NCI CA-16672 from
the National Cancer Institute.

Address all correspondence and reprints request to
András Kónya, MD, PhD,
Section of Vascular and Interventional Radiology,
Division of Diagnostic Imaging, Unit 057,
The University of Texas M. D. Anderson Cancer Center,
1515 Holcombe Blvd., Houston, TX 77030;
Phone: (713) 792-2733; Fax: (713) 745-3034.
E-mail: akonya@mdanderson.org

Introduction

Percutaneous management of thrombosed hemodialysis access, both synthetic and native, is an accepted standard of care supported by published guidelines.[1] The use of percutaneous techniques for declotting along with treatment of underlying stenotic lesions prolongs access life, diminishes costs, allows continuation of dialysis and is well tolerated by patients. Formerly, general agreement was held that the dialysis graft declotting depended more on the treatment of the underlying stenosis than on the technique of removal of the clot. However, recent trials have suggested that certain techniques of clot removal may be superior to others in regard to long-term outcomes.[2–6] The basic principle of percutaneous graft declotting involves complete thrombus removal from the access as well as treatment of the underlying venous stenosis. Attempts should be made to eliminate the clots in their entirety using clot fragmentation, maceration, and/or lysis and aspiration. Such attempts also include the removal of adherent clots and treatment of intragraft stenosis. Among the several approved mechanical thrombectomy devices the wall-contact devices (Arrow-Trerotola PTD, Arrow; Cragg Brush, MicroTherapeutics Inc.) are capable of removing the most residual thrombi.[7] The maceration of adherent clots with the other non-wall-contact devices can be supplemented with use of a special device dedicated to adherent clot removal (Fogarty Adherent Clot Catheter, Edwards Lifesciences, 8), which adds to the cost of the procedure. The wall-contact mechanical devices, however, need a costly motor drive for operation. There is a need for a mechanical declotting device that is able to effectively clean synthetic grafts with ease without using a motor unit, has adequate torque control, and allows for fluid injection.

The purpose of this preliminary study was to compare a new 6-F non-rotational basket thrombectomy device (AKónya Eliminator™, AKE, IDev Technologies, Inc., Houston, TX) to the 5-F Arrow-Trerotola PTD™ (PTD, Arrow International, Reading, PA) with regard to clot maceration and torque control in a swine arterial model. Fluid injection capabilities (saline and contrast) were also compared on the bench top. Both devices are FDA approved for declotting of synthetic hemodialysis access grafts.

Methods

Device Description   The AKE is composed of a 6-F woven mesh basket at the end of a 4-F flexible shaft consisting of a coaxially arranged stainless steel inner microtube and an outer catheter with a fexible tip (Fig 1). The lumen of the catheter is accessible via a Touhy-Borst adapter equipped with side arm, which allows for fluid administration. The dimensions (length and diameter) of the mesh basket are continuously adjustable between complete elongation (to minimize profile) and maximum unconstrained expansion (10 mm) by moving the Touhy-Borst connector and device handle axially (Fig 2, 3). The microtube and catheter are interconnected and capable of being locked with the Touhy-Borst locking mechanism. The device requires the use of a 6-F or larger introducer sheath. Both ends of the mesh basket have radiopaque markers for fluoroscopic visualization, and the soft, flexible tip at the end of the shaft is highly maneuverable.

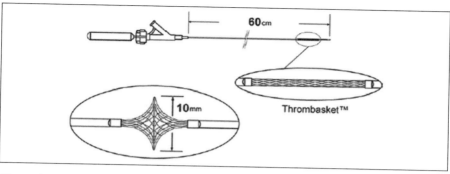

Figure 1:   Drawings showing the parts and dimensions of the device.

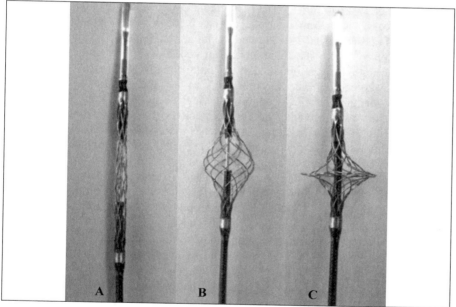

Figure 2:   Photographs showing the adjustable basket (A) completely elongat-
             ed, (B) partially deployed (8-mm) , and (C) maximally deployed.

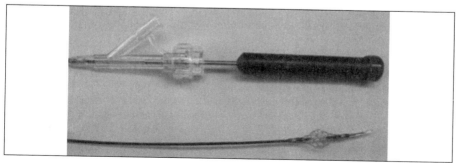

Figure 3:   Photograph showing the proximal and the distal ends of the device:
             the Touhy-Borst adapter with side port attached to the 4-F outer
             catheter and the handle attached to the inner microtubing.

Animal Studies   All experimentation involving animals was approved by the Institutional Animal Care and Use Committee. Animals were maintained in facilities approved by the American Association for Accreditation of Laboratory Animal Care and in accordance with current U.S. Department of Agriculture, Department of Health and Human Services, and National Institutes of Health regulations and standards.

Six domestic pigs weighing 50.7- 80.4 kg (median 56.5 kg) were used. The anesthesia was initiated by an intramuscular injection of solution containing ketamine hydrochloride, acepromazine (0.15 mg/kg), and atropine sulfate (0.04 mg/kg). Anesthesia was induced with isoflurane (5%) via mask. Once the pig was anesthetized, an endotracheal tube was inserted and anesthesia was maintained with isoflurane (1.5%) and oxygen (0.8 L/min). In a bilateral/unilateral thrombosis model, the arteries of the hind limbs were used for mechanical thrombolysis.

Creation of Test Conduits   The right carotid artery was surgically isolated and an 11-F Check-Flo Performer introducer (Cook Incorporated, Bloomington, IN) was inserted and advanced into the abdominal aorta. Heparin (100 units/kg) was administered through the sheath, and was repeated in every hour thereafter. Lower abdominal aortograms were obtained by injecting contrast (Conray 60, iothalamate meglumine, Mallinckrodt Inc., St. Louis, MO; 15 ml/s for a total of 35 ml).

To reduce the number of test conduit side branches, a 5-F multipurpose catheter (Cook Inc.) was advanced into the deep circumflex iliac and medial circumflex femoral arteries, respectively, and these branches were occluded with stainless steel macrocoils (Cook Inc.). Contrast injections were used to confirm branch occlusions. To compare the devices in a straight conduit, the right femoral artery was surgically isolated and a 6-F 5-cm long introducer sheath (Arrow International, Inc.) was inserted. To compare the devices in a curved conduit, the right femoral artery was surgically isolated and a 7-F 40-cm long Check-Flo Performer Balkin contralateral introducer sheath (Cook Inc.) was inserted and advanced into the left iliac artery.

After finishing preparation of the test conduit, the 11-F carotid sheath was positioned into the vessel to be used for thrombectomy and 1-7 day-old clots were injected until complete occlusion was achieved. To avoid fragmentation, the clots were preloaded into a 5-cc Luer Lok syringe that had had the tip within the Luer Lok mechanism removed. In addition, a 6-cm-long piece of 12-F thin-walled stainless steel tubing with a metal hub was fabricated and attached to the syringe to inject the clots through the sheath check-flow valve. Once the conduit was prepared with the clots, the thrombectomy procedure was initiated using either the AKE or the 5-F Arrow-Trerotola rotational percutaneous thrombectomy device (PTD). All procedures were performed by the same interventional radiologist (A.K.).

Clot maceration   For the PTD, the manufacturer's instructions were followed. The PTD was flushed with saline then the function of the rotator drive unit was verified by pressing the on/off switch of the unit. The PTD in compressed position was inserted through the valve of the introducer and advanced to the distal end of the test conduit. Once the desired position of the catheter was achieved, the rotator drive unit was attached to the PTD catheter. The 9-mm self-expanding nitinol basket (Fig. 4) was exposed by retracting the outer catheter cover. Contrast was injected through the outer cover sheath to visualize clots. The deployed fragmentation basket was activated by depressing the switch of the motor (3000 rpm) and slowly withdrawn to the tip of the introducer sheath to perform a 30-second pass.

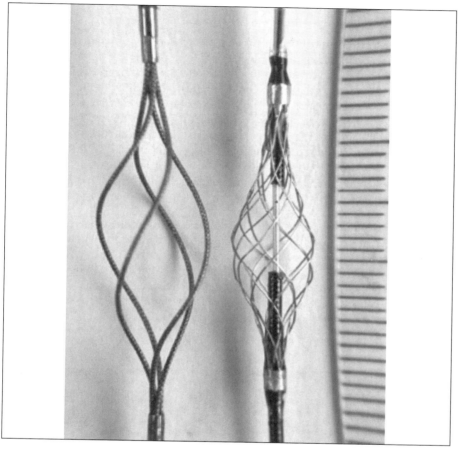

Figure 4:   Photograph showing the structural differences between the two
              baskets. The AKE (top) is partially deployed (6-mm) while the PTD
              assumed its unconstrained 9-mm diameter.

Before using the AKE, the device was flushed with saline and the basket was
deployed and re-elongated to check it for functionality. The flexible tip of the device
was inserted through the check-flow valve of the introducer sheath and the device
was advanced to the distal end of the test conduit. Contrast was injected to visualize clots and the basket was then deployed. The diameter of the basket was selected so that it could move freely within the vessel. The basket was moved back-and-
forth axially (with 3-5 mm strikes) while being slowly withdrawn through the test
conduit to the tip of the sheath. One pass through the conduit lasted 30 seconds.

Each device was passed twice through the test conduit. The device was then
removed, the clot slurry was aspirated and contrast was injected through the carotid
sheath and/or the femoral sheath to evaluate the degree of clot removal. If residual
thrombi were detected, the device was re-inserted into the test conduit and additional

passes were conducted followed by additional aspirations until complete removal of the clots was achieved. The number of aspirations and the amount of aspirated blood slurry were recorded. The size and number of larger fragments in the aspirate were also noted.

Branch selection ability   The portion of the curved test conduit where the medial femoral circumflex artery branched off from the iliofemoral artery (Figure 5) was used to test the ability of the devices to select side branches. This part of the study was conducted to compare the torque control / steerability of the test devices. The test device was advanced via the Balkin contralateral sheath from the right femoral artery. The tip of the devices spontaneously took either the femoral artery or the medial circumflex branch. Attempts were made to direct the device in the alternate direction. The number of attempts required for selection of the desired vessel was recorded.

During device manipulation in the test conduit, the motor unit was not attached to the PTD catheter.

Injection capability   To test the injection capability of the devices, a uniform amount (5 cc) of saline or contrast (Conray-60, iothalamate meglumine) at room temperature (20 C) was injected through the AKE and PTD prior to using the devices for clot maceration. The time required for the saline/contrast to pass through the lumen of the devices was measured in full seconds and recorded. The contrast and saline injections were repeated six times for both devices. The AKE was used with a partially deployed basket, while the fragmentation basket of the PTD was unsheathed prior to injection.

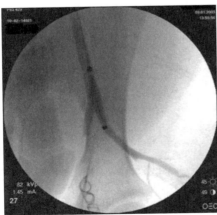

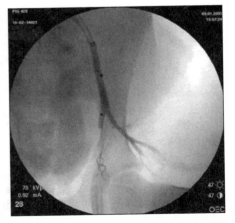

Figure 5A: Curved conduit, accessed from the contralateral femoral artery (not shown), used for testing the branch selection ability of the devices. (A) The AKE selected the iliofemoral artery.

Figure 5B: The tip of AKE was redirected into the medial circumflex femoral artery. Note the occlusion coils placed in the medial circumflex femoral artery.

Statistical analysis   The data was analyzed using the two-sample Student t-test assuming equal variances and assuming unequal variances. The results were considered significant when p value was < 0.05.

Results

Clot maceration   In the straight conduit, six declotting treatments were performed with each device. In the curved conduit, three treatments were accomplished with both AKE and PTD.

Table 1 summarizes the data with regard to the number of passes required to achieve complete clot removal from the test conduits. Aspiration of clot slurry was attempted after the second pass and each additional passes using either AKE or PTD. The amount of aspirated slurry was measured as 0-10 cc (mean 4.4 cc) for both AKE and PTD. In 5 of 22 attempts, minimal or immeasurable amount of aspirate was recorded (4 with PTD, 1 with AKE). The aspirated slurry was mainly fluid with occasionally small fragments of clots after using either AKE or PTD. With AKE, two fragments were aspirated in two of nine procedures (one in the straight, and one in the curved conduit). With PTD, 10 fragments measuring from 1x1 mm to 10x8 mm were found in four of nine procedures. In one of these procedures, 6 fragments measuring 1-3x3-5 mm were aspirated. All fragments associated with PTD procedures resulted from aspirations from the straight test conduit.

There was no difference in clot maceration and declotting efficiency between the two devices in the straight conduit, but a statistically significant difference existed between AKE and PTD in the curved conduit. AKE required less treatment passes and was superior to PTD in that respect (p=0.013).

Branch selection ability   The curved test conduit created in two animals was used to redirect the tip of the devices from either the femoral artery to the medial circumflex femoral artery or vice versa (Table 2). In pig 429, to achieve the desired position, it required 1-5 attempts (mean 2.8) for the AKE and 8-12 attempts (mean 9.3) for the PTD, respectively, with a significant difference between the two devices (p=0.002). In pig 426, AKE required 1-5 attempts (mean 2.5) while PTD required 3-8 attempts (mean 6). These results were also statistically different (p=0.037).

Table 1.   Comparison of AKE and PTD in efficiency of declotting in the straight and the curved test conduits.

Treatment passes required in the straight conduits (n=6)		
AKE	PTD	
2.5 mean (2-3)	3 mean (2-5)	p=0.34

Treatments required in the curved conduits (n=3)		
AKE	PTD	
2.7 mean (2-3)	4.7 mean (4-5)	p=0.013

Table 2.   Comparison of branch selection ability of the test devices: Redirection of the device tips from femoral artery to medial circumflex femoral branch or vice versa.

No of pig	Number of attempts w/AKE	Mean	Number of attempts w/PTD	Mean	P value
429	1		8		
	3		9		
	2		12		
	5	2.8	8	9.3	0.002
426	5		6		
	3		3		
	1		8		
	3		7		
	2				
	1	2.6		6	0.037
Total		2.7		7.6	0.0004

Combining the data from both pigs, the number of attempts with the AKE (mean 2.6) was significantly less than that with the PTD (mean 7.62; p=0.0004).

Injection capability   There was no statistically significant difference between the fluid injection capabilities of the tested devices. The calculated flow rates for the saline injection were 1.94 cc/sec (AKE) and 2.0 cc/sec (PTD), and for contrast 0.81 cc/sec (AKE) and 0.97 cc/sec (PTD), respectively.

Conclusions

In comparison to pharmacomechanical thrombolysis, purely mechanical declotting techniques of thrombosed dialysis access offer reduced procedure time, reduced bleeding complications, and, at least for some devices and techniques, reduced costs. Mechanical techniques include balloon stripping alone[9] in combination with angioplasty,[10] and the use of latex balloons.[11] High-speed recirculation devices such as the Amplatz Clot Bluster (Microvena),[12] and more recently the Helix (eV3),[13] as well as hydrodynamic (rheolytic) catheters such as the Hydrolyser (Cordis)[14] have also been used to declot thrombosed hemodialysis accesses. The rotational motor-driven wall-contact devices (Arrow-Trerotola PTD; Cragg / Castaneda brushes, MicroTherapeutics) have been proven to be the most efficient to remove residual thrombi from the synthetic grafts.[8] A simple device, the mini pigtail catheter, was found comparable to more sophisticated and expensive devices in declotting both synthetic grafts as well as native fistulas.[15]

As for its mechanism of clot maceration, the AKónya Eliminator™ is a wall-contact device; the adjustable mesh basket has the ability to adapt its entire circumference to the graft or vessel wall even in curved segments.

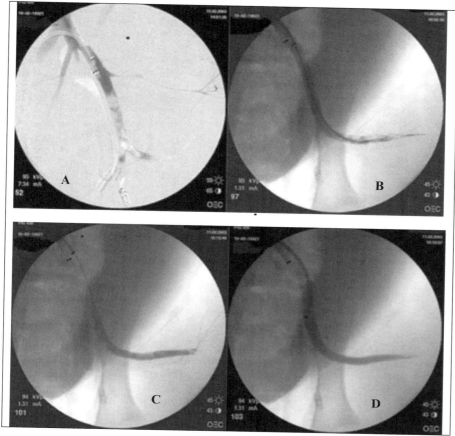

Figure 6:   (A) Pre-procedure arteriogram reveals complete occlusion of the left iliofemoral segment. Note the carotid and the contralateral sheaths in the left iliac artery side by side. (B) After two passes with the PTD partial occlusion of the segment is shown. (C) After 3 passes and aspiration some residual clots are still observed. (D) Following 4 passes and aspiration of 10 cc of clot slurry the conduit is completely clean.

With respect to device construction, the AKE is similar to the "mesh basket" device,[16] which was constructed by securing a 7-mm Wallstent to a 0.035-inch steerable guide wire with two sleeves. The wire with the completely folded basket was introduced coaxially through a 6-F OD – 4F ID polytetrafluoroethylene (PTFE) catheter so that the floppy end of the guide wire tip with the distal sleeve protruded. The proximal end of the catheter was sealed by an adapter with a hemostasis valve and a side port. Once in position, the mesh basket was expanded partially or completely by withrawing the introducer catheter. Partial basket release with fixation of the wire in the tightened hemostasis valve allowed adjustment of the basket size to the vessel size.

However, unlike the "mesh basket", the Thrombasket™ of AKE is shorter and continously adjustable between its elongated profile and its maximum 10-mm diameter,

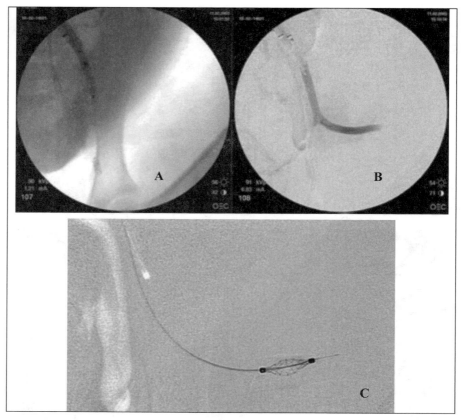

Figure 7:   (A) Pre-procedure arteriogram reveals complete occlusion of the test conduit. (B) AKE basket is adjusted to the diameter of the vessel. (C) After 2 passes and aspiration of 8 cc of clot slurry the conduit is devoid of thrombi. The conduit was reused after a thrombectomy session with PTD (see Figures 6 A-D).

and the device provides for fluid injection. In addition, the Thrombasket™ exerts adjustable lateral force to the graft or vessel wall, which aids in maceration and removal of firmly adhered clots.

The Thrombasket™ can be activated by retracting the handle from the Touhy-Borst connector while holding the connector stationary or by pushing the Touhy-Borst connector away from the handle while holding the handle stationary. The basket can be used by different axial back-and-forth movement, rotation, and/or a pulsating technique. The latter is produced by moving the two ends of the basket relative to each other in rapid succession. The axial movements can be combined with rotation. In the present study, short (3-5mm) axial back-and-forth strikes were utilized for clot maceration. The pulsating technique requires at least a 10-mm diameter conduit to be performed without traumatizing the wall, therefore it was not tested in the vascular models used in the reported studies.

The present study showed that with regard to clot maceration, AKE was similar to PTD in the straight conduit, but superior to PTD in the curved conduit. The difference seemed to reside not in the clot maceration capability of the devices in general, but rather in the clot maceration ability of the devices when in close proximity to the end of the introducer sheath. Since the manufacturer does not recommend rotation of the PTD within the guiding sheath, rotation of the device was stopped when the proximal end of basket reached the tip of the sheath. This limitation coupled with longer length of the tapered segment at each end of the PTD basket resulted in larger clots remaining close to the tip of the sheath after treatment with the PTD compared to the AKE. Contrast injection and the advancement of the PTD for the successive pass carried these clots back toward the center of the test conduit, and subsequent pass(es) of the device were required to finally macerate these clot fragments. Furthermore, the presence of large clots close to the end of the introducer sheath might explain why aspiration attempts were unsuccessful more often after PTD treatment passes (4 with PTD vs. 1 with AKE). This speculation is supported by the fact that larger clots were more often aspirated after PTD treatment passes than AKE passes in the straight conduit even if the mean amount of the aspirated clot slurry was identical for the two devices.

The branch selection ability of AKE was significantly better than that of PTD. PTD was designed to work "in-axis" with limited directional capabilities. AKE's better tracking and torque control seems to be an advantageous feature for utilization in native vessels that are usually more tortuous than a synthetic graft.

Both devices showed similar fluid injection capabilities. AKE, however, allows for fluid injection in any phase of basket deployment except for the maximal deployment when a stopper located inside the basket occludes the distal end of the 4-F outer catheter. The self-expanding basket of PTD must be uncovered (unsheathed) first to use the covering sheath for fluid injection. AKE allows for fluid injection without deployment of the basket as well as at any point of a treatment session. Consequently, simultaneous or subsequent fluid injections (e.g., contrast, saline, heparin, lytic agents, etc.) can be made through both the device and the introducer sheath prior to, during and after clot maceration. The 4-F shaft of the AKE device offers ample room for injection through the 6-F introducer sheath. Conversely, some aspiration through a 6-F sheath can be accomplished even if the device is within the sheath.

Mechanical thrombectomy procedures can cause blood loss by several different mechanisms. These include bleeding from access entry sites, aspiration of blood, and mechanical hemolysis. Several thrombectomy devices such as the Hydrolyser (Cordis), the Oasis (Boston Scientific), and the EndoVac (Neovascular Technologies) have powerful aspiration capabilities. Prolonged inattentive activation of these devices can lead to substantial intraprocedural blood loss. Since AKE utilizes controlled hand-aspiration through the introducer sheath(s), use of the AKE is not limited by the need to minimize device activation time. Furthermore, AKE does not appear to produce mechanical hemolysis.

The rotational speed of devices with a mechanical drive shaft like the PTD as well as the Cragg and Castaneda brushes may be reduced when used around sharp corners. Devices with guide wire compatibility and lack of a rotating drive shaft, such as Xpeedior (Possis Medical), the Oasis (Boston Scientific) and the Hydrolyzer (Cordis) are advantageous for use around sharp corners an/or through intragraft stenoses. Use in the curved test conduit showed that the functionality of the AKE is preserved even at sharp angulations.

The AKónya Eliminator™ is devised to efficiently macerate and declot thrombosed sites in the body. The ability of the device to exert adjustable radial force improves its capability of removing adherent as well as mature clots. The AKE also allows fluid injection at almost any stage of basket deployment. The next generation of the device will be equipped with guide wire access, which can also be used as an additional venue for fluid administration. Further experimental and clinical studies are warranted to address the safety and utility of the AKE device.

References

1. NKF-DOQI clinical practice guidelines for vascular access. National Kidney Foundation - Dialysis Outcomes Quality Initiative. *Am J Kidney Dis.* 1997; (Suppl 3):S150-191.
2. Trerotola SO, Vesely TM, Lund GB, et al. Treatment of thrombosed hemodialysis access grafts: Arrow-Trerotola percutaneous thrombolytic device versus pulsepray thrombolysis. Arrow-Trerotola Percutaneous Thrombolytic Device Clinical Trial. *Radiology.* 1998; 206. 403-414.
3. Vesely TM, Williams D, Weiss M, et al. Comparison of the angiojet rheolytic catheter to surgical thrombectomy for the treatment of thrombosed hemodialysis grafts. Peripheral AngioJet Clinical Trial. *J Vasc Interv Radiol.* 1999; 10. 1195-1205.
4. Dolmatch BL, Casteneda F, McNamara TO, et al. Synthetic dialysis shunts: thrombolysis with the Cragg thrombolytic brush catheter. *Radiology.* 1999; 213. 180-184.
5. Sofocleous CT, Cooper SG, Schur I, et al. Retrospective comparison of the Amplatz thrombectomy device with modified pulse-spray pharmacomechanical thrombolysis in the treatment of thrombosed hemodialysis access grafts. *Radiology.* 1999; 213. 561-567.
6. Barth KH, Gosnell MR, Palestrant AM, et al. Hydrodynamic thrombectomy system versus pulse-spray thrombolysis for thrombosed hemodialysis grafts: a multicenter prospective randomized comparison. *Radiology.* 2000; 217. 678-684.
7. Vesely TM, Hovsepian DM, Darcy MD, et al. Angioscopic observations after percutaneous thrombectomy of thrombosed hemodialysis grafts. *J Vasc Interv Radiol.* 2000; 11. 971-977.
8. Trerotola SO, Harris VJ, Snidow JJ, Johnson MS. Percutaneous use of the Fogarty adherent clot catheter. *J Vasc Interv Radiol.* 1995; 6. 578-580.
9. Trerotola SO, Lund GB, Scheel PJ Jr, et al. Thrombosed dialysis access grafts: percutaneous mechanical declotting without urokinase. *Radiology.* 1994; 191. 721-726.
10. Middlebrook MR, Amygdalos MA, Soulen MC, et al. Thrombosed hemodialysis grafts: percutaneous mechanical balloon declotting versus thrombolysis. *Radiology.* 1995; 196. 73-77.
11. Soulen MC, Zaetta JM, Amygdalos MA, et al. Mechanical declotting of thrombosed dialysis grafts: experience in 86 cases. *J Vasc Interv Radiol.* 1997; 8. 563-567.

12. Uflacker R, Rajagopalan PR, Vujic I, et al. Treatment of thrombosed dialysis access grafts: randomized trial of surgical thrombectomy versus mechanical thrombectomy with the Amplatz device. *J Vasc Interv Radiol.* 1996; 7. 185-192.

13. Qian Z, Kvamme P, Raghed D, et al. Comparison of a new recirculation thrombectomy catheter with other devices of the same type: in vitro and in vivo evaluations. *Invest Radiol.* 2002; 37. 503-511.

14. Vorwerk D, Sohn M, Schurmann K, et al. Hydrodynamic thrombectomy of hemodialysis fistulas: first clinical results. *J Vasc Interv Radiol.* 1994; 5. 813-821.

15. Schmitz-Rode T, Wildberger JE, Hubner D, et al. Recanalization of thrombosed dialysis access with use of a rotating mini-pigtail catheter: follow-up study. *J Vasc Interv Radiol.* 2000; 11. 721-727.

16. Schmitz-Rode T, Bohndorf K, Gunther RW. New "mesh basket" for percutaneous removal of wall-adherent thrombi in dialysis shunts. *Cardiovasc Intervent Radiol.* 1993; 16. 7-10.

35

PATCH ANGIOPLASTY OF STENOSED AUTOGENOUS ARTERIOVENOUS FISTULAS USING HARVESTED VEINS

Fahim Zaman[1] MD, Aslam Pervez[1] MD, Sara Murphy[1] RN, Kenneth Abreo[1] MD and Warren Maley[2] MD

*Departments of Medicine[1] and Surgery[2];
Louisiana State University Health Sciences Center; Shreveport LA*

Address correspondence to:
Fahim Zaman MD
Department of Medicine
Division of Nephrology
Louisiana State University Health Sciences Center
1501 Kings Highway
Shreveport, LA 71130
Phone: (318) 675 7402
Fax: (318) 675 5913
E mail: fzaman @ lsuhsc.edu

Introduction

Vascular access creation and maintenance remain two of the most important and difficult issues in the management of patients on hemodialysis.[1, 2] Recent publication of the Dialysis Outcome Quality Initiative (K/DOQI) guidelines have focused on the need for increasing use of autogenous fistulas (AVF) and reducing creation of synthetic grafts (SG) for permanent vascular access for hemodialysis.[3] Even though there is general agreement amongst nephrologists and surgeons over the superiority of AVF over SG, the 1999 data from the Health Care Finance Administration (HCFA) clinical performance measures project revealed 27% fistula rate in prevalent patients and a 28% rate in the incident patients on hemodialysis.[4] Angioplasty remains the primary endovascular technique for the treatment of AVF related stenoses. However, in a small number of cases, the underlying lesion is unresponsive to angioplasty. Herein, we describe our experience with the use of vein patch angioplasty to salvage stenosed AVF in our hemodialysis patients.

Methods

Five patients were referred to the interventional vascular laboratory for malfunction of their AVF from 1/1/03 to 12/31/03. These patients underwent fistulograms and percutaneous transluminal angioplasty (PTA) of stenosed lesions using standard techniques. However, these lesions were resistant to PTA and subsequently were referred to our vascular access surgeon. The location of AVF and segment of venous patch angioplasty used are in Table 1. Medical records of all patients who underwent patch angioplasty were reviewed. Excellent results were obtained with the use of patch angioplasty of these stenosed AVF using harvested veins.

Results

Table 1.

PATIENT	LOCATION OF AVF	VEIN PATCHED	VEIN USED	COMPLICATION
1	Right Wrist	CEPHALIC	CEPHALIC	NONE
2	Right Upper Arm	CEPHALIC	SAPHENOUS	NONE
3	Left Upper Arm	CEPHALIC	SAPHENOUS	NONE
4	Left Upper Arm	CEPHALIC	SAPHENOUS	NONE
5	Left Upper Arm	AXILLARY	AXILLARY	NONE

Discussion

The importance of vascular access in the care of dialysis patients was recognized in the of DOQI guidelines by the National Kidney Foundation. Autogenous arteriovenous fistulas remain the vascular access of choice for ESRD patients on hemodialysis due to better long-term patency and morbidity.[5, 6] Many centers have focused their attention on creating and maintaining AVF in their hemodialysis patients.[6]

The reasons for early vascular access failure are: 1) technical problems at the anastomosis and positioning of the artery and vein relative to another including rotation and angulation 2) a sclerotic vein segment 3) calcification of the arterial wall causing difficulty at the anastomosis 4) hypotension from recent dialysis. Thrombosis with access dysfunction after maturation is usually due to the following: 1) anastomotic or outflow vein stenosis 2) repeated puncture of AVF at same site with extravasation of blood and hematoma may lead to stenosis and fibrosis 3) anastomotic intimal hyperplasia 4) hypotension 5) hypercoagulable state.

The primary choice of treatment of short segment outflow stenosis is PTA.[7] A surgical venous patch angioplasty may be used after failed PTA in some cases.[8] Vein strictures or areas of elastic stenosis resistant to TPA were successfully surgically revised by an experienced vascular access surgeon at our institution. This form of repair is advisable due to the risk of venous rupture with balloon angioplasty at the site of the cephalic vein entering the subclavian vein, as noted in 3 of our patients. Patch angioplasty remains a technically difficult procedure, but is safe in experienced hands with excellent results and salvage of the current vascular access. Patch angioplasty should be considered in patients with AVF malfunction due to stenosed segments resistant to PTA as it may prolong the life of the vascular access. All the AVF undergoing patch angioplasty were functional at 90 days post procedure, and required no further intervention. Patch angioplasty is a safe and effective method of correcting these lesions. A team approach with nephrologists, interventionalists and vascular access surgeons working together will result in better outcome for access for patients and reduce morbidity.

References

1. Schwab SJ, Harrington JT, King AJ, Singh A, Levey AS, Roher R, Al Shohaib S, Meyer K, Rohrer, Perrone RD. Vascular access for hemodialysis. *Kidney Int.* 1999, Vol.55: p2078-2090.
2. Hakim R, Himmelfarb J. Hemodialysis access failure: A call to action. *Kidney Int.* 1999,vol.54: p1029-1040.
3. National Kidney Foundation. K/DOQI Clinical Practice Guidelines for vascular access. *Am J Kidney Disease.* 2001.37 (S1): S137-S181.
4. ESRD Clinical performance Measures Project 2000 Annual Report. Washington DC: Department of Health and Human Services, Health Care Financing Administration Office of Clinical Standards and Quality, 2000.
5. Zibari GB, Rohr MS, Landreneau MD, Bridges RM, DeVault GA, Petty FH, Costley KJ, Brown ST. Complications from permanent hemodialysis vascular access. *Surgery.* 1988; 104:681-686.
6. Sands JJ. Increasing AV fistulas: revisiting a time-tested solution. *Semin Dial.* 2000;13: 351- 353.
7. Oakes DD, Sherck JP, Cobb LF. Surgical salvage of failed radiocephalic arteriovenous fistulae: techniques and results in 29 patients. *Kidney Int.* 1998; 53: 480-487.

8. Tordoir JHM. Surgical management of autologous fistulae. Early and late thrombosis,maturation failure, and other complications. In: Gray RJ, ed. *Dialysis Access: A multidisciplinary approach.* Lippincot Williams and Wilkins; 2002; 242-249.

Index